Recent Progress in Emergency Surgery

Recent Progress in Emergency Surgery

Editor: Gideon Allen

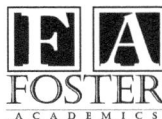

FA FOSTER ACADEMICS

www.fosteracademics.com

www.fosteracademics.com

FA FOSTER ACADEMICS

Cataloging-in-Publication Data

Recent progress in emergency surgery / edited by Gideon Allen.
    p. cm.
Includes bibliographical references and index.
ISBN 978-1-63242-639-0
1. Surgical emergencies. 2. Medical emergencies. 3. Surgery. 4. Emergency medicine. I. Allen, Gideon.
RD93 .R43 2019
617.1--dc23

Foster Academics,
118-35 Queens Blvd., Suite 400,
Forest Hills, NY 11375, USA

ISBN 978-1-63242-639-0 (Hardback)

Contents

Preface

This book has been a concerted effort by a group of academicians, researchers and scientists, who have contributed their research works for the realization of the book. This book has materialized in the wake of emerging advancements and innovations in this field. Therefore, the need of the hour was to compile all the required researches and disseminate the knowledge to a broad spectrum of people comprising of students, researchers and specialists of the field.

The medical condition, which poses an immediate risk to a person's life, is known as medical emergency. The type of non-elective surgery performed in the case of a medical emergency, where immediate surgery is the only possible way to solve the problem successfully, is called an emergency surgery. It is done immediately in order to save life, organ or functional capacity. Some of the acute emergencies that can be managed surgically include abdominal emergencies, respiratory obstructions and pleural diseases, urinary obstructions, intestinal obstruction or perforation, etc. Without early treatment and surgical care, mortality rates for these conditions are high. Different approaches, evaluations, methodologies and advanced studies on emergency surgery have been included in this book. It presents researches and studies performed by experts across the globe. This book will prove to be immensely beneficial to students and researchers in this field.

At the end of the preface, I would like to thank the authors for their brilliant chapters and the publisher for guiding us all-through the making of the book till its final stage. Also, I would like to thank my family for providing the support and encouragement throughout my academic career and research projects.

Editor

Grading operative findings at laparoscopic cholecystectomy- a new scoring system

Michael Sugrue[1*], Shaheel M Sahebally[1], Luca Ansaloni[2] and Martin D Zielinski[3]

Abstract

Introduction: Variation in outcomes from surgery is a major challenge and defining surgical findings may help set benchmarks, which currently do not exist in laparoscopic cholecystectomy. This study outlines a new surgical scoring system incorporating key operative findings.

Methods: English language studies (from January 1965 to July 2014) pertaining to severity scoring and predictors of difficult laparoscopic cholecystectomy were searched for in PubMed, Embase and Cochrane databases using the search terms 'Laparoscopic cholecystectomy or Lap chole' and/or 'Scoring Index or Grading system or Prediction of difficulty or Conversion to open' in various combinations. Cross-referencing from papers retrieved in the original search identified additional articles.

Results: Sixteen published papers report a gallbladder (GB) scoring system, but all relate to pre-operative clinical and imaging findings, rather than operative findings. The current scoring system, using operative findings incorporates the appearance of the GB, presence of GB distension, ease of access, potential biliary complications and time taken to identify cystic duct and artery. A score of <2 would imply mild difficulty, 2–4 moderate, 5–7 severe and 8–10 extreme.

Conclusion: This paper reports one of the first operative classifications of findings at laparoscopic cholecystectomy. It has the potential to allow benchmarks for international collaboration of operative and patient outcomes in patients undergoing laparoscopic cholecystectomy.

Keywords: Cholecystitis, Cholecystectomy, Laparoscopic, Operative severity scoring system, Conversion to open

Introduction

Gallbladder-related disease is now one of the commonest indications for elective and emergency surgery. Management of cholecystitis and its complications has evolved dramatically [1] and there have been significant paradigm shifts in the management of patients since the introduction of laparoscopic cholecystectomy in the mid 1990 [2]. Recently the importance of index admission laparoscopic cholecystectomy has been highlighted [3]. In many large series and meta-analyses detailed patient demographics and imaging findings have been recorded. A number of international guidelines recommend pathways of care [4,5]. Attempts have been made to standardize definitions particularly relating to cholecystitis [6]. Understanding outcomes is key to advancing health care, and while conversion to open cholecystectomy will always be an essential part of safe surgical practice, a greater understanding of the factors leading to conversion and potential post-operative complications would be essential.

Despite these advances, significant variability in approaches to care and outcomes in gall-bladder disease management are reported [7]. While a number of pre-operative scoring systems are reported there is no operative classification of findings at laparoscopic surgery [8,9]. This limits the ability to compare outcomes or provide a common benchmark for future research. This paper outlines a new scoring system for operative findings at laparoscopic cholecystectomy, to allow grading of the findings and standardize the degree of cholecystitis.

Methods

A literature review was undertaken of PubMed, Embase and Cochrane databases between January 1965 and July 2014 for publications relating to difficulty prediction in laparoscopic cholecystectomy using the search terms

* Correspondence: michael.sugrue@hse.ie
[1]Department of Surgery, Letterkenny Hospital and Donegal Clinical Research Academy, National University Ireland Galway, Letterkenny, Donegal, Ireland
Full list of author information is available at the end of the article

'Laparoscopic cholecystectomy or Lap chole' and/or 'Scoring Index or Grading system or Prediction of difficulty or Conversion to open' in various combinations. Cross-referencing from papers retrieved in the original search identified additional articles. All studies had to be published in English literature. Case reports and data from abstracts were excluded.

Results

In total 16 papers were found relating to difficulty prediction in laparoscopic cholecystectomy. These are summarised in Table 1. All papers focused on the ability to predict conversion to open surgery using preoperative parameters. No operative grading system was found. Our study provides a preliminary scoring system to enable key aspects of the surgical findings to be documented.

The current scoring system proposed is based on the severity of cholecystitis and degree of potential difficulty with a score from 1 to 10. The key aspects of the score include access to the gallbladder including patient body mass index (BMI), the degree of pericholic and right upper quadrant adhesions particularly in patients who have had previous abdominal surgery, the presence of complicated cholecystitis and the time taken by the surgeon to achieve the triangle of safety [10] with identification of the cystic artery and duct. With this scoring system a score of <2 would be considered easy, 2 to 4 moderate, 5–7 very difficult, and 8 to 10, extreme.

Fistulation of the gallbladder which would be associated with extreme difficulty and a high rate of conversion was not included in the score, given its rarity and potential to skew a simple scoring system. The five key aspects include: 1) gallbladder appearance and amount of adhesions, 2) degree of distension/contracture of the gallbladder, 3) ease of access, 4) local/septic complications, and, 5) time taken to identify the cystic artery and duct (Table 2). Where there are no adhesions, a score of zero is given. The maximum achievable score for adhesions is 3, which would occur if the gallbladder were completely buried in adhesions. A distended gallbladder receives a score of 1. Failure to grasp the gallbladder with a standard, atraumatic laparoscopic forceps scores a further point. This applies either with or without adhesions present. If decompression is performed to allow grasping then a point is still awarded. Further points are awarded for access difficulties (i.e. port placement difficulties using Hasson's technique) and complicated cholecystitis with perforation. The different grades and points are shown in Figures 1, 2, 3, 4, 5. The patient in Figure 5 would get a total of 7 points: 3 for adhesions, 1 for distended gallbladder, 1 for obesity, 1 for free fluid and 1 for a large (>1 cm) stone impacted in Hartmann's pouch. If you could not grasp the gallbladder with a standard forceps a further point would be given.

Discussion

Cholecystectomy is currently one of the commonest reasons for admission to hospital with an associated mortality of 0.45 to 6% depending on severity of gallbladder disease [11]. It accounts for a significant workflow in gastrointestinal surgery and emergency care [4,12]. Optimising care and care pathways requires an understanding of the underlying disease [13,14]. Not only can the natural history of gallbladder disease vary with patient cohorts but surgical findings can be surprising, with somewhat unexpected degrees of surgical difficulty (or ease) [15]. It is one of the more unpredictable operations in general surgery, due to the variable operative findings. Publications reporting outcomes, including conversion to open surgery, are hard to compare as currently there is no grading or scoring of operative findings at surgery [16,17].

There are some well-reported models of grading and classification systems that have laid the foundation for collaborative research and improved outcomes [18,19]. The importance of disease classification is increasingly recognised. Crandall and colleagues [20] provide a grading system for measuring anatomic severity of several Emergency General Surgery (EGS) diseases based on the American Association for the Surgery of Trauma (AAST) uniform grading system. Grading and scoring surgical conditions provide a uniform tool for reporting disease severity. As many have only been recently developed, they need validation as does the current scoring system.

The aetiology underlying variable outcomes from laparoscopic cholecystectomy is complex in origin, relating to disease severity, surgical experience, and available instrumentation. Laparoscopic cholecystectomy is now the gold standard replacing open cholecystectomy. It is accepted that recovery is delayed, and risk of complications compounded by both delayed emergency cholecystectomy and excessive conversion from laparoscopic to open surgery. Account needs to be taken, however, that a specialist hepatobiliary surgeon may have a lower conversion rate than general surgeons. However, comparisons between surgeons, institutions and published series are currently impossible as the denominator of the severity of cholecystitis is not only not standardized but also rarely reported.

Lal [15] and colleagues suggest that a difficult cholecystectomy is one taking longer that 90 minutes, tearing the gallbladder, spending more that 20 minutes dissecting the gallbladder adhesions, or more than 20 minutes dissecting Calot's triangle. While time to dissection of Calot's triangle will vary on surgical skills and level of experience, it will generally be longer in patients with increasing access difficulty, inflammation and adhesions. Predicting a difficult cholecystectomy is possible with some degree of accuracy, using patient demographics, BMI, presence of a palpable gallbladder, and pre-

Table 1 Summary of studies reporting severity scoring system for laparoscopic cholecystectomy

Study details	Statistically significant clinical parameters	Statistically significant radiological parameters	Statistically significant intra-operative parameters	Comments
Vivek et al. Prospective (n = 323)	Male gender, Previous attacks of AC, Previous upper abdominal surgery	Multiple stones Peripancreatic fluid collection	Cirrhotic liver Contracted/ distended GB Inflamed GB Ductal anomalies Adhesions	Max score of 44 (with 9 predicting difficult LC), sensitivity of 85% & specificity of 97.8%. ROC of 0.96.
Gupta et al. Prospective (n = 210) All underwent elective LC.	History of previous hospitalization due to AC, Palpable GB	Thickened (≥4 mm) GB wall, Impacted stone	N/A	Min score 0 (easy) Max score 15 (very difficult). Conversion rate 4.28% ROC of 0.86. PPV for easy and difficult LC were 90% and 88% respectively.
Randhawa et al. Prospective (n = 228)	BMI >27.5, Previous hospitalization due to AC, Palpable GB	Thickened (≥4 mm) GB wall	N/A	Conversion rate of 1.31%. ROC of 0.82. PPV for easy and difficult LC were 88.8% and 92.2% respectively.
Kanakala et al. Initially retrospective then prospective (n = 2117)	Male gender, ASA II and III	N/A	N/A	Conversion rate of 6.3%.
Bouarfa et al. Retrospective (n = 337) All underwent elective LC.	Male gender, High BMI	GB wall thickening (>2 mm), GB wall inflammation	N/A	Classification algorithms based on preoperative patient data to predict intraoperative complexity, with an accuracy of 83%.
Kama et al. Retrospective (n = 1000)	Age ≥ 60 (p = 0.052), Male gender, Abdominal tenderness, Previous upper abdominal operation	Thickened GB wall (>4 mm), Previous attacks of AC	N/A	Conversion rate of 4.8%. Both a constant and coefficient were calculated for each parameter; the sum of both gives a score for the patient
Kologlu et al. Prospective (n = 400)				This was a validation of the study by Kama et al. using the RSCLO score. Increasing RSCLO scores correlated with higher conversion rates. Conversion rate of 3%.
Lal P et al. Prospective (n = 73) All underwent elective LC.	N/A	GB wall thickness (>4 mm), Contracted GB, Stone impaction at Hartmann's pouch.	Total operating time (>90mins), Time taken to dissect GB bed/Calot's triangle (>20 mins), Spillage of stones, Tear of GB during dissection, Conversion to open were chosen as parameters describing a difficult LC.	Conversion rate of 23.3%. PPV of GB thickness, stone impaction and contracted GB to predict conversion to open were 70%, 63.6% and 45.4%, respectively, with a combined overall ultrasonographic PPV of 61.9%.
Schrenk et al. Prospective with 2 arms (n = 640 altogether)	RUQ pain, Rigidity in RUQ, Previous upper abdominal surgery, biliary colic in last 3 weeks, WCC > 10 x 10⁹/L	GB wall thickening (>5 mm), Hydroptic GB, Pericholecystic fluid, Shrunken GB, No GB filling on preoperative IV cholangiography/incarcerated cystic duct stone (on U/S)	N/A	Conversion rate of 8.2%. 5 possible scores, ranging from 0–9 (with 0 = easy LC and ≥4 = conversion to open expected). PPV of 80%.
Rosen et al. Retrospective (n = 1347) undergoing both elective and non-elective LC.	Age, BMI, AC	GB wall thickness	N/A	Conversion rate of 5.3%. For elective LC, BMI >40 and GB wall thickness > 4 mm predicted conversion. For non-elective LC, ASA >2 predicted conversion.
Nachnani et al. Prospective (n = 105)	Male gender, Previous abdominal surgery, BMI > 30, Previous AC/ acute pancreatitis	GB wall thickness > 3 mm	N/A	Conversion rate of 11.4%.
Abdel-Baki et al. (n = 40)	N/A	GB wall thickness (≥3 mm), Liver fibrosis	N/A	Conversion rate of 0.42%.
Daradkeh et al. Prospective (n = 160)	N/A	GB wall thickness (>3 mm), CBD diameter (≥7 mm)	N/A	Conversion rate of 2.5%. Adjusted r^2 for U/S parameters was 0.25.

Note on the WCC value: $WCC > 10 \times 10^9/L$

Table 1 Summary of studies reporting severity scoring system for laparoscopic cholecystectomy (Continued)

Bulbuller et al. Prospective (n = 571)	N/A	N/A	N/A	Conversion rate of 3.3%. Evaluation of RSCLO score showed good correlation with conversion to open, with a PPV of 43%, NPV of 100%, sensitivity of 100% and specificity of 96%.
Kwon et al. Retrospective (n = 305) All patients underwent ERCP and EST prior to LC (acute or elective).	See comments	See comments	See comments	This study evaluated risk factors for conversion to open surgery in patients who underwent prior ERCP and EST for choledochocystolithiasis. Cholecystitis, mechanical lithotripsy and ≥ 2 CBD stones predicted open surgery. Conversion rate of 15.7%.
Lipman et al. Retrospective (n = 1377)	Male gender, Elevated WCC (≥11,000/µL), Low serum albumin (<3.5 g/dL), Diabetes Mellitus, Elevated total bilirubin (≥1.5 g/dL)	Pericholecystic fluid	N/A	Conversion rate of 8.1%. ROC of model was 0.83.

AC: acute cholecystitis; LC: laparoscopic cholecystectomy; GB: gallbladder; ASA: American Society of Anaesthesiologists; BMI: body mass index; RUQ: right upper quadrant; WCC: white cell count; ERCP: endoscopic retrograde cholangiopancreatography; EST: endoscopic sphincterotomy.

Table 2 Operative Grading System for Cholecystitis Severity

Gallbladder appearance		
Adhesions < 50% of GB		1
Adhesions burying GB		3
	Max	3
Distension/Contraction		
Distended GB (or contracted shrivelled GB)		1
Unable to grasp with atraumatic laparoscopic forceps		1
Stone ≥1 cm impacted in Hartman's Pouch		1
Access		
BMI >30		1
Adhesions from previous surgery limiting access		1
Severe Sepsis/Complications		
Bile or Pus outside GB		1
Time to identify cystic artery and duct >90 minutes		1
	Total Max	10
Degree of difficulty		
A Mild	<2	
B Moderate	2–4	
C Severe	5–7	
D Extreme	8–10	

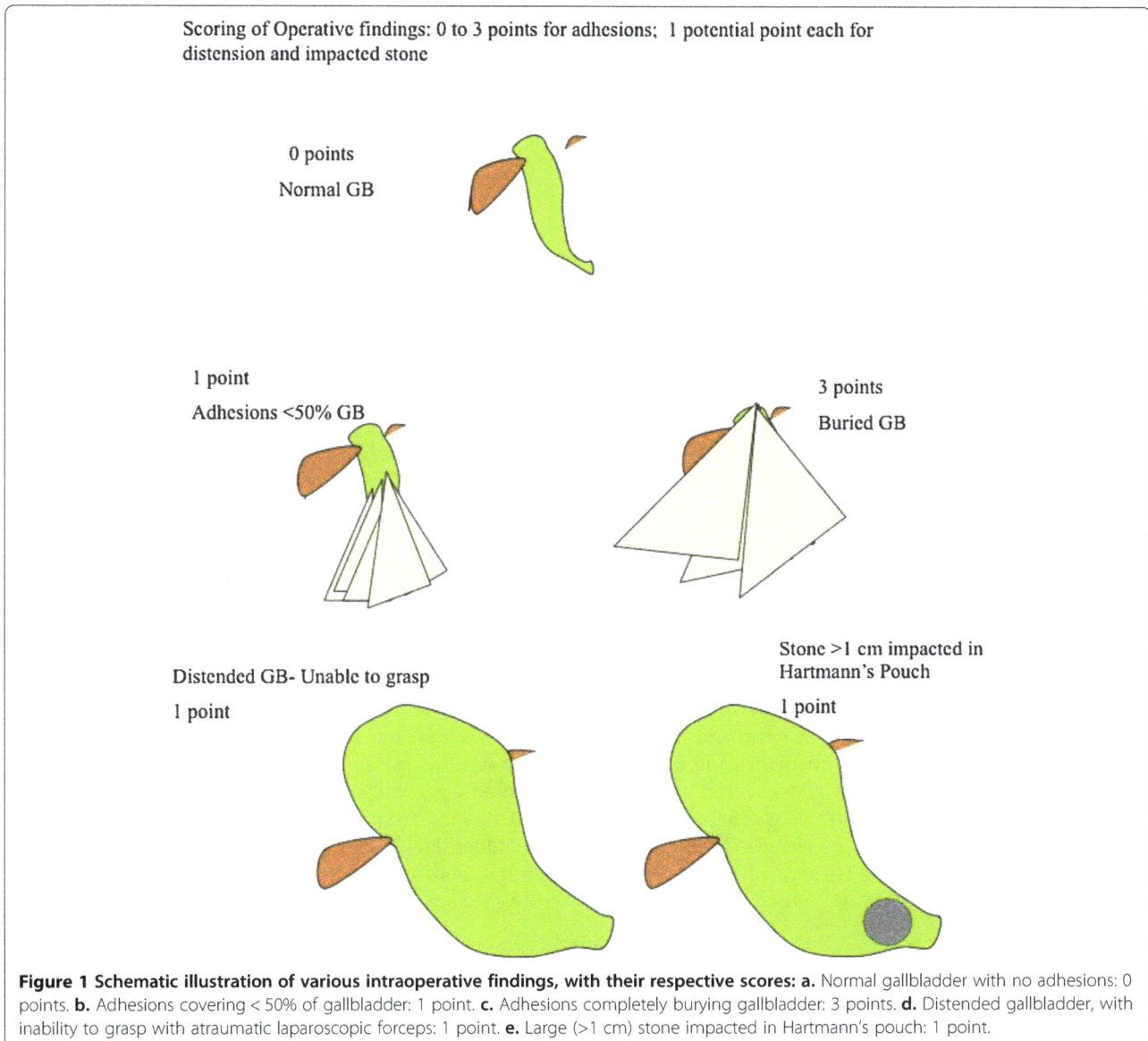

Scoring of Operative findings: 0 to 3 points for adhesions; 1 potential point each for distension and impacted stone

0 points
Normal GB

1 point
Adhesions <50% GB

3 points
Buried GB

Distended GB- Unable to grasp
1 point

Stone >1 cm impacted in Hartmann's Pouch
1 point

Figure 1 Schematic illustration of various intraoperative findings, with their respective scores: a. Normal gallbladder with no adhesions: 0 points. **b.** Adhesions covering < 50% of gallbladder: 1 point. **c.** Adhesions completely burying gallbladder: 3 points. **d.** Distended gallbladder, with inability to grasp with atraumatic laparoscopic forceps: 1 point. **e.** Large (>1 cm) stone impacted in Hartmann's pouch: 1 point.

operative ultrasound (US) or computed tomography (CT) findings [8,9]. In addition, previous cholecystitis or lithotripsy has been shown to increase the likelihood of a difficult procedure [21].

With increasing pressure to perform acute index admission laparoscopic cholecystectomy, an intraoperative-based scoring system will potentially allow meaningful comparison of outcomes [22]. In addition it may provide a trigger to prompt earlier conversion or link specific outcomes measures such as bile leaks to specific operative scores.

However, the current scoring system has some limitations. It has not been validated in a large series and has some subjectivity in terms of the percentage of the gallbladder covered by adhesion. Also, it is difficult to objectively define the amount of adhesions from previous abdominal surgery. In addition adhesions may vary in tenacity and vascularity. However these are difficult to define objectively and as such have omitted from the scoring system. It is, however, simple to calculate and provides a score out of ten. Another limitation is that it does not particularly take into account intra-operative bleeding. The actual amount of bleeding is hard to measure objectively outside a clinical trial.

Other international scoring systems have facilitated advances in clinical and research into different areas of surgery [18-20,23]. Some scoring systems, like some of the previously published gallbladder related reports, have focused on prediction of outcomes from clinical and pre-operative investigations rather than operative findings.

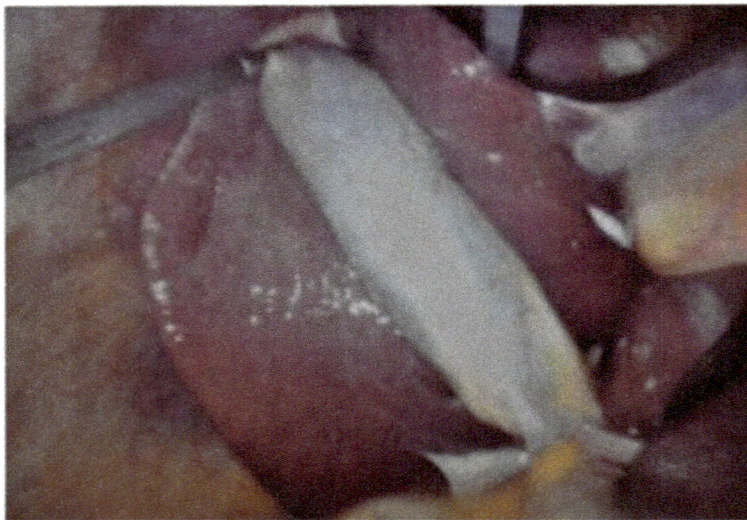

Figure 2 Intraoperative image demonstrating < 50% of gallbladder covered by adhesions (1 point).

Vivek *et al.* [9] recently reported scoring assessment of difficulty in over 300 patients undergoing laparoscopic cholecystectomy and were accurate in predicting the difficulty and need for conversion. Vivek's grading system, however, is complex using 22 parameters including 4 intra-operative parameters (distended/contracted or inflamed gallbladder, overhanging liver edge, and cirrhosis). Their scoring system has a sensitivity of 85% and specificity of 97.8% with a maximum score of 44, with a score of 9 predicting a difficult procedure. Their grading systems incorporated many other surgical challenges, including ease or difficulty with umbilical port entry, gall bladder grasping, adhesiolysis, or dissection of Calot's triangle and duct clipping. However, these are objectively difficult to measure and score. The presence of a cholecystoenteric fistula will invariably indicate severe inflammation and complexity inevitably resulting in conversion. While the absence of fistula in our scoring system may be viewed as a limitation, this phenomenon is rare enough, and if encountered intraoperatively, may warrant a maximal difficulty score.

Gupta et al. [8] in a validation of the scoring system proposed by Randhawa and colleagues [24] allocated a score ranging from 0 (easy) to 15 for the very difficult gallbladder. However, Gupta describes very few operative features- only an ultrasonographically thickened (≥4 mm) GB wall, and an impacted stone in their scoring system.

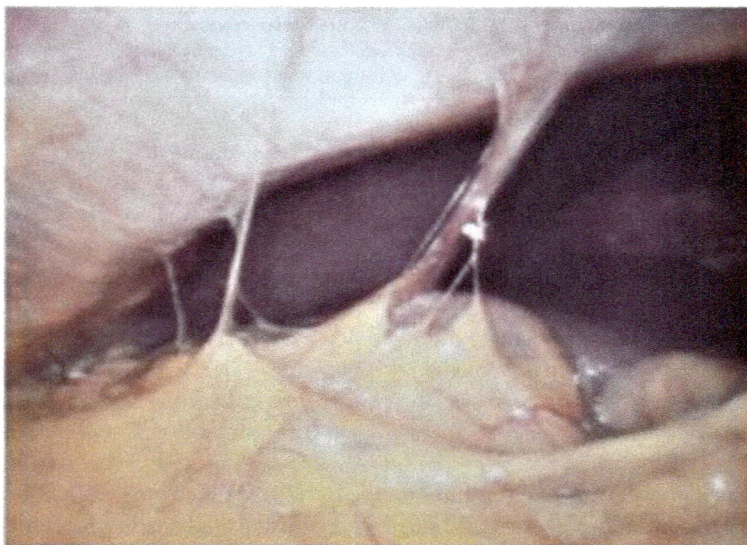

Figure 3 Intraoperative image demonstrating gallbladder completely buried in adhesions (3 points).

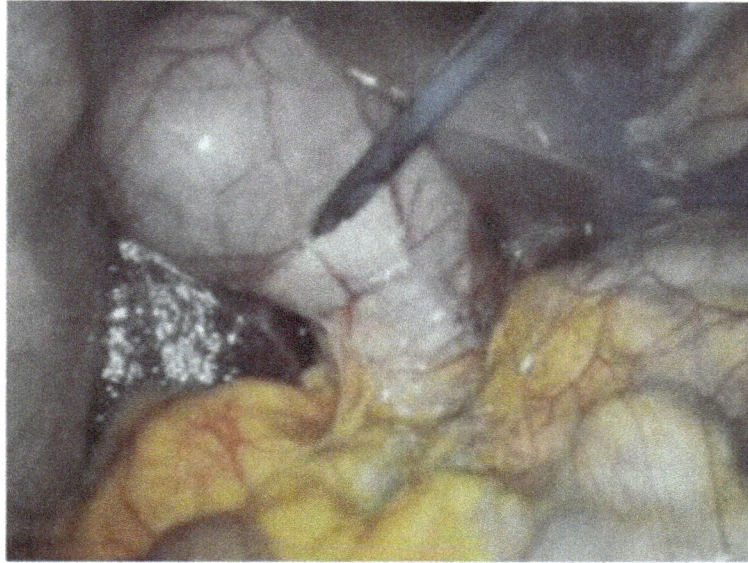

Figure 4 Intraoperative image demonstrating a distended gallbladder (1 point), with < 50% of its surface area covered by adhesions (1 point).

Gallbladder wall thickness is easily measured preoperatively on US and has been widely used in scoring systems [15,25,26]. Intra-operative measurement of thickness, while technically possible, is not practical in day-to-day surgery and has not been incorporated into our scoring system. Classification of cholecystitis such as the Tokyo Consensus [27] are used to help determine outcomes in studies evaluating treatment modalities in cholecystitis defined as the presence of local inflammation (Murphy sign or right upper quadrant mass, or tenderness) and systemic inflammation (temperature >38°C, elevated C-reactive protein [CRP] levels [>5 mg/L] or an elevated white blood cell count >10 000/μL) and imaging findings (gallstone or biliary debris with a gallbladder wall thickness >4 mm , enlarged gallbladder (long-axis diameter >8 cm and short-axis diameter >4 cm), pericholecystic fluid collection, or linear high density areas in the pericholecystic fat tissue. Severe acute calculous cholecystitis (grade III) is defined as being accompanied by dysfunctions in any one of the following organs or systems: cardiovascular dysfunction with hypotension requiring treatment, neurological dysfunction (decreased level of consciousness), respiratory dysfunction (PaO$_2$/FIO$_2$ ratio <300), renal dysfunction (oliguria, creatinine > 2.0 mg/dL liver dysfunction (prothrombin time > 3, international normalized ratio > 2) or platelet count <100 000/μL. Moderate acute calculous cholecystitis (grade II) is accompanied by any of the following parameters: white blood cell count greater than 18 000/μL, a palpable tender mass in the right upper abdominal quadrant, duration of complaints for more than 72 hours, or marked local inflammation (gangrenous cholecystitis, pericholecystic abscess, hepatic abscess, biliary peritonitis, or emphysematous cholecystitis). Cases not meeting criteria for severe or moderate acute calculous cholecystitis are classified as mild (grade I). This classification is not surgical based however, and rather broad.

Regimbeau's [28] open-label, noninferiority, randomized clinical trial utilises these recognised criteria, however, greater emphasis needs to be paid to the actual degree of operative difficulty as this reflects the degree of inflammation and potential for complications. Solomkin [29] rightly emphasizes the importance of

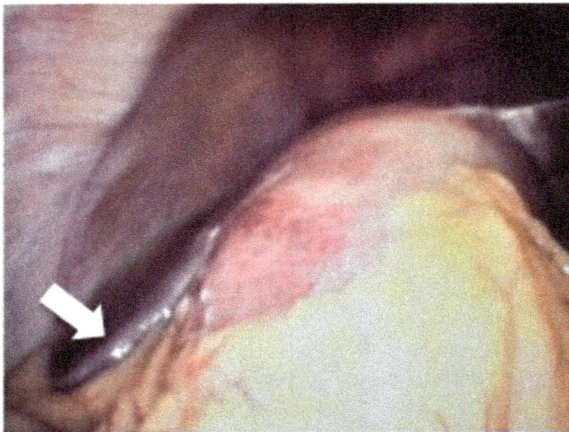

Figure 5 Intraoperative image demonstrating severe sepsis/complications, with free bile (1 point, arrow) outside a distended (I point) gallbladder, covered by adhesions (3 points).

evaluating care and outcomes in cholecystitis but we need to go a step further and recognise the importance of documenting the surgical findings to make outcome analysis more meaningful.

The current scoring system is one of the first to outline key operative findings at laparoscopic cholecystectomy. Its validity needs to be tested in future large prospective series before potentially serving as a template for future database and research into patient outcomes.

Competing interests
The authors declare that they have no competing interests.

Authors' contributions
MS: drafting of manuscript, development of scoring system, final authorization of manuscript for submission. SMS: literature search and summary of existing scoring systems, drafting of manuscript, proofreading. LA: drafting of manuscript, proofreading, critical appraisal. MDZ: drafting of manuscript, proofreading, critical apprasial. All authors read and approved the final manuscript.

Author details
[1]Department of Surgery, Letterkenny Hospital and Donegal Clinical Research Academy, National University Ireland Galway, Letterkenny, Donegal, Ireland. [2]Department of Surgery, Papa Giovanni XXIII Hospital, Bergamo, Italy. [3]Department of Surgery, Mayo Clinic, Rochester, Minnesota, USA.

References
1. Murphy JB. The diagnosis of gallstones. Am Med News 1903:825–833.
2. Litynski GS. Erich Muhe and the rejection of laparoscopic cholecystectomy (1985): a surgeon ahead of his time. JSLS : Journal of the Society of Laparoendoscopic Surgeons/Society of Laparoendoscopic Surgeons. 1998;2:341–6.
3. Gutt CN, Encke J, Koninger J, Harnoss JC, Weigand K, Kipfmuller K, et al. Acute cholecystitis: early versus delayed cholecystectomy, a multicenter randomized trial (ACDC study, NCT00447304). Ann Surg. 2013;258:385–93.
4. Takada T, Strasberg SM, Solomkin JS, Pitt HA, Gomi H, Yoshida M, et al. TG13: Updated Tokyo Guidelines for the management of acute cholangitis and cholecystitis. J Hepatobiliary Pancreat Sci. 2013;20:1–7.
5. Committee AT, Adler DG, Conway JD, Farraye FA, Kantsevoy SV, Kaul V, et al. Biliary and pancreatic stone extraction devices. Gastrointest Endosc. 2009;70:603–9.
6. Yokoe M, Takada T, Strasberg SM, Solomkin JS, Mayumi T, Gomi H, et al. TG13 diagnostic criteria and severity grading of acute cholecystitis (with videos). J Hepatobiliary Pancreat Sci. 2013;20:35–46.
7. Pitt HA. Patient value is superior with early surgery for acute cholecystitis. Ann Surg. 2014;259:16–7.
8. Gupta N, Ranjan G, Arora MP, Goswami B, Chaudhary P, Kapur A, et al. Validation of a scoring system to predict difficult laparoscopic cholecystectomy. Int J Surg. 2013;11:1002–6.
9. Vivek MA, Augustine AJ, Rao R. A comprehensive predictive scoring method for difficult laparoscopic cholecystectomy. Journal of minimal access surgery. 2014;10:62–7.
10. Strasberg SM, Hertl M, Soper NJ. An analysis of the problem of biliary injury during laparoscopic cholecystectomy. J Am Coll Surg. 1995;180:101–25.
11. de Mestral C, Rotstein OD, Laupacis A, Hoch JS, Zagorski B, Alali AS, et al. Comparative operative outcomes of early and delayed cholecystectomy for acute cholecystitis: a population-based propensity score analysis. Ann Surg. 2014;259:10–5.
12. Stromberg C, Nilsson M. Nationwide study of the treatment of common bile duct stones in Sweden between 1965 and 2009. Br J Surg. 2011;98:1766–74.
13. Sheffield KM, Ramos KE, Djukom CD, Jimenez CJ, Mileski WJ, Kimbrough TD, et al. Implementation of a critical pathway for complicated gallstone disease: translation of population-based data into clinical practice. J Am Coll Surg. 2011;212:835–43.
14. Okamoto S, Nakano K, Kosahara K, Kishinaka M, Oda H, Ichimiya H, et al. Effects of pravastatin and ursodeoxycholic acid on cholesterol and bile acid metabolism in patients with cholesterol gallstones. J Gastroenterol. 1994;29:47–55.
15. Lal P, Agarwal PN, Malik VK, Chakravarti AL. A difficult laparoscopic cholecystectomy that requires conversion to open procedure can be predicted by preoperative ultrasonography. JSLS : Journal of the Society of Laparoendoscopic Surgeons/Society of Laparoendoscopic Surgeons. 2002;6:59–63.
16. Singh K, Ohri A. Difficult laparoscopic cholecystectomy: a large series from North India. Ind J Surg. 2006;68:205e208.
17. Nachnani J, Supe A. Pre-operative prediction of difficult laparoscopic cholecystectomy using clinical and ultrasonographic parameters. Indian journal of gastroenterology : official journal of the Indian Society of Gastroenterology. 2005;24:16–8.
18. Bjorck M, Bruhin A, Cheatham M, Hinck D, Kaplan M, Manca G, et al. Classification–important step to improve management of patients with an open abdomen. World J Surg. 2009;33:1154–7.
19. Coccolini F, Ansaloni L, Manfredi R, Campanati L, Poiasina E, Bertoli P, et al. Peritoneal adhesion index (PAI): proposal of a score for the "ignored iceberg" of medicine and surgery. World journal of emergency surgery : WJES. 2013;8:6.
20. Crandall ML, Agarwal S, Muskat P, Ross S, Savage S, Schuster K, et al. Application of a uniform anatomic grading system to measure disease severity in eight emergency general surgical illnesses. Journal of Trauma and Acute Care Surgery. 2014;77:703–8.
21. Kwon YJ, Ahn BK, Park HK, Lee KS, Lee KG. What is the optimal time for laparoscopic cholecystectomy in gallbladder empyema? Surg Endosc. 2013;27:3776–80.
22. Pisano M, Ceresoli M, Campanati L, Coccolini F, Falcone C, Capponi MG, et al. Should We must Push for Primary Surgery Attempt in Case of Acute Cholecystitis? A Retrospective Analysis and a Proposal of an Evidence based Clinical Pathway. Emegency Medicine. 2014;4:201.
23. Alvarado A. A practical score for the early diagnosis of acute appendicitis. Ann Emerg Med. 1986;15:557–64.
24. Randhawa JS, Pujahari AK. Preoperative prediction of difficult lap chole: a scoring method. Indian J Surg. 2009;71:198–201.
25. Bouarfa L, Schneider A, Feussner H, Navab N, Lemke HU, Jonker PP, et al. Prediction of intraoperative complexity from preoperative patient data for laparoscopic cholecystectomy. Artif Intell Med. 2011;52:169–76.
26. Kama NA, Kologlu M, Doganay M, Reis E, Atli M, Dolapci M. A risk score for conversion from laparoscopic to open cholecystectomy. Am J Surg. 2001;181:520–5.
27. Hirota M, Takada T, Kawarada Y, Nimura Y, Miura F, Hirata K, et al. Diagnostic criteria and severity assessment of acute cholecystitis: Tokyo Guidelines. J Hepatobiliary Pancreat Surg. 2007;14:78–82.
28. Regimbeau JM, Fuks D, Pautrat K, Mauvais F, Haccart V, Msika S, et al. Effect of postoperative antibiotic administration on postoperative infection following cholecystectomy for acute calculous cholecystitis: a randomized clinical trial. JAMA. 2014;312:145–54.
29. Solomkin JS. Clinical trial evidence to advance the science of cholecystectomy. JAMA. 2014;312:135–6.

2

Surgical treatment of multiple rib fractures and flail chest in trauma: a one-year follow-up study

Eva-Corina Caragounis[1][*] [iD], Monika Fagevik Olsén[1,2], David Pazooki[1] and Hans Granhed[1]

Abstract

Background: Multiple rib fractures and unstable thoracic cage injuries are common in blunt trauma. Surgical management of rib fractures has received increasing attention in recent years and the aim of this 1-year, prospective study was to assess the long-term effects of surgery.

Methods: Fifty-four trauma patients with median Injury Severity Score 20 (9–66) and median New Injury Severity Score 34 (16–66) who presented with multiple rib fractures and flail chest, and underwent surgical stabilization with plate fixation were recruited. Patients responded to a standardized questionnaire concerning pain, local discomfort, breathlessness and use of analgesics and health-related quality of life (EQ-5D-3 L) questionnaire at 6 weeks, 3 months, 6 months and 1 year. Lung function, breathing movements, range of motion and physical function were measured at 3 months, 6 months and 1 year.

Results: Symptoms associated with pain, breathlessness and use of analgesics significantly decreased from 6 weeks to 1 year following surgery. After 1 year, 13 % of patients complained of pain at rest, 47 % had local discomfort and 9 % used analgesics. The EQ-5D-3 L index increased from 0.78 to 0.93 and perceived overall health state increased from 60 to 90 % ($p < 0.0001$) after 6 weeks to 1 year. Lung function improved significantly with predicted Forced vital capacity and Peak expiratory flow increasing from 86 to 106 % ($p = 0.0002$) and 81 to 110 % ($p < 0.0001$), respectively, from 3 months to 1 year after surgery. Breathing movements and range of motion tended to improve over time. Physical function improved significantly over time and the median Disability rating index was 0 after 1 year.

Conclusions: Patients with multiple rib fractures and flail chest show a gradual improvement in symptoms associated with pain, quality of life, mobility, disability and lung function over 1 year post surgery. Therefore, the final outcome of surgery cannot be assessed before 1 year post-operatively.

Keywords: Trauma, Rib fractures, Flail chest, Surgery, Lung function, Quality of life

Background

Multiple rib fractures occur in 10 % of poly-traumatized patients due to blunt, high-energy trauma [1] and can lead to unstable thoracic cage injuries or flail chest [2] with respiratory insufficiency. Whilst conservative management with analgesics and ventilator support has been the conventional treatment for flail chest, this can entail long hospitalization with immobilization, which leads to complications, such as pulmonary infections and long-term disability with chronic pain [3, 4]. Recently, a number of new fixation devices and better techniques have been developed for surgical treatment of rib fractures [5]. Three small, prospective, Randomized Controlled Trials (RCTs) suggest that surgical management of flail chest may decrease the need for ventilator support and intensive care [6–8]. In our clinical setting, we have found plate fixation of rib fractures to be a safe method with a low rate of complications and a reduced time and need for ventilator treatment in comparison to

* Correspondence: eva-corina.caragounis@gu.se
[1]Department of Surgery, Institute of Clinical Sciences, Sahlgrenska Academy, University of Gothenburg, Gothenburg, Sweden
Full list of author information is available at the end of the article

conservatively-managed, historical controls [9]. Our patients were reported to have experienced mild disability, decreased range of motion and lung function, and 35 % of patients had enduring pain after 6 months [10]. Long-term studies concerning lung function, mobility, pain and Quality of Life (QoL) after surgery are lacking. Two studies have reported significantly better lung function in surgically-managed patients 1 month after surgery [6, 7], whereas Marasco et al. [8] found no significant difference between operated and conservatively-managed patients after 3 months. There is a disparity in the surgical techniques used in these studies, which makes comparison difficult.

The aim of this prospective study was to examine the long-term patient outcomes associated with pain, physical function, QoL and lung function after surgical stabilization of multiple rib fractures or flail chest.

Methods

A consecutive series of 60 patients who underwent surgical fixation of multiple rib fractures as a result of blunt trauma were included in a prospective study during the period 2010–2013 [9]. The inclusion criteria for this study were: (i) Flail chest defined as three or more adjacent ribs each fractured in more than one location [2], with respiratory insufficiency (ii) Multiple rib fractures (>4) with respiratory insufficiency and also in need of a thoracotomy due to bleeding or air leakage. Respiratory insufficiency was defined as failing arterial oxygenation despite oxygen administration. Additional information on the 60 patients can be found in a previously published feasibility study [9]. Patients with severe head injury and spinal cord injury were excluded from this follow-up study.

Pre-operative Three-Dimensional (3D) reconstructions of Computer Tomography (CT) images of the thorax were used for planning the surgical procedure. The 3D reconstructions were based on images with 0.625 mm slice thickness and produced in the program AW Volume Share™ 5 (GE Healthcare). Patients were intubated with a double lumen endotracheal tube. A non-muscle sparing thoracotomy was performed to clean out hematoma and debris, identify and, if necessary, manage intra-thoracic injuries. The reason for a non-muscle sparing approach was to gain good access to the chest wall and the multiple fractured ribs. The MatrixRIB® (DePuy Synthes) Fixation System consisting of pre-shaped angular locked plates in titanium and intra-medullary splints was used to stabilize rib fractures. Post-operative pain was managed using either an intra-pleural or epidural catheter with adjunct, oral pain medication. Intravenous broad-spectrum antibiotic therapy was given prophylactically until the chest tubes had been removed. Low-molecular weight heparin was given

subcutaneously as thrombotic prophylaxis. A surgeon assessed patients at 6 weeks, 3 months, 6 months and 1 year post-operatively using a standardized questionnaire concerning pain, local discomfort, breathlessness and analgesics and QoL according to EQ-5D-3 L [11]. Pain was defined as a strong distressing sensation whereas local discomfort was defined as an unpleasant or abnormal sense to touch. The EQ-5D-3 L results were converted to a single summary index using the Time Trade-Off (TTO) technique with a Swedish reference value set [12]. A chest X-ray was taken 6 weeks post-operatively to assess the presence of lung disease and implant dysfunction or migration. A physiotherapist assessed a subgroup of patients ($n = 16$) at 3 months, 6 months and 1 year post-operatively. The selected patients all had flail chest, no co-morbidities and spoke Swedish. Standardized lung function tests [13] were performed and Forced Vital Capacity (FVC), Forced Expiratory Volume in one second (FEV1) and Peak Expiratory Flow (PEF) were recorded using an EasyOne® Spirometer (ndd Medical Technologies Inc., MA, Us). Breathing movements were measured at rest and during maximal breathing by using a Respiratory Movement Measuring Instrument, RMMI® (ReMo Inc. Keldnaholt, Reykjavik, Iceland) [14]. The range of motion in the thorax was assessed by measuring thoracic excursion (at the level of the 4th costae and the xiphoid process), flexion and lateral flexion in a standardized manner [10]. Physical function was estimated by using the Disability Rating Index (DRI) questionnaire [15] where 100 is the worst possible outcome and 0 is the best.

The SAS® statistical software package (NC, USA) was used for all statistical analyses. Results are presented as median with range or mean with standard deviation (SD) for continuous variables and n and % for categorical variables. For comparison over time, the Wilcoxon Signed Rank test was used for continuous variables and Sign test was used for categorical variables. The significance level was considered $p < 0.05$.

Results

Of the 60 patients operated six were excluded from this follow-up. Two patients died during the immediate post-operative period due to multiple organ system failure and respiratory insufficiency. Four patients were excluded due to concomitant injuries resulting in tetraplegia in one case and severe head injury in three patients. Of the 54 patients included in the study 49 patients participated while 5 patients were lost to follow-up (Fig. 1). Nineteen patients were on ventilator pre-operatively and 24 patients were on ventilator 24 h post-operatively. The mechanism of injury was in 92 % of cases either traffic accidents (59 %) or falls (33 %). The indication for surgery was flail chest in 51 patients,

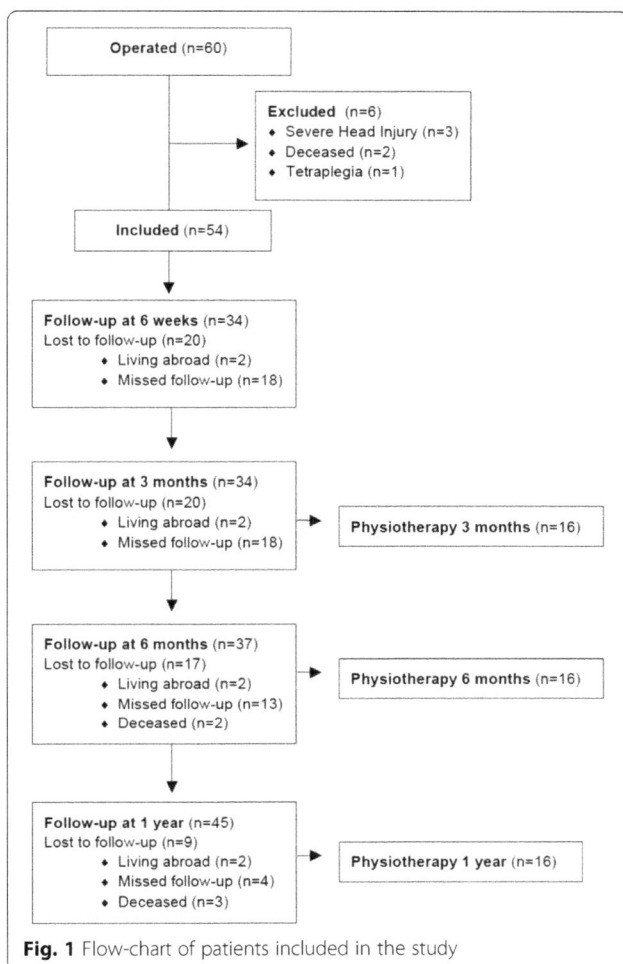

```
┌──────────────────────────┐
│     Operated (n=60)      │
└──────────────────────────┘
            │
            │       ┌─────────────────────────────────┐
            ├──────▶│ Excluded (n=6)                   │
            │       │ ◆ Severe Head Injury (n=3)       │
            │       │ ◆ Deceased (n=2)                 │
            │       │ ◆ Tetraplegia (n=1)              │
            │       └─────────────────────────────────┘
            ▼
┌──────────────────────────┐
│     Included (n=54)      │
└──────────────────────────┘
            │
            ▼
┌──────────────────────────────┐
│ Follow-up at 6 weeks (n=34)  │
│ Lost to follow-up (n=20)     │
│   ◆ Living abroad (n=2)      │
│   ◆ Missed follow-up (n=18)  │
└──────────────────────────────┘
            │
            ▼
┌──────────────────────────────┐      ┌──────────────────────────────┐
│ Follow-up at 3 months (n=34) │      │ Physiotherapy 3 months (n=16)│
│ Lost to follow-up (n=20)     │─────▶│                              │
│   ◆ Living abroad (n=2)      │      └──────────────────────────────┘
│   ◆ Missed follow-up (n=18)  │
└──────────────────────────────┘
            │
            ▼
┌──────────────────────────────┐      ┌──────────────────────────────┐
│ Follow-up at 6 months (n=37) │      │ Physiotherapy 6 months (n=16)│
│ Lost to follow-up (n=17)     │─────▶│                              │
│   ◆ Living abroad (n=2)      │      └──────────────────────────────┘
│   ◆ Missed follow-up (n=13)  │
│   ◆ Deceased (n=2)           │
└──────────────────────────────┘
            │
            ▼
┌──────────────────────────────┐      ┌──────────────────────────────┐
│ Follow-up at 1 year (n=45)   │      │ Physiotherapy 1 year (n=16)  │
│ Lost to follow-up (n=9)      │─────▶│                              │
│   ◆ Living abroad (n=2)      │      └──────────────────────────────┘
│   ◆ Missed follow-up (n=4)   │
│   ◆ Deceased (n=3)           │
└──────────────────────────────┘
```

Fig. 1 Flow-chart of patients included in the study

bleeding in two patients and air leakage in one patient. The included patients consisted of 40 (74 %) men and 14 (26 %) women with the median age of 57 years (20–86), median Injury Severity Score (ISS) 20 (9–66) and median New Injury Severity Score (NISS) 34 (16–66). Between 63–83 % of included patients in our study attended each follow-up but only 22 patients attended all dates. A physiotherapist assessed 16 patients; ten men and six women, at 3 months, 6 months and 1 year post-operatively. There was a larger proportion of women in the subgroup assessed by a physiotherapist, otherwise age, ISS and NISS was comparable to the overall study group.

The proportion of patients seen at follow-up with pain at rest decreased with 26 % ($p = 0.039$) between 6 weeks and 3 months after surgery. Problems associated with pain on breathing and breathlessness decreased progressively by 21 % ($p = 0.039$) and 27 % ($p = 0.022$), respectively, during the first post-operative year. After 1 year, 13 % of patients complained of pain at rest, 9 % experienced pain on breathing and 16 % experienced breathlessness. Local discomfort did not decrease with time, but remained constant and affected approximately 47 % of patients. Despite enduring pain, there was a significant, 49 % ($p < 0.0001$) decrease in the proportion of patients using analgesia, with 9 % on pain medication after 1 year (Table 1).

Patients' QoL measured with EQ-5D-3 L showed median index values that progressively increased from 0.78 at 6 weeks to 0.93 after 1 year, with the greatest improvement occurring between 6 weeks and 3 months after surgery (Fig. 2). There was a significant decrease in the proportion of patients experiencing problems with mobility (27 %, $p = 0.022$), self-care (36 %, $p = 0.0005$), performance of usual activities (55 %, $p = 0.0001$), and pain or discomfort (27 %, $p = 0.035$) from 6 weeks to 1 year after surgery. There was no significant improvement in symptoms of anxiety or depression over time. The QoL measured by Visual Analogue Scale (VAS) improved significantly over time: median VAS was 60 % (20–96) at 6 weeks, 76 % (40–97) at 3 months, 80 % (20–100) at 6 months and 90 % (30–100) after 1 year. Quality of life significantly increased (30 %, $p < 0.0001$) between 6 weeks to 1 year following surgery.

Percent predicted FVC improved by 6.88 % (SD 5.84; $p = 0.0002$) from 3 to 6 months and by 19.8 % (SD 14.1; $p = 0.0002$) from 3 months to 1 year after surgery. There was no significant improvement in FEV1 over time. There was no significant improvement in mean predicted PEF between 3 and 6 months, but PEF significantly increased by 28.5 % (SD 20.4; $p < 0.0001$) from 3 months to 1 year. After 1 year the mean FVC was 106 %, PEF was 110 % and FEV1 was 80 % compared to predicted values (Table 2).

Breathing movements were decreased on the operated side of the thorax as compared to the non-operated side 3 months after surgery. The operated side showed a tendency towards improved movement over time and better results at 1-year follow-up as regards movements of the upper thorax at rest as compared to the non-operated side (Table 3). Ranges of motion at different levels in the thorax were measured at 3 months, 6 months and 1 year after surgery. Lower level thoracic excursion improved significantly between 3 and 6 months, thoracic flexion and thoracic extension improved significantly between 3 months and 1 year, otherwise movement stayed unchanged (Table 3). Physical function increased significantly over time (Table 3). Between 3 and 6 months, there was an 8.7 mm ($p = 0.047$) decrease in median DRI and between 3 months and 1 year, there was an 18.4 mm ($p = 0.013$) decrease with a median DRI of 0. Of the subset of 16 patients, the number who experienced no disability was three at 3 months, six at 6 months and 10 after 1 year (Table 3).

Table 1 Proportion of patients at follow-up with subjective symptoms after rib fracture surgery

Symptoms	6 weeks (n = 34)	3 months (n = 34)	6 months (n = 37)	1 year (n = 45)
Pain at Rest	12 (35.3 %)	4[a]* (11.8 %)	6 (16.2 %)	6[c]* (13.3 %)
Pain on Breathing	8 (23.5 %)	5 (14.7 %)	3 (8.1 %)	4[c]* (8.9 %)
Local Discomfort	14 (41.2 %)	17 (50.0 %)	19 (51.4 %)	21 (46.7 %)
Breathlessness	14 (41.2 %)	12 (35.3 %)	10 (27.0 %)	7[c]* (15.6 %)
Analgesia Usage	18 (52.9 %)	13 (38.2 %)	5[b]** (13.5 %)	4[c]*** (8.9 %)

* p-value <0.05
** p-value <0.01
*** p-value <0.001
[a] Difference from 6 weeks to 3 months (n = 27)
[b] Difference from 6 weeks to 6 months (n = 27)
[c] Difference from 6 weeks to 1 year (n = 33)

One patient developed osteomyelitis and underwent a re-operation with plate extraction after 7 months with cessation of infection as a result. A second re-operation was performed on a professional athlete who experienced local pain at the site of a protruding plate when practicing his sport. One patient had a loose screw on the plate, whilst another patient had a loose intra-medullary splint on chest X-rays 6 weeks post-operatively; however neither patient experienced clinical symptoms and they were not re-operated. Three patients (5.6 %) died within 1 year after surgery; one patient died after 65 days due to cardiac arrest, one patient died after 137 days due to complications of Chronic Obstructive Lung Disease (COPD) and the third patient died after 277 days due to osteomyelitis in the tenth thoracic vertebra.

Discussion

In this prospective study of 54 trauma patients who underwent stabilizing surgery of rib fractures, we found progressive improvement in pain, mobility, activity, QoL, lung function and disability during the first, post-operative year.

The primary end-point in previous studies of surgical treatment of flail chest has mainly focused on aspects associated with respiratory insufficiency. Although acute pain can contribute to respiratory problems, chronic pain can be debilitating and lead to decreased QoL. We found that 13 % of our patients experienced enduring chest pain at rest after 1 year. In contrast, a previous observational study of conservatively-managed patients with flail chest showed that 49 % experienced enduring pain after a mean follow-up of 5 years [4]. It is probable that surgery decreases chronic pain. In the prospective RCT of Tanaka et al., symptoms of chest tightness, thoracic cage pain and dyspnea on effort were more frequent in conservatively-managed patients [6]. Surgery *per se* is associated with morbidity, however, and 47 % of our patients experienced some form of local discomfort, although it was unclear whether this was due to the trauma or surgery. Despite enduring pain and discomfort, only 9 % of patients used analgesics, suggesting mild and not particularly disabling symptoms. Patient

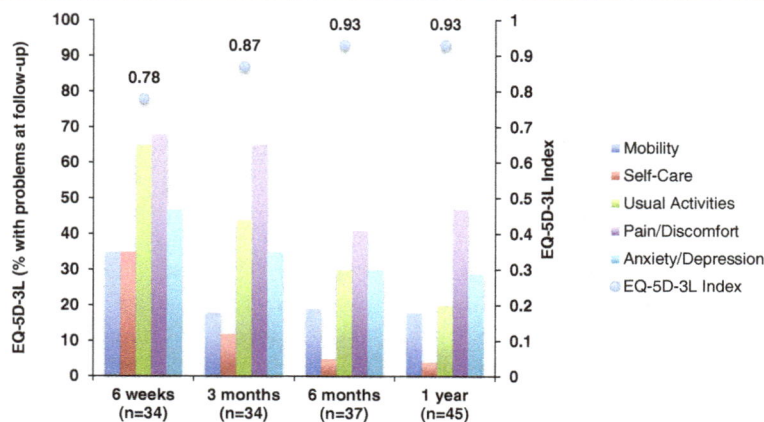

Fig. 2 Quality of life measured by EQ-5D-3 L, showing the percentage of patients with some or extreme difficulties and median EQ-5D-3 L index values at 6 weeks, 3 months, 6 months and 1 year follow-up

Table 2 Lung function of patients with flail chest ($n = 16$) at 3, 6 and 12 months after surgery

Lung Function	3 months % Predicted	6 months % Predicted	Δ 3–6 months % Predicted	Δ 3–6 months P-value	12 months % Predicted	Δ 3–12 months % Predicted	Δ 3–12 months P-value
FVC (L)	86.2 ± 19.4	93.1 ± 20.7	6.9 ± 5.8	$p = 0.0002$	105.9 ± 17.5	19.8 ± 14.1	$p = 0.0002$
FEV1 (L)	79.4 ± 22.7	81.8 ± 25.3	2.3 ± 7.5	$p = 0.100$	80.4 ± 29.6	0.95 ± 31.9	$p = 0.74$
PEF (L/min)	81.4 ± 19.5	83.7 ± 24.3	2.3 ± 16.5	$p = 0.50$	109.9 ± 24.8	28.5 ± 20.4	$p < 0.0001$

QoL improved gradually after surgery; the median EQ-5D-3 L VAS was 90 % after 1 year, which is higher than that of a Swedish population study, which showed a mean VAS of 77.4 and 75.8 % for men and women, respectively [16]. The median EQ-5D-3 L index was 0.93 in our patients 1 year after surgery, which is higher than that of healthy individuals in the population study mentioned [16], where men had 0.84 and women 0.80. We found that our patients did not improve significantly in the dimension concerning anxiety or depression. It is possible that these were pre-existing problems since trauma patients are often afflicted with psychiatric problems and substance abuse [17], but it is also probable that the trauma itself is a cause of persisting anxiety and depression. The only RCT to compare QoL in operated and conservatively managed patients found no difference between the groups at 6 months follow-up [8].

Lung function in a subgroup of patients improved significantly over time and patients reached FVC and PEF values of greater than 100 % of predicted values after 1 year. The FEV did not improve over time and was approximately 80 % of the predicted value, which indicates a remaining obstructive component. Tanaka et al. [6] found progressive improvement in FVC during a follow-up period of 1 year, where patients stabilized with Judet struts had consistently significantly better results compared to conservatively-managed patients. These patients, however, did not reach the 100 % and above values in predicted lung function, as seen in our study. Granetzny et al. [7] used Kirschner wires to stabilize patients and also showed better lung function compared to conservatively-managed patients, 2 months after surgery, whereas Marasco et al. used biodegradable inion plates and found no difference in lung function after 3 months [8]. Whilst it takes the inion plate 18–24 months to

Table 3 Breathing movements, range of motion and disability rating index (DRI) of patients with flail chest ($n = 16$) 3, 6 and 12 months after surgery

Breathing Movements ($n = 16$)	3 months Mean Δ Operated vs Non-Operated side	6 months Mean Δ Operated vs Non-Operated side	1 year Mean Δ Operated vs Non-Operated side
Rest			
Upper Thorax (mm)	-0.76 ± 1.12	-0.40 ± 0.68	0.49 ± 1.32[b]**
Lower Thorax (mm)	-0.22 ± 0.88	0.10 ± 0.56	0.27 ± 0.82
Abdominal (mm)	-0.20 ± 1.67	0.43 ± 1.63	0.14 ± 1.40
Maximal Breathing			
Upper Thorax (mm)	-3.04 ± 5.24	-1.24 ± 1.77	0.10 ± 4.88
Lower Thorax (mm)	-0.05 ± 4.57	1.48 ± 3.62	1.05 ± 4.46
Abdominal (mm)	-0.91 ± 4.92	-0.58 ± 2.64	0.65 ± 5.09
Range of Motion ($n = 16$)	3 months Mean	6 months Mean	1 year Mean
Upper level Thoracic Excursion (cm)	3.84 ± 1.71	4.09 ± 1.53	3.98 ± 1.58
Lower level Thoracic Excursion (cm)	3.41 ± 1.29	4.38 ± 1.70[a]*	3.82 ± 1.61
Thoracic Flexion (cm)	1.75 ± 0.88	2.06 ± 1.03	2.25 ± 0.75[b]*
Thoracic Extension (cm)	0.66 ± 0.47	0.88 ± 0.43	1.17 ± 0.45[b]**
Lateral Flexion towards injured side (cm)	14.50 ± 3.80	15.50 ± 5.30	14.10 ± 6.20
Lateral Flexion from injured side (cm)	14.80 ± 5.40	15.90 ± 4.20	14.40 ± 6.40
DRI ($n = 16$)	3 months Median	6 months Median	1 year Median
(0–100 mm)	23.0 (0.0–78.1)	15.3[a]* (0.0–65.3)	0.0[b]* (0.0–66.9)

* p-value <0.05
** p-value <0.01
[a] Difference from 3 months to 6 months
[b] Difference from 3 months to 1 year

resorb, it gradually loses most of its strength within 18–36 weeks and might weaken before the bone is fully healed. Considering the very different approaches to surgical stabilization in the aforementioned studies, comparison of results is difficult. Based on our studies [9, 10], we believe that surgical stabilization using the MatrixRIB® (DePuy Synthes) Fixation System is superior since the plates mimic the biodynamic characteristics of the ribs and are fixed with angular locked screws creating stability in movement without losing strength over time.

None of the RCTs have studied breathing movements and range of motion at follow-up. We found that breathing movements were decreased on the operated side, but tended to improve gradually over time, and whilst a statistically significant improvement was found in movements of the upper thorax at rest, these changes were not clinically significant and there was no major difference between operated and non-operated side. The range of motion was statistically improved as regards the lower level thoracic excursion, flexion and extension but the changes were small and of little clinical relevance. Physical function, assessed by DRI, improved gradually and significantly with time; the median was 0 after 1 year, indicating no loss of function. However, the range of 0–67 suggests a spread, with some patients experiencing some difficulty (≥25) or difficulty (≥50) in function. The results may also reflect long-term outcome of concomitant injuries; however, we found that at least 50 % of trauma patients who have undergone surgical fixation of flail chest have no remaining disability after 1 year. Previous studies of conservatively-managed patients with flail chest have shown that 66 and 38 % of them experienced persistent disability after 2 months [3] and during a mean follow-up period of 5 years (6 months-12 years) [4], respectively. Marasco et al. found that 71 % of conservatively managed patients experienced daily limitations and disabilities after 3 months compared to 48 % of operated patients, suggesting that surgical management of flail chest decreases prolonged disability, although this may be particularly evident in cases of isolated thoracic injuries.

Late complications were seen in four out of 60 patients with two undergoing re-operations due to deep wound infection and subjective symptoms from a protruding plate. We consider this a low rate of complications considering these were among the first patients operated at our centre.

The results of this study are limited as this was an uncontrolled study. The patients included were mostly subjected to poly-trauma, as demonstrated by a median ISS of 20. Poly-trauma patients are an inherent, heterogeneous group with associated injuries in addition to their thoracic trauma, which serve as confounding factors influencing the perception of pain, function, activity and QoL. Results from patients with isolated thoracic injury are likely to have been more homogenous and easier to interpret, but such a group would not have been representative of the population at large. Even in isolated thoracic injury, however, there are confounding factors due to commonly associated clavicle and scapular fractures that influence the mobility, function and pain of the thoracic cage. Moreover, the pre-existing pain, function and disability were unknown for patients in this study. Between 63–83 % of patients in our study attended each follow-up but only 22 patients attended all dates, which poses a weakness and a potential bias in the results. However, the age, sex, ISS and NISS values compared between included patients and those at each follow-up were similar.

Surgical treatment of rib fractures has received increasing attention in recent years. While previous studies have largely focused on the treatment of flail chest, it is not clearly defined if patients with multiple rib fractures or dislocated ribs also benefit from surgery. We chose to study the long-term results of patients with flail chest as this group has been the main focus of previous studies. However, patients with multiple rib fractures that required surgery for other reasons, such as air leakage or bleeding, were also stabilized and therefore included in this study. With the development of minimally invasive approaches to rib fixation more will be gained from surgery and the indications may well include multiple rib fractures in the future. A muscle-sparing approach to the ribs and a selective usage of thoracotomy would presumably decrease post-operative pain. However, muscle-sparing techniques minimize access to the injured chest wall making it difficult to fixate multiple rib fractures. Video-assisted thoracoscopic surgery (VATS) could be used to clear out hematoma and resect leaking lung tissue. However, the technique does require lung deflation to some extent, which may not be possible in all trauma patients with severe lung contusions.

The method used for stabilizing ribs varies between different studies, making comparison difficult as the biomechanical properties of the implants differ. There is a need for larger prospective RCTs that compare not only the outcome of surgery concerning ventilator support and Intensive Care Unit (ICU) care, but also the long-term outcomes associated with pain, function, activity and QoL, as well as cost-benefit of such surgical management.

Conclusions

Patients who underwent surgical plate fixation of multiple rib fractures and flail chest showed a gradual improvement in symptoms associated with pain, physical function, lung function and QoL, which continued throughout the first post-operative year. Breathing movements, range of motion, symptoms of anxiety or depression, and local discomfort did not improve significantly over time. We conclude that the final outcome after plate fixation of rib fractures cannot be assessed before 1 year post-operatively.

Abbreviations
3D, Three-Dimensional; COPD, Chronic Obstructive Lung Disease; CT, Computer Tomography; DRI, Disability Rating Index; FEV1, Forced Expiratory Volume in One second; FVC, Forced Vital Capacity; ICU, Intensive Care Unit; ISS, Injury Severity Score; NISS, New Injury Severity Score; PEF, Peak Expiratory Flow; QoL, Quality of Life; RCT, Randomized Controlled Trial; RMMI, Respiratory Movement Measuring Instrument; SD, Standard Deviation; TTO, Time Trade-Off; VAS, Visual Analogue Scale.

Acknowledgements
We would like to thank Sahlgrenska University Hospital, Gothenburg, Sweden for supporting this study.

Funding
The study was supported by funds administered by Sahlgrenska University Hospital and Sahlgrenska Academy, University of Gothenburg, Gothenburg, Sweden. The funding source had no involvement in the design of the study, analyses of the results or in the writing and submission of the manuscript for publication.

Authors' contributions
ECC acquired and analyzed the data and drafted the manuscript. MFO, DP and HG participated in designing the study and collecting data. All authors read and approved the final manuscript for submission.

Competing interests
The authors declare that they have no competing interests.

Author details
[1]Department of Surgery, Institute of Clinical Sciences, Sahlgrenska Academy, University of Gothenburg, Gothenburg, Sweden. [2]Department of Physical Therapy, Institute of Neuroscience and Physiology, Sahlgrenska Academy, University of Gothenburg, Gothenburg, Sweden.

References
1. Ziegler DW, Agarwal NN. The morbidity and mortality of rib fractures. J Trauma. 1994;37(6):975–9.
2. Gennarelli TA, Wodzin E, Barrington IL. Association for the Advancement of Automotive Medicine: The Abbreviated Injury Scale 2005 - Update 2008. 2008.
3. Fabricant L, Ham B, Mullins R, Mayberry J. Prolonged pain and disability are common after rib fractures. Am J Surg. 2013;205(5):511–5. discusssion 515-516.
4. Landercasper J, Cogbill TH, Lindesmith LA. Long-term disability after flail chest injury. J Trauma. 1984;24(5):410–4.
5. Bemelman M, Poeze M, Blokhuis TJ, Leenen LP. Historic overview of treatment techniques for rib fractures and flail chest. Eur J Trauma Emerg Surg. 2010;36(5):407–15.
6. Tanaka H, Yukioka T, Yamaguti Y, Shimizu S, Goto H, Matsuda H, Shimazaki S. Surgical stabilization of internal pneumatic stabilization? A prospective randomized study of management of severe flail chest patients. J Trauma. 2002;52(4):727–32. discussion 732.
7. Granetzny A, Abd El-Aal M, Emam E, Shalaby A, Boseila A. Surgical versus conservative treatment of flail chest. Evaluation of the pulmonary status. Interact Cardiovasc Thorac Surg. 2005;4(6):583–7.
8. Marasco SF, Davies AR, Cooper J, Varma D, Bennett V, Nevill R, Lee G, Bailey M, Fitzgerald M. Prospective randomized controlled trial of operative rib fixation in traumatic flail chest. J Am Coll Surg. 2013;216(5):924–32.
9. Granhed HP, Pazooki D. A feasibility study of 60 consecutive patients operated for unstable thoracic cage. J Trauma Manag Outcomes. 2014;8(1):20.
10. Fagevik Olsén M, Pazooki D, Granhed H. Recovery after stabilising surgery for "flail chest". Eur J Trauma Emerg Surg. 2013;39(5):501–6.
11. Group TE. EuroQol-a new facility for the measurement of health-related quality of life. Health Policy. 1990;16(3):199–208.
12. Burstrom K, Sun S, Gerdtham UG, Henriksson M, Johannesson M, Levin LA, Zethraeus N. Swedish experience-based value sets for EQ-5D health states. Qual Life Res. 2014;23(2):431–42.
13. Quanjer PH, Tammeling GJ, Cotes JE, Pedersen OF, Peslin R, Yernault JC. Lung volumes and forced ventilatory flows. Report Working Party Standardization of Lung Function Tests, European Community for Steel and Coal. Official Statement of the European Respiratory Society. Eur Respir J Suppl. 1993;16:5–40.
14. Ragnarsdottir M, Kristinsdottir EK. Breathing movements and breathing patterns among healthy men and women 20-69 years of age. Reference values. Respiration Int Review Thorac Dis. 2006;73(1):48–54.
15. Salén B, Spangfort E, Nygren A, Nordemar R. The Disability Rating Index: an instrument for the assessment of disability in clinical settings. J Clin Epidemiol. 1994;47:1423–35.
16. Burstrom K, Johannesson M, Rehnberg C. Deteriorating health status in Stockholm 1998-2002: results from repeated population surveys using the EQ-5D. Qual Life Res Int J Qual Life Asp Treat Care Rehab. 2007;16(9):1547–53.
17. Brattstrom O, Eriksson M, Larsson E, Oldner A. Socio-economic status and co-morbidity as risk factors for trauma. Eur J Epidemiol. 2015;30(2):151–7.

3

Focused abdominal sonography for trauma in the clinical evaluation of children with blunt abdominal trauma

Offir Ben-Ishay[*], Mai Daoud, Zvi Peled, Eran Brauner, Hany Bahouth and Yoram Kluger

Abstract

Introduction: In pediatric care, the role of focused abdominal sonography in trauma (FAST) remains ill defined. The objective of this study was to assess the sensitivity and specificity of FAST for detecting free peritoneal fluid in children.

Methods: The trauma registry of a single level I pediatric trauma center was queried for the results of FAST examination of consecutive pediatric (<18 years) blunt trauma patients over a period of 36 months, from January 2010 to December 2012. Demographics, type of injuries, FAST results, computerized tomography (CT) results, and operative findings were reviewed.

Results: During the study period, 543 injured pediatric patients (mean age 8.2 ± 5 years) underwent FAST examinations. In 95 (17.5 %) FAST was positive for free peritoneal fluid. CT examination was performed in 219 (40.3 %) children. Positive FAST examination was confirmed by CT scan in 61/73 (83.6 %). CT detected intra-peritoneal fluid in 62/448 (13.8 %) of the patients with negative FAST results. These findings correspond to a sensitivity of 50 %, specificity of 88 %, positive predictive value (PPV) of 84 %, and a negative predictive value (NPV) of 58 %. In patients who had negative FAST results and no CT examination (302), no missed abdominal injury was detected on clinical ground. FAST examination in the young age group (<2 years) yielded lower sensitivity and specificity (36 and 78 % respectively) with a PPV of only 50 %.

Conclusions: This study shows that although a positive FAST evaluation does not necessarily correlate with an IAI, a negative one strongly suggests the absence of an IAI, with a high NPV. These findings are emphasized in the analysis of the subgroup of children less than 2 years of age. FAST examination tempered with sound clinical judgment seems to be an effective tool to discriminate injured children in need of further imaging evaluation.

Background

Focused abdominal sonography for trauma (FAST) was first described in the early 1970s as an adjunct for injured evaluation in the emergency department. FAST has demonstrated its advantages as an easily comprehended examination, which is performed quickly, entails no radiation dose and has a reasonable sensitivity and specificity in adults.

FAST was first abandoned soon after its emergence, only to resurface in the 1990's [1, 2] For adults, the use of FAST rapidly flourished, and in 1999, 80 % of the level I adult trauma centers reported its routine use [3].

Fast is used to detect fluid in the Morison and splenorenal pouch, pelvis and around the pericard, recently eFAST (Extended FAST) was introduced and included also the evaluation of both hemithoraxes. FAST has not gained popularity among pediatric trauma care providers. A national survey published in 2009 revealed that only 15 % of pediatric trauma centers in the United States adopted FAST as part of a blunt abdominal injury assessment protocol, compared to 96 % of the adult centers [4]. Therefore, the body of evidence for the use of FAST in the pediatric population is limited and mostly extrapolated from studies in adults. Furthermore, data on the sensitivity and specificity of FAST in toddlers

* Correspondence: o_ben-ishay@Rambam.health.gov.il
Department of General of Surgery, Division of Surgery Rambam Health Care Campus, 8 Ha'Aliyah St, Haifa 35254, Israel

under the age of 2 years is particularly deficient. Negus et al. addressed this issue and emphasized the need for pediatric separate guidelines [5].

The use of FAST as a triage tool for further investigation is important in an effort to reduce unnecessary exposure to ionizing radiation. Menaker et al. showed the use of FAST increases with the physician's suspicion for IAI (Intraabdominal injury), and in patients with low and medium risk for IAI the use of FAST decreased the use of abdominal computed tomography [6].

The purpose of the current study was to assess the sensitivity and specificity of FAST for detecting free peritoneal fluid and abdominal injury in the pediatric population, with a particular focus on toddlers.

Methods

We performed a retrospective analysis of prospectively collected data of the trauma registry of a single level I pediatric trauma center. Patients under the age of 18 years who underwent FAST during the period January 2010 through December 2012 were identified. Results of FAST, CT scan and operative findings were collected from patients' electronic files. The primary outcome measure was the presence of free fluid in the peritoneal cavity, confirmed by CT scan. Secondary outcome measures were intra-abdominal injury (IAI), confirmed by CT scan or at laparotomy. The absence of IAI was defined either by a normal CT scan in patients that underwent one, or a clinical follow-up in patients who did not. Sensitivity, specificity, accuracy, and positive and negative predictive values were calculated for the primary and secondary outcome measures. Further subgroup analysis was undertaken for patients ≤ 2 years of age.

FAST technique

According to hospital protocol, FAST examination was performed upon admission for all patients who sustained blunt abdominal injury, regardless of their hemodynamic status. Initial FAST examination was performed by a radiology resident, who in our institution is a trauma team member. The examiner routinely evaluated the presence of free fluid in the hepato-renal, spleno-renal, pelvis, and pericardial spaces. Results are reported as positive or negative without any further interpretation of intra-abdominal injury. FAST was performed with a Sonosite Ultrasound Machine M-Turbo, (FujiFilm). Using a Micromax abdominal curved array transducer 2-5MHZ. During the time frame of the study no protocol existed regarding the use of CT scan in this cohort of patients, decisions regarding the patient's management were taken by the trauma attending in charge of the case, patients would either go to the OR, further imaging modalities or observation. The decision was taken namely according to the mechanism of injury and associated injuries.

CT technique

The CT was performed with a Siemens Somatom definition flash, 128 channels. Iodine based IV contrast material (Iomeron 300, Dexxon, Or akiva, Israel) was injected intravenously in all patients. Our abdominal CT trauma protocol include a first scan that is performed with a delay of 70 s and a second delayed scan (5 min) for nephrographic delination. All scans were evaluated by a radiology resident and further re-evaluated by a radiology attending.

Results

During the study, 543 children with suspected blunt abdominal injury were evaluated with FAST examination. The mean age was 8.2 ± 5 years. Ninety- five (17.5 %) had a positive FAST examination. CT scan was performed in 219 (40.3 %). A total of 22 (4 %) patients had abdominal injuries: 11 (50 %) had splenic injuries, 11 (50 %) liver injuries and 3 (13.6 %) small bowel injuries. One patient (4.5 %) sustained renal trauma. Exploratory laparotomy was performed in 9 (1.7 %) patients. One (0.2 %) succumbed to a severe head injury. Indications for laparotomy were hemodynamic instability in 5 (55.6 %) patients, failure of non-operative management of a grade IV liver injury in 1 (11.1 %), and a CT finding that suggested small bowel injury in 3 (33.3 %) patients.

Of the 95 patients with positive FAST results, CT was performed in 73 (76.8 %) and free fluid was detected in 61 (64.2 %) (Fig. 1). Thus, the use of FAST for the detection of free peritoneal fluid yielded a sensitivity of 50 %, specificity of 88 %, and a positive predictive value (PPV) of 84 % (Table 1).

Intra abdominal injury (IAI) was detected in 12 of the 73 patients who had positive FAST results and underwent CT (Fig. 2). None of the patients with a positive FAST result who did not undergo CT had a clinically significant missed IAI, based on clinical findings and follow-up of these patients. The 5 who had an IAI were operated based on the positivity of the FAST examination and their hemodynamic status. Thus, the detection by FAST of IAI yielded a sensitivity of 77 %, specificity of 70 %, and a negative predictive value (NPV) of 97 % (Table 1).

In a subgroup analysis of the 89 (16.4 %) toddlers under the age of 2 years, 13 (14.6 %) had positive FAST results (Fig. 3). CT was performed in 8/13 (61.5 %) of them, and free fluid detected in 4/8 (50 %). Thus, the use of FAST for the detection of free peritoneal fluid in children aged < 2 years yielded a sensitivity of 37 % and a specificity of 78 %, with a fairly low PPV and NPV (50 and 67 % respectively). Two of the patients with a positive FAST result had an IAI (Fig. 4) and were transferred directly to the operating room due to hemodynamic instability. None of the 76 patients with a negative FAST had an IAI. Thus, the correlation of FAST with

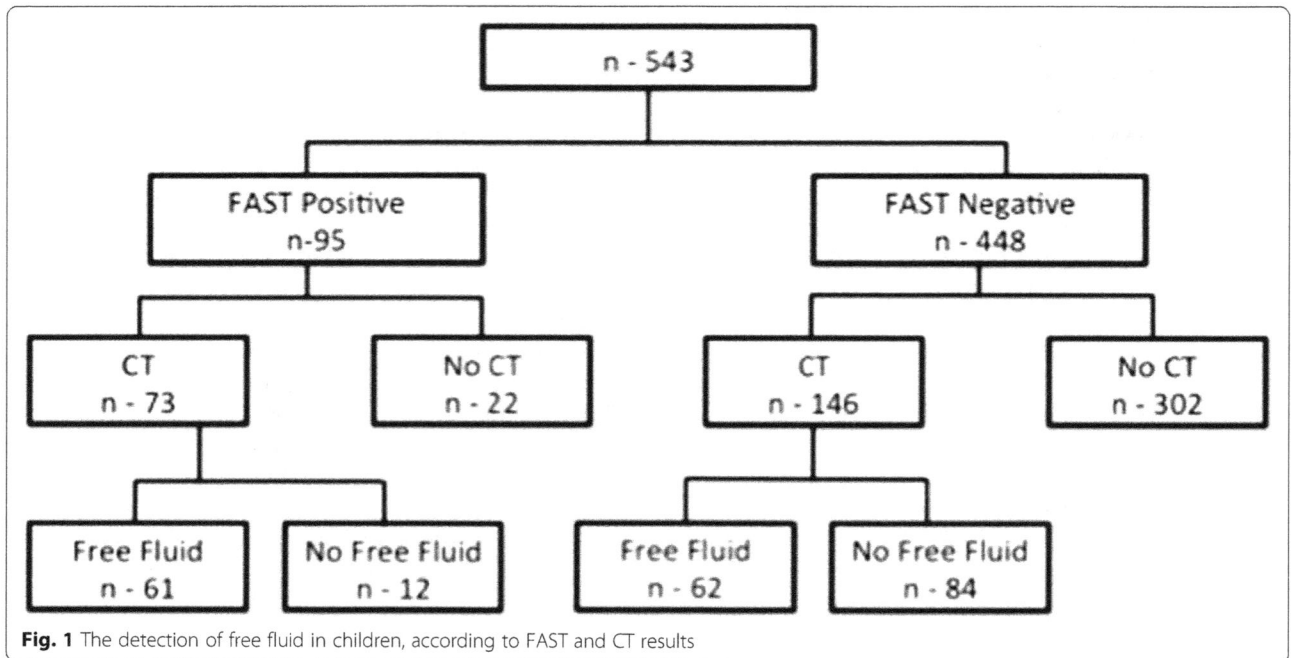

Fig. 1 The detection of free fluid in children, according to FAST and CT results

IAI yielded a sensitivity of 100 % and specificity of 72 % with a low PPV but a fairly high NPV (20 and 100 % respectively).

Discussion

In recent years most adult trauma centers have integrated the FAST examination into an assessment protocol of blunt abdominal injury. However, pediatric trauma centers have responded tepidly to the incorporation of this technology. We believe that the main reason for the low adoption of FAST in the evaluation of children is the rare occurrence of unstable children with IAI. In adults FAST has almost eliminated the need for deep peritoneal lavage (DPL) that was used extensively in the past. Although rarely used DPL have the advantage of not only detecting free fluid in the abdominal cavity but also to elaborate on its quality (blood, bowel content, urine etc.).

Table 1 Sensitivity, specificity, PPV, NPV, and accuracy all of the groups

| | Overall (n-543) | | >2 years (n-454) | | <2 years (n-89) | |
	Free fluid	IAI[a]	Free fluid	IAI[a]	Free fluid	IAI[a]
Sensitivity	50 %	77 %	51 %	75 %	37 %	100 %
Specificity	88 %	70 %	90 %	69 %	78 %	72 %
PPV	84 %	22 %	88 %	22 %	50 %	20 %
NPV	58 %	97 %	56 %	96 %	67 %	100 %
Accuracy	66 %	66 %	64 %	70 %	62 %	74 %

PPV positive predictive value, *NPV* Negative Predictive value, *IAI* Intra-abdominal injury
[a]IAI: intra-abdominal injury

Previous studies reported a wide range of sensitivity and specificity of the use of FAST in the pediatric population (30-97 % and 50-97 % respectively) [7–11]. The low sensitivity is partially due to the supposition that only one third of the children with IAI present without free fluid in the abdomen [12]. Furthermore, there is a severe paucity of evidence regarding the use of FAST in children younger than 2 years of age. The current study clarifies the contemporary use of FAST in a level I pediatric trauma center. We calculated sensitivity, specificity, accuracy, PPV, and NPV, not only for the presence of free fluid in the abdomen but also for the actual correlation IAI diagnosed either by CT scan or at laparotomy. No IAI was defined on clinical bases during the child's admission and follow-up in the outpatient clinic.

Reported ranges of sensitivity and specificity for FAST in adults are: 73 - 88 % and 96 - 98 % respectively [13–15]. Our results are consistent with previous studies reporting low sensitivity (50 %) and reasonable specificity (88 %) of FAST in children [11]. Accuracy in the current study is significantly lower (66 %) than values reported for adults (96-98 %). Our results showed greater sensitivity and somewhat lower specificity (77 and 70 % respectively) for anticipating IAI than for the detection of free fluid. Although the presence of free fluid in the abdomen did not directly correlate with IAI (PPV - 22 %), the absence of fluid strongly suggests the absence of IAI (NPV - 97 %). These data contradict the previous assumption that one third of children with abdominal blunt trauma are without free fluid in the abdomen [12].

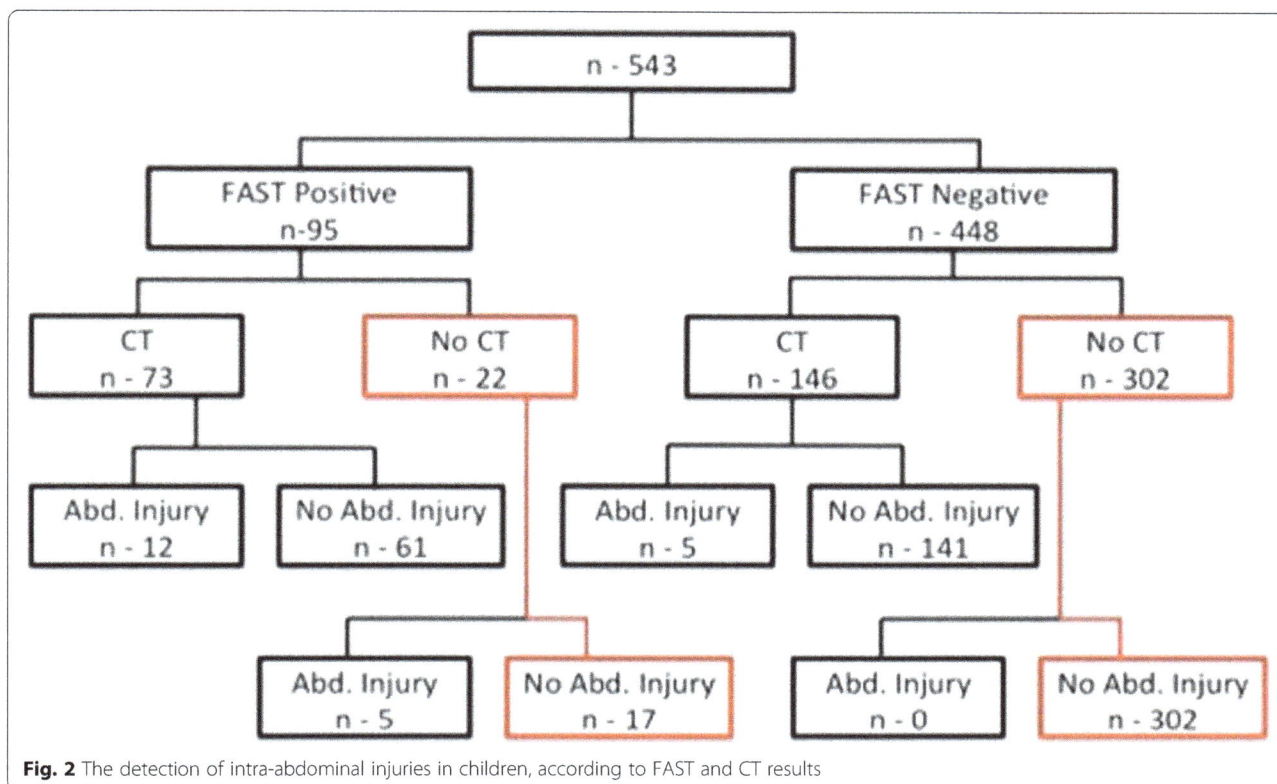

Fig. 2 The detection of intra-abdominal injuries in children, according to FAST and CT results

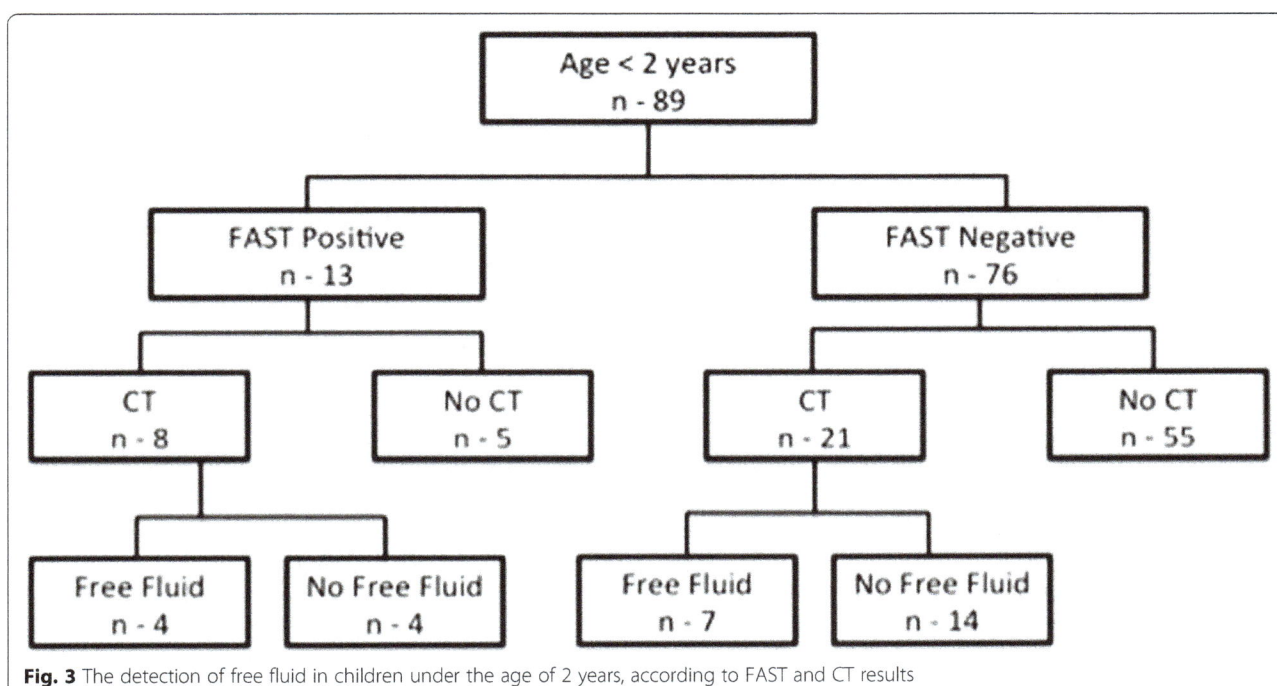

Fig. 3 The detection of free fluid in children under the age of 2 years, according to FAST and CT results

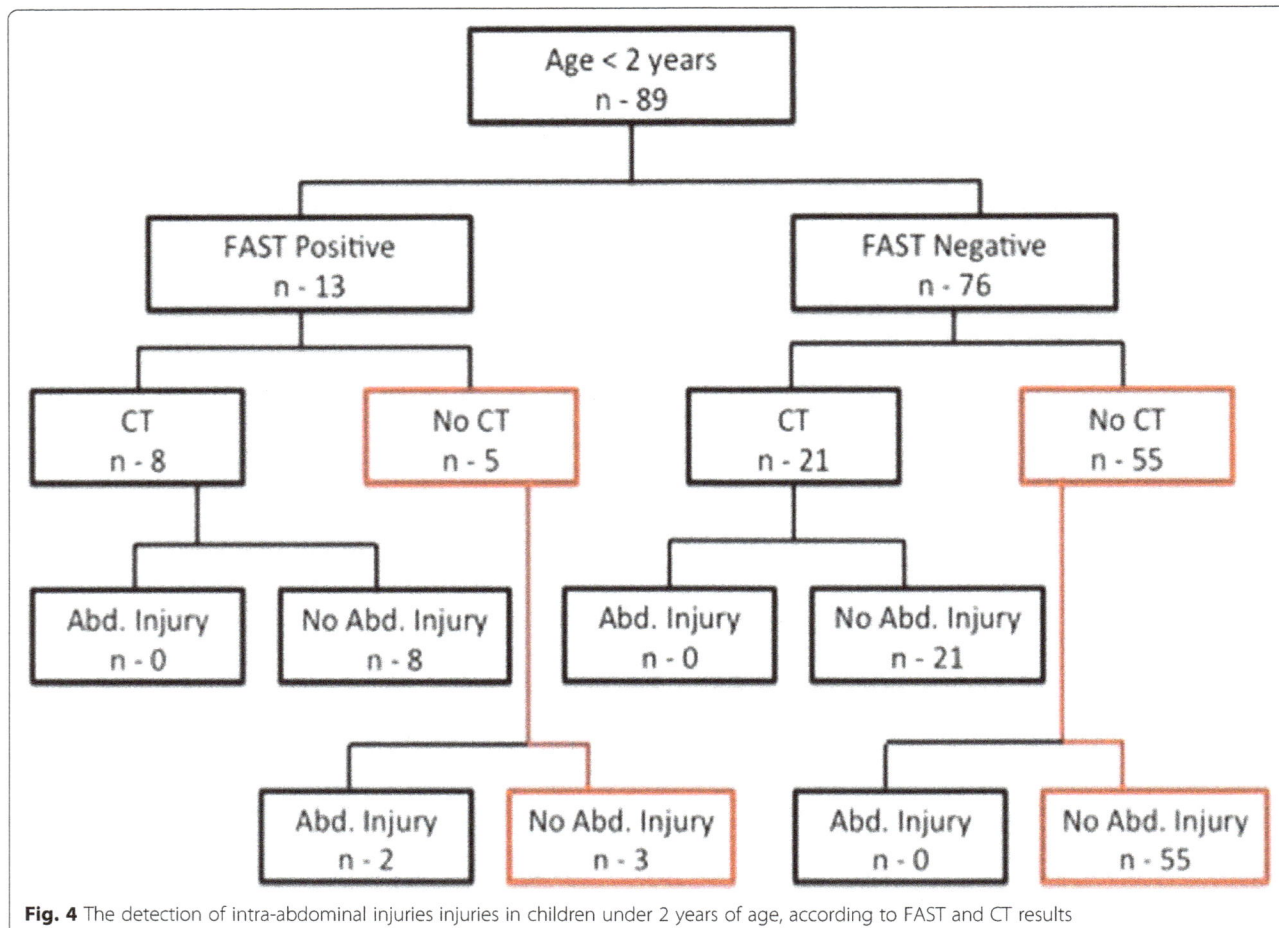

Fig. 4 The detection of intra-abdominal injuries injuries in children under 2 years of age, according to FAST and CT results

FAST was able to predict the need for an exploratory laparotomy in 89 % (*n* = 8) of the injured children in the current study. The only child who needed a laparotomy and had a negative FAST examination was a 16 year old with a handle bar injury. He presented with peritonitis of the upper abdomen. A CT scan showed a minimal amount of free fluid in the pelvis and a loop of small bowel with thickened wall and haziness of the fat around it. Therefore, he underwent an exploratory laparotomy that revealed small bowel injury. The ability to predict the need for laparotomy in our study is limited but the small number of patients who needed surgery all together.

In the subgroup analysis of children under age of 2 years, sensitivity and specificity for the presence of free fluid did not markedly differ from that of the whole cohort (37 and 78 % respectively). However, for IAI, sensitivity and NPV were both 100 % (Table 1). These findings suggest that FAST examination tempered with sound clinical judgment may reduce the need for further imaging and therefore reduce the radiation exposure of children under the age of 2 years.

In most centers in North America, the FAST examination is performed by a surgery resident. A number of studies showed equivalent accuracy when FAST is performed by surgeons, emergency medicine physicians, ultrasound technicians, and radiologists [16–19]. More recently, a Canadian survey showed that only 39 % of the surgical residents felt comfortable to make treatment decisions based on FAST examinations that they performed [20]. Although surgical residents are trained to perform FAST examinations in our institution, these exams are traditionally performed by radiology residents and subsequently evaluated by radiology attending physicians. The current study does not evaluate the differences between the two and therefor no conclusions could be extracted.

Conclusions

This study shows that although a positive FAST evaluation does not necessarily correlate with an IAI, a negative one strongly suggests the absence of an IAI, with a high NPV. These findings are emphasized in the analysis of the subgroup of children less than 2 years of age.

FAST appears to be best used for the detection of free fluid in the abdomen, as a surrogate of IAI in the unstable patient. It may be used as an adjunct in the assessment of the stable patient, to reduce the use of radiation, especially in children. Our findings support the integration of FAST into an assessment protocol of blunt abdominal injury in children. The prospective assessment of the impact of such protocol on the clinical outcome and the actual reduction of the use of unnecessary radiation emitting exams is needed.

Competing interests
The authors declare that they have no competing interests.

Authors' contributions
OBI conception and design of the study, data Collection, data analysis, drafting of the manuscript. MD data collection. ZP data collection. HB critical review of the manuscript. YK conception and design of the study, data analysis, critical review of the manuscript. All authors read and approved the final manuscript.

References
1. Sivit CJ, Kaufman RA. Commentary: sonography in the evaluation of children following blunt trauma: is it to be or not to be? Pediatr Radiol. 1995;25:326–8.
2. Thomas B, Falcone RE, Vasquez D, Santanello S, Townsend M, Hockenberry S. Ultrasound evaluation of blunt abdominal trauma: program implementation, initial experience, and learning curve. J Trauma. 1997;42:384–8 [discussion 388–390].
3. Boulanger BR, Kearney PA, Brenneman FD, Tsuei B, Ochoa J. Utilization of FAST (focused assessment with sonography for trauma) in 1999: results of a survey of North American trauma centers. Am Surg. 2000;66:1049–55.
4. Scaife ER, Fenton SJ, Hansen KW, Metzger RR. Use of focused abdominal sonography for trauma at pediatric and adult trauma centers: a survey. J Pediatr Surg. 2009;44:1746–9.
5. Negus S, Danin J, Fisher R, Johnson K, Landes C, Somers J, et al. Paediatric trauma imaging: why do we need separate guidance? Clin Radiol. 2014;69(12):1209–13.
6. Menaker J, Blumberg S, Wisner DH, Dayan PS, Tunik M, Garcia M, et al. Use of the focused assessment with sonography for trauma (FAST) examination and its impact on abdominal computed tomography use in hemodynamically stable children with blunt torso trauma. J Trauma Acute Care Surg. 2014;77(3):427–32.
7. Mutabagani KH, Coley BD, Zumberge N, McCarthy DW, Besner GE, Caniano DA. Preliminary experience with Focused Abdominal Sonography for Trauma (FAST) in children: is it useful? J Pediatr Surg. 1999;34:48–52 [discussion 52–44].
8. Patel JC, Tepas 3rd JJ. The efficacy of Focused Abdominal Sonography for Trauma (FAST) as a screening tool in the assessment of injured children. J Pediatr Surg. 1999;34:44–7 [discussion 52–44].
9. Emery KH, McAneney CM, Racadio JM, Johnson ND, Evora DK, Garcia VF. Absent peritoneal fluid on screening trauma ultrasonography in children: a prospective comparison with computed tomography. J Pediatr Surg. 2001;36:565–9.
10. Soudack M, Epelman M, Maor R, Hayari L, Shoshani G, Heyman-Reiss A. Experience with Focused Abdominal Sonography for Trauma (FAST) in 313 pediatric patients. J Clin Ultrasound. 2004;32(2):53–61.
11. Holmes JF, Gladman A, Chang CH. Performance of abdominal ultrasonography in pediatric blunt trauma patients: a meta-analysis. J Pediatr Surg. 2007;42:1588–94. Review.
12. Taylor GA, Sivit CJ. Posttraumatic peritoneal fluid: is it a reliable indicator of intraabdominal injury in children? J Pediatr Surg. 1995;30:1644–8.
13. Healey MA, Simons RK, Winchell RJ, Gosink BB, Casola G, Steele JT, et al. A prospective evaluation of abdominal ultrasound in blunt trauma: is it useful? J Trauma. 1996;40(6):875–83. discussion 883–5.
14. Boulanger BR, Brenneman FD, McLellan BA, Rizoli SB, Culhane J, Hamilton P. A prospective study of emergent abdominal sonography after blunt trauma. J Trauma. 1995;39:325–30.
15. Smith RS, Kern SJ, Fry WR, Helmer SD. Institutional learning curve of surgeon-performed trauma ultrasound. Arch Surg. 1998;133:530–6.
16. Branney SW, Wolfe RE, Moore EE, Albert NP, Heinig M, Mestek M, et al. Quantitative sensitivity of ultrasound in detecting free intraperitoneal fluid. J Trauma. 1995;39:375–80.
17. Kern SJ, Smith RS, Fry WR, Helmer SD. Sonographic examination of abdominal trauma by senior surgical residents. Am Surg. 1997;63:669–74.
18. Rozycki GS, Ochsner MG, Schmidt JA, Frankel HL, Davis TP, Wang D. A prospective study of surgeon-performed ultrasound as the primary adjuvant modality for injured patient assessment. J Trauma. 1995;39:492–500.
19. McKenney M, Lentz K, Nunez D, Sosa JL, Sleeman D, Axelrad A. Can ultrasound replace diagnostic peritoneal lavage in the assessment of blunt trauma? J Trauma. 1994;37:439–41.
20. Dubois L, Leslie K, Parry N. FACTS survey: focused assessment with sonography in trauma use among Canadian residents training in general surgery. J Trauma. 2010;69:765–9.

4

Surgeon agreement at the time of handover, a prospective cohort study

Richard Hilsden[1,3*], Bradley Moffat[1,3], Sarah Knowles[1,3], Neil Parry[1,2] and Ken Leslie[1]

Abstract

Background: Acute Care Surgical Teams are responsible for emergent surgical patients, and as such require regular handover and coordination between different surgeons. Despite the recent emergence of this model of care, minimal research has been conducted on the quality of patient handover and no research has attempted to determine the rate of clinical agreement or disagreement among surgeons participating in these teams.

Methods: A prospective cohort study was carried out with our acute care surgical service at a tertiary care teaching hospital from January 2 to March 31 2012. At the conclusion of the daily morning handover, receiving surgeons were asked to indicate, on provided handover sheets, whether they agreed with the proposed management plan for each patient that was discussed. The specific aspects of care over which they disagreed were also described, and disagreements were classified a priori as major or minor. The primary outcome was the rate of disagreement over the handed over management plan.

Results: Six staff surgeons agreed to participate and a total of 417 unique patients were handed over during the study period. For the primary outcome, a total of 41 disagreements were recorded for a disagreement rate of 9.8 %. 15 of the 41 disagreements were classified as major, for a major disagreement rate of 3.6 %. Consultant to consultant disagreements were classified as major disagreements 63 % of the time, whereas consultant to resident disagreements were classified as major 31 % of the time ($P = 0.217$). On average, the age of patients for which a clinical disagreement occurred were older; 63 vs. 57 ($P < 0.05$).

Conclusions: Despite the frequency of handovers in clinical practice, little research has been conducted to determine the rate of disagreement over patient management among surgeons participating working in academic centers. This study demonstrated that the rate of clinical disagreement is low among surgeons working in an tertiary care teaching hospital.

Keywords: Acute care surgery, Handover, Patient safety

Background

Acute care surgical teams represent an emerging model of surgical care in large hospitals and teaching institutions. These teams are tasked with the specific mandate to care for patients with urgent surgical issues. In high-volume hospitals, the acute care surgical service is frequently called upon by emergency departments, trauma services, and intensive care units [1, 2]. These teams differ from the traditional emergency surgical model: where a single surgeon was responsible for all acute general surgical emergencies over a period of 12–24 h, while simultaneously managing busy elective surgical lists and outpatient responsibilities [3]. The main weakness of this traditional model is the inherent conflict of responsibilities that occurs between the surgeon's elective and emergency patients [4, 5].

Acute care surgical teams afford several advantages over the traditional model of emergency surgical care in that they allow for clear lines of responsibility to be established in the treatment of emergent surgical patients; they ensure that hospital resources are

* Correspondence: richard.hilsden@londonhospitals.ca
Presented at: The Eastern Association for the Surgery of Trauma Annual Scientific Assembly, Scottsdale Arizona, January 2013.
[1]Department of Surgery, University of Western Ontario, London Health Sciences Centre, University Hospital, 339 Windermere Road, P.O. Box 5339, London, ON N6A 5A5, Canada
[3]Schulich School of Medicine and Dentistry, Western University, London, ON, Canada
Full list of author information is available at the end of the article

consistently being allocated to the sickest patients in a timely fashion without drawing focus away from elective patients [6]. At the same time, the decision to shift from the traditional model of surgical care to an acute care surgical model places significant time demands on clinical staff. To manage these demands, regular handover from staff surgeon to staff surgeon is required [1]. As a result, those who administrate acute care surgical services have made continuity of care a priority for these teams [3]. In this context, an appropriate definition of "continuity of care" is the degree to which a patient's management proceeds along the same care trajectory from admission to discharge [7]. For continuity of care to be maintained throughout the handover process, information must be adequately passed from one party to another, agreement over the patients' care plans must be met between the incoming and outgoing clinicians, and finally the care plan must ultimately be followed [7].

Until now, research in the realm of patient handover has focused mainly on the frequency and quality of communication during handovers [8–10]. On this issue, an evaluation of sentinel events leading to litigation by the Joint Commission on Accreditation of Healthcare Organization demonstrated that miscommunication of one form or another could be identified in nearly 70 % of medical misadventure cases [11]. Of these, miscommunication was considered to be contributory to a negative outcome in 49 % of cases [11].

It has been shown that over the course of several unique patient encounters different physicians often arrive at different clinical conclusions [12, 13]. Despite this, the medical literature on continuity of care has not addressed the role of clinical agreement in shared health care models. In particular, little research has been done to outline the degree to which surgeons disagree over specific patient management decisions, and no research has been conducted to determine the frequency of concurrence among surgeons during patient handover in a teaching hospital. The primary objective of this study was to determine the frequency of agreement at the time of patient handover among surgeons participating in the acute care surgery team at an academic tertiary care hospital.

Methods

A prospective cohort design was used to evaluate the rate of clinical agreement by the receiving surgeon regarding the patient management plan at the time of handover. Local institutional ethics board approval was obtained. The surgeons who participate in the general surgery acute care surgical service (ACCESS) at Victoria Hospital, London Health Sciences Centre in London, Ontario were approached via email, and in person (by KL, RH and NP) inviting them to participate. All

surgeons who were approached agreed to participate in this study. Surgeons who had privileges at the institution but did not regularly participate as members of the acute care surgery team were excluded. The study period ran from January 9th 2012 to March 24th 2012. During this period there were six different consultant surgeons who covered ACCESS.

The acute care surgical service at our institution consists of a single consultant who leads a team of house staff and is responsible for daytime emergencies from Monday to Sunday. During weeknights, different surgeons from the call pool are responsible for emergency care. On a daily basis, the post-call staff surgeon and house staff meet face to face to hand over all of the overnight surgical patients to the daytime team. The acute care surgery consultant changes on a weekly basis with a face-to-face handover occurring on Monday mornings. All patients on the ACCESS team are discussed during these daily handover sessions. During these meetings patient histories, physical exam findings, investigation results, and patient care plans are discussed in detail between the receiving team and the providers handing off. The receiving consultants are encouraged to question the handing over team members to ensure understanding of all active clinical issues and to clarify the management plans previously set in place. The purpose of these daily handover meetings is to clearly communicate patient care plans and maintain continuity of care as the clinical providers for these patients.

As part of routine care in this institution, the patient handover lists are generated from the electronic medical record so that all the participants in the handover process can discuss patient issues. These patient lists contain names, basic demographics such as gender and age, as well as an admission diagnosis, and are standardized for all patients. These handover sheets provide a platform for the discussion of patient care plans; however, all clinical information is communicated verbally face to face between clinicians participating in the acute care surgery handover.

On a daily basis, the receiving surgeon was given a second copy of the ACCESS patient list upon which he/she was asked to indicate whether he/she agreed or disagreed with the previously established patient management plan. The surgeons were instructed to keep their agreement decisions and all study patient lists confidential. For each patient, where the receiving surgeon felt there was a disagreement, that surgeon was asked to indicate (in point form on the provided handover sheets) the aspects of patient care upon which he/she disagreed. As residents at this institution are given graduated level of responsibility for patient care, the receiving consultants at handover were asked to indicate whether they felt the

Recent Progress in Emergency Surgery

management plan for which they disagreed originated with the resident or previous consultant. Participating surgeons were encouraged to indicate a disagreement for any situation where they felt their opinion differed over a specific issue, even if they felt the issue was trivial. Participating surgeons were blinded as to how disagreements would be classified in the final analysis.

Each day, following handover, the patient lists containing the surgeon's indications of agreement were placed in opaque envelops and securely stored at an on campus location. At the end of the research period these patient lists were compiled in a database stored on a secure hospital computer in an anonymous fashion.

The primary outcome was the rate of agreement at the time of handover, expressed as a percentage of all handovers. Clinical disagreements were defined either as major or minor. A major disagreement was considered to be any disagreement event that fell into one of four pre-specified categories: (1) delay to operating room, (2) disagreement over diagnosis, (3) disagreement over operative technique, and (4) disagreement over disposition decisions. These categories were defined a priori. All other disagreements were considered minor. Post-hoc analysis of patient outcomes was explored by examining patients' electronic records as well as morbidity and mortality records. Additional outcomes included rate of disagreement by age, gender, and disease type. Morbidity and mortality data were collected prospectively on a daily basis.

T-test, chi-square, and Mann-Whitney U tests were used based on data type to determine statistical significance within 95 % confidence. Statistics were calculated using SPSS Statistics version 20.0.0.

Results

Receiving surgeons completed the required study patient list data for 55 of a possible 76 handover days resulting in a 72 % completion rate. A total of 417 unique patients were handed over during this period giving an average of 7.6 patients handed over daily. For the "Monday morning" handover days, (which the entire team was handed over to a new consultant of the week) there was an average of 13.1 patients handed over. For regular weekdays where another consultant may have been covering overnight, the average number of patients handed over was 5.5. Among the patients handed over, 41 disagreements were identified (Table 1). This represented an overall disagreement rate of

9.8 %. Of these disagreements, 15 were identified as major resulting in a major disagreement rate of 3.6 % (Fig. 1). There was a trend toward an increased frequency of minor disagreements (6.2 % minor vs. 3.6 % major); however, this did not reach statistical significance ($p = 0.086$).

Of the patients handed over for which there was a major disagreement, 3 involved a delay to the operating room, 4 were the result of disagreement over diagnosis, 3 represented a disagreement over the operative technique, and 5 represented a disagreement over disposition (Table 2). Among the patients for whom there was a major disagreement, 33 % carried a diagnosis of large bowel obstruction and among patients for whom a minor disagreement was identified the most frequent diagnosis was small bowel obstruction at 23 %. However, none of the major disagreement categories were statistically over-represented compared to another.

The level at which the disagreement occurred could be determined for 27 of 41 disagreements. Consultant to consultant disagreements were classified as major disagreements 63 % of the time and consultant to resident disagreements were major 31 % of the time ($P = 0.217$) (Fig. 2).

The mean age of patients for whom there was a disagreement was 63 years compared to 57 for those whom no disagreement was indicated ($p < 0.05$) (Table 3). Length of stay for those patients for whom there was a disagreement was an average of 3.5 days compared to 5.2 days for those whom no disagreement was identified ($p = 0.649$).

There were a total of 4 deaths among patients handed over for a mortality rate of 0.96 %. There were 25 morbidities identified resulting in a morbidity rate of 6.0 %. Among patients for whom there was a disagreement, there was one death leading to a mortality rate of 2.4 %. This compared to 3 deaths, and a mortality rate of 0.80 %,

Table 1 Handover agreement rate

Primary Outcome Category	Number	Rate
Total	417	-
Agree	376	90.2 %
Major Disagreement	15	3.4 %
Minor Disagreement	26	6.4 %

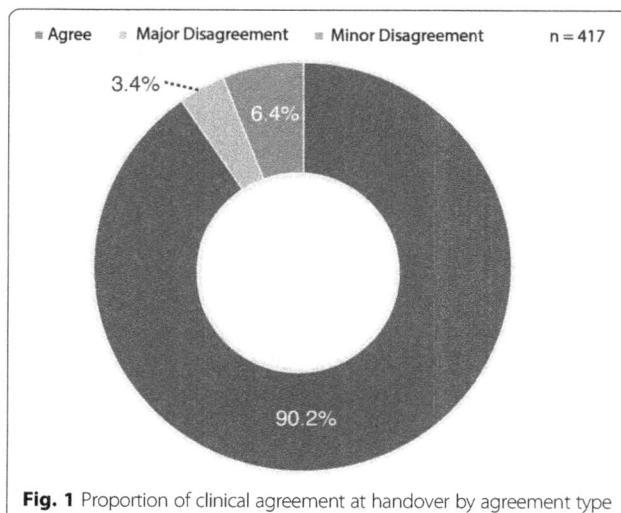

Fig. 1 Proportion of clinical agreement at handover by agreement type

Table 2 Disagreements by diagnosis and indication

Major Disagreement Diagnosis	Number
Small Bowel Obstruction	1
Large Bowel Obstruction	5
Trauma	0
Appendicitis	1
Biliary Disease	2
Other	6
Minor Disagreement Diagnosis	Number
Small Bowel Obstruction	6
Large Bowel Obstruction	2
Trauma	2
Appendicitis	2
Biliary Disease	2
Other	12
Reason for Major Disagreement	Number
Delay to OR	3
Wrong Diagnosis	4
Wrong Operative Technique	3
Disposition	5

Table 3 Patient characteristics by agreement type

	Agree	Disagree	P
N	376	41	
Age (mean)	57	63	<0.05
Length of stay (mean)	5.2	3.5	=0.649

among patients for whom there was full agreement ($p = 0.307$). There were 4 morbidities among patients whom there was clinical disagreement giving a morbidity rate of 9.8 % compared to a morbidity rate of 5.6 % ($p = 0.462$) for patients for whom there was full agreement.

Discussion and conclusions

Due to the diverse and complex nature of clinical decision making, the occasional clinical disagreement between providers is understood to be an expected feature of modern medical practice [14]. The wide range of training and experience embodied by the various providers involved in a patient's hospital course inevitably leads to differences of opinion. In the traditional model of surgical care, a single surgeon was ultimately responsible for all aspects of patient care throughout the patient's admission, and could dictate the overall trajectory of patient care [1]. The authority of a single surgeon over the patient's course in this practice model made differences of opinion unlikely to have an impact on continuity of care [1]. However, this model of care is changing, and the emergence of acute care surgery teams has made multiple surgeons primarily responsible for a single patient's care at different points during an admission. In such an environment, disagreements over clinical management have the potential to significantly impact patient care – positively or negatively. A recent evaluation of acute care surgery handover practices indicated that problematic handovers could have a negative impact on patient outcomes, and the experience of learners [15]. In that study residents felt, that on average, inadequate handover contributed to at least a minor harm in 2.7 individual patients, and a major harm in 0.6 individual patients over the course of their training [15]. With this evidence in mind, we feel that the clinical disagreements which occur when key patient care providers change over have the greatest potential to impact continuity of care, and ultimately affect patient outcomes.

Clinical disagreement among attending surgeons has previously been described in contexts other than patient handover. In one example, when evaluating the same group of patients to determine whether surgery for peptic ulcer disease had been effective, 2 senior surgeons agreed on the patient outcome less than two thirds of the time [16]. Despite the known occurrence of clinical disagreements and the potential implications these

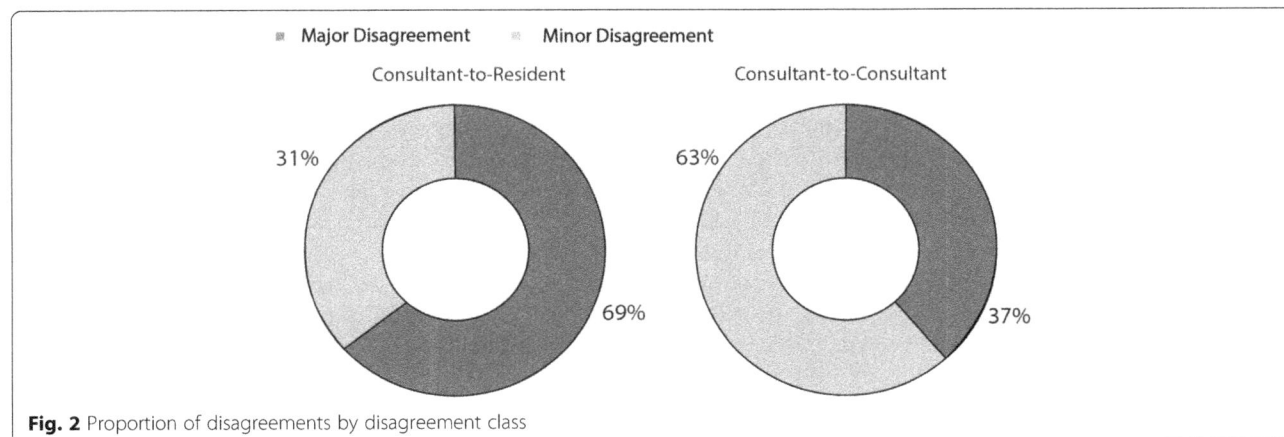

Fig. 2 Proportion of disagreements by disagreement class

disagreements have on patient care continuity, until now no research has been conducted to determine the frequency to which such disagreements occur. We found an absolute clinical disagreement rate between surgeons at a single tertiary care institution to be 9.8 %. Since no previous research has attempted to estimate clinical disagreement under similar conditions, it is difficult to imply how this disagreement level might compare to other institutions. As such, we believe that this level of disagreement has the potential to represent a benchmark for the evaluation of handover practices of other academic institutions.

Of the 9.8 % of handovers identified as clinical disagreements, 3.4 % fell into the category of major disagreement. The pre-specified major disagreement categories (diagnosis, time to OR, disposition, and operative technique) were felt to represent 4 broad categories where a disagreement would most likely result in a change to the patient care plan. Some of the more common examples of minor disagreements included disagreements over specific diagnostic tests ordered, antibiotic choice, involvement of consulting medical services, and the timing of drain/tube removal. In many cases, no clearly established clinical guideline exists for these issues, and as a result the clinical choices surrounding the more frequent minor disagreements are influenced heavily by clinical judgment and experience.

Although not statistically significant, there was a trend toward consultant to consult disagreements more frequently being classified as major compared to consultant to resident disagreements (63 % vs 31 %). This potential difference is likely explained by the fact that in our institution the 4 major disagreement categories tended to represent consultant level decisions, whereas the more frequent minor disagreements tended to occur over issues which a resident may be encouraged to exercise some autonomy. Finally, we demonstrated a trend toward an increased mortality (2.4 % vs 0.8 %, $p = 0.307$) and increased morbidity (9.8 vs 5.6 %, $p = 0.462$) among patients for whom there was a disagreement. The intention of this study was to look at the thought process of surgeons during handover and not to evaluate patient outcomes; however, this trend certainly supports the authors' belief that among patients in whom there is a clinical disagreement, there may be associated poor clinical outcomes. Also, patients in the disagreement group were older (57 vs 63) which may suggest that they have more complex conditions that could generate more clinical disagreements. We were unable to differentiate if indeed it was the more complex medical issue or the concerns with continuity of care that were responsible for differences in clinical outcomes. A larger prospective study would be required to determine that relationship.

The fact that clinical disagreements occurred between surgeons at handover also raises the question of the source of these disagreements. On this issue, the literature has previously demonstrated that the process of acquiring clinical information is subject to a number of influences, which may lead one clinician to have different information than another about the same patient [13]. A unique aspect of this research, is the fact that the surgeon (and the resident team) handing the patient over represents the source of the information being utilized by the receiving surgeon to make a clinical judgment [12].

Our study has several limitations. This study was limited to a single institution, and a relatively small number of surgeons ($n = 6$). In addition, these surgeons have worked closely together for a number of years in a teaching hospital environment; which, may have lead to relatively homogenous practice patterns, and consequently low levels of disagreement. As a result, it is reasonable to expect that larger institutions with a greater number of surgeons who have a wider variety of clinical experience and training may have higher disagreement rates.

It is also possible that the 9.8 % disagreement rate may underestimate the actual frequency of disagreements at our institution, since it relied on the careful consideration and effort of the receiving surgeon to indicate that a disagreement had actually occurred. It may have simply been easier for surgeons to indicate an agreement as opposed to offering a short written explanation, as was required of the study protocol, for all disagreements. Additionally, concern about the possibility of offending a clinical partner could have entered into the minds of participants potentially influencing their behavior despite assurances that no identifying data would be collected, and that participants were blinded to the responses of their colleagues. These factors could have potentially reduced the number of disagreements identified by participants increasing the risk of a type II error in this study.

This research sheds a unique light on clinical judgments at the time of handover by providing a unique estimate of clinical agreement between surgeons. With a 90.2 % agreement rate, this study demonstrates a high degree of concurrence among surgeons caring for patients in acute care surgical teams. Further research, with larger volumes, is required to elucidate the underlying reasons for the disagreements that do occur as well as to further elucidate the role of clinical disagreements on patient outcomes.

Competing interests
The authors declare that they have no competing interests.

Authors' contributions

RH designed the study, collected data, performed the statistical analysis and drafted the manuscript. BM contributed to data collection, data analysis and assisted in manuscript preparation. SK contributed to data collection, data analysis and assisted in manuscript preparation. NP contributed to design of the study, statistical analysis, data interpretation, and assisted in manuscript preparation. KL conceived of the study, obtained ethics approval for the research, contributed to the data analysis, and assisted in manuscript preparation. All authors read and approved the final manuscript.

Author details

[1]Department of Surgery, University of Western Ontario, London Health Sciences Centre, University Hospital, 339 Windermere Road, P.O. Box 5339, London, ON N6A 5A5, Canada. [2]Department of Critical Care, London, On, Canada. [3]Schulich School of Medicine and Dentistry, Western University, London, ON, Canada.

References

1. Hameed M, Breneman F, Ball C, Pagliarello P, Razek T, Parry N, et al. General Surgery 2.0: the emergence of acute care surgery in Canada. Can J Surg. 2010;53:79–83.
2. The Committee to Develop the Reorganized Specialty of Trauma, Surgical Critical Care, and Emergency Surgery. Acute care surgery: trauma, critical care, and emergency surgery. J Trauma. 2005;58:614–6.
3. Ball C, Hameed S, Breneman F. Acute care surgery: a new strategy for the general surgery patients left behind. Can J Surg. 2010;53:84–5.
4. Lamiri M, Grimaud F, Xie X. Optimization methods for a stochastic surgery problem. Int J Production Economics. 2009;120:400–10.
5. Velmahos GC, Jurkovich GJ. The concept of acute care surgery: a vision for the not-so-distant future. Surgery. 2007;141:288–90.
6. Victorian government department of health. Good practice management of emergency surgery: a literature review. 2010.
7. Donaldson M. Continuity of care: a reconceptualization. Med Care Res Rev. 2001;58:255–90.
8. Nagpal K, Vats A, Lamb B, Sevdalis N, Vincent C, Moorthy K. Information transfer and communication in surgery: a systematic review. Ann Surg. 2010;25:225–39.
9. Kitch BT, Cooper JB, Zapol WM, Marder JE, Karson A, Hutter M, et al. Handoffs causing patient harm: a survey of medical and surgical house staff. Jt Comm J Qual Patient Saf. 2008;34:563–70.
10. Patterson ES, Roth EM, Woods DD, Chow R, Gomes JO. Handoff strategies in settings with high consequences for failure: lessons for health care operations. Int J Qual Health Care. 2004;15(2):125–32.
11. Greenberg C, Regenbogen S, Studdert D, Lipsitz S, Rogers S, Zinner M, et al. Patterns of communication breakdowns resulting in injury to surgical patients. J Am Coll Surg. 2007;204:533–40.
12. Department of Clinical Epidemiology and Biostatistics, McMaster University. Clinical disagreement I: How often it occurs and why. Can Med Assoc J. 1980;20(123):499–504.
13. Koran L. The reliability of clinical methods, data and judgments. N Engl J Med. 1975;293:642–6.
14. Kljakovic M. Clinical disagreement: a silent topic in general practice. NZ Fam Physician. 2003;30:358–60.
15. Johner A, Merchant S, Aslani N, Planting A, Ball C, Widder S, et al. Acute care general surgery in Canada: a survey of current handover practices. Can J Surg. 2013;56:E24–8.
16. Hall R, Horrocks I, Clamp S, De Dombali F. Observer variation is assessment of results of surgery for peptic ulceration. Br Med J. 1976;1(6013):814.

5

Emergency right colectomy: which strategy when primary anastomosis is not feasible?

Hugo Teixeira Farinha, Emmanuel Melloul, Dieter Hahnloser*, Nicolas Demartines and Martin Hübner

Abstract

Background: Primary anastomosis is considered the standard strategy after right emergency colectomy. The present study aimed to evaluate alternative treatment strategies when primary anastomosis is not possible to prevent definitive ostomy.

Methods: This retrospective study included all consecutive patients who underwent right emergency colectomy between July 2006 and June 2013. Demographics, surgical data, and postoperative outcomes were entered in an anonymized database. Comparative analysis was performed between patients with primary anastomosis (PA group) and those where alternative strategies were employed (no-PA group). Outcomes were 30 days complications rate and rate of bowel continuity restoration.

Results: One hundred forty-eight patients (57 % male) with a median age of 65 years (15–96) were included. One hundred and sixteen patients underwent PA (78 %) and 32 were in the no-PA group (22 %). No-PA group patients had more comorbidities (Carlson comorbidity index >3: 98 % vs. 54, $p < 0.001$). Major complications rate (Dindo-Clavien III to IV) was 24 % in PA group, 88 % in no-PA group ($p < 0.001$). The 30-day mortality rate was 6 % ($n = 7$) in PA group versus 25 % ($n = 8$) in no-PA group ($p = 0.004$). Fourteen patients in the no-PA group had a split stoma and 18 had a two-staged procedure. Five patients had continuity restoration after initial split stoma (36 %) compared to 10 after a two-staged procedure (55 %; $p = 0.265$). Anastomotic leak occurred in 10 patients of the PA group (9 %) versus 0 in the no-PA group, where 15 out of 32 patients (47 %) had continuity restoration.

Conclusion: Eighty percent of patients requiring emergency right colectomy were anastomosed primarily. For the remaining a two-staged procedure might facilitate bowel continuity restoration in the long-term.

Background

Elective right colectomy entails a risk for postoperative complications and mortality around 22 and 1 % respectively [1, 2]. In the emergency setting, these rates grow up to 50 and 10 %, especially if risk factors are present. [3–5], Patient-related risk factors are age >70 years, male, malnutrition, ASA score >3, diabetes, tobacco smoking or immunosuppression. Procedure-related risk factors other than emergency include intra-operative blood transfusion, surgeon experience, operative duration or operations performed during night-shift [6–8].

Safety strategies are useful for emergency procedures if several risk factors are present. For *left*-sided emergency colonic resections, valuable options are creation of an end colostomy or primary anastomosis with diverting ileostomy

[9, 10]. However, safety strategies have not been established for emergency *right*-sided resections. Resection with primary anastomosis remains the standard of care also in the emergency setting [11, 12]. Nevertheless, overall morbidity and mortality rates raise the question whether safer strategies are needed.

Therefore, the aim of the present study was to assess our institutional practice and outcome for emergency right colectomy and to evaluate alternative treatment to primary anastomosis and if definitive ostomy rate can be reduced.

Methods
Patients

This retrospective audit analysis included all consecutive patients who underwent a right-sided emergency colectomy from July 2006 to June 2013 in the department of visceral surgery, in Lausanne University Hospital. Right emergency

* Correspondence: dieter.hahnloser@chuv.ch
Department of Visceral Surgery, University Hospital of Lausanne (CHUV), Lausanne 1011, Switzerland

colectomy included formal right colectomy including resection of up to 20 cm of small bowel. Transverse colic resections or extended right colonic resections were excluded. Emergency operation was defined as being performed during an unplanned hospital admission. Indication for surgery was given by the surgeon on call. Surgeries were performed by a board certified surgeon. Although this is a retrospective study, Swiss law demands that we submit the project to an Ethics Committee. The study was approved by the local Ethics Committee (University of Lausanne, Switzerland).

Data collection

Demographics and risk factors as well as outcome measures were defined *a priori* and entered in an anonymized database. All data were collected retrospectively after the last included patient was operated.

Demographic data and patients' co-morbidities (diabetes, obesity, chronic renal failure, cirrhosis, cardiopathy, tobacco smoking or immunosuppressive drugs consumption including corticoids, anti-TNF and chemotherapy) were included in the database. Co-morbidities and patient preoperative health were prospectively graded using the Charlson co-morbidity Index and *American Society of Anesthesiology* (ASA) score [13]. Surgical data included operative time, blood loss, as well as intraoperative vasopressor requirements (Noradrenalin >10ug/min intravenously) or surgeon's expertise (junior or senior consultant)[14–16]. Junior staff are within 5 years after surgical graduation. Senior consultants have completed surgical training at least 5 years ago and/or have done a fellowship.

The retrospective cohort was divided into two groups. The first group included all patients with non-protected primary anastomosis (PA group) at the time of the intervention. All types of anastomotic techniques (end-to-end, side-to-end, side-to-side; hand-sewn or mechanical) were included. The second group without primary anastomosis (No-PA group) included patients who received either primary split stoma or who had just resection without primary anastomosis and a planned second look (so called two-staged procedure). Split stoma was defined by exteriorisation of both ends of the bowel through the same hole. The proximal end formed the functioning stoma and with faeces pass. The distal end of bowel was brought out through the abdominal wall and formed a non-functioning stoma. Split stoma procedure may permit a bowel continuity restoration without performing a laparotomy.

Outcomes

Overall postoperative 30-day complications rate including mortality and the rate of bowel continuity restoration were the main outcomes. Complications were classified according to the Clavien-Dindo grading of surgical complications [17].The complication with the highest severity for each patient was considered for the analysis.

Other outcomes included length of intensive care unit (ICU) stay (days), length of hospital stay (days), destination after discharge (home or rehabilitation) and time to stoma reversal (months).

The study included all cases of stoma reversal after split stoma at fist intention, or after split stoma performed during a planned second-look following a two-stage procedure. Reasons not to close the stoma were entered in the database.

Statistical analysis

Descriptive statistics for categorical variables were reported as frequency (%), while continuous variables were reported as median (interquartile range: IQR). Chi-square was used for comparison of categorical variables and the Wilcoxon test for continuous data. All statistical tests were two-sided and a level of 0.05 was used to indicate statistical significance. Data analyses were performed using SPSS Inc. released 2012.for Mac, Version 21.0. Chicago: SPSS Inc.

Results

Patients

One hundred and forty-eight patients underwent emergency right-sided colectomy during the study period. Primary anastomosis (PA group) was performed in 116 (78 %) patients. Of the remaining 32 patients (=no-PA group), 14 (9.5 %) received a primary split stoma, while 18 (12.5 %) had a two-stage procedure (Fig. 1).

Demographic information for the two comparative groups are displayed in Table 1. Patients in the PA group were younger and had a lower BMI and ASA score as well as less co-morbidities.

Surgical data

The most frequent indication for emergency right colectomy was mechanical obstruction ($n = 52$). Seventy-one percent ($n = 37$) overall obstructions were due to malignant obstruction. Other causes of obstruction were ileus due to adhesions ($n = 7$), obstruction due to inflammatory disease ($n = 4$), caecal volvulus ($n = 3$), and one hernia. All obstructions in the no-PA group were due to malignant lesions. In the no-PA group, perforation and ischemia were the prominent underlying pathologies. Obstruction and ischemia were indications that significantly differ between the groups. Patients in the PA group received significantly less intraoperative Noradrenalin than the others during surgery. Estimated blood losses (ml) were comparable between both groups Table 1.

There was no difference in the surgical management regarding surgeon expertise or between day and night-shift. Out of 116 anastomosis in the PA group, 28 (25 %) were stapled. The median operation time was 166 min (55–400 min) in PA group versus 107 min (47–338 min) for no-PA group ($p = 0.003$) Table 1.

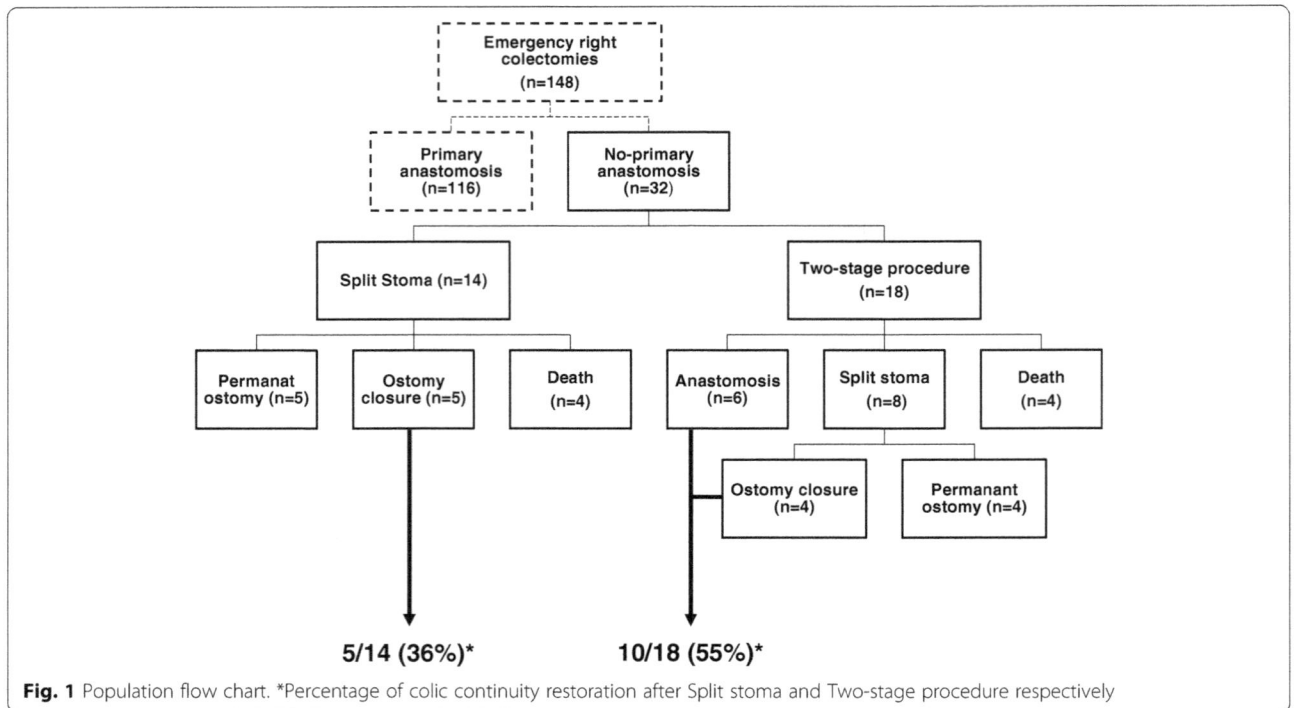

Fig. 1 Population flow chart. *Percentage of colic continuity restoration after Split stoma and Two-stage procedure respectively

Outcomes

There were significantly more major complications (Clavien-Dindo III-IV) including more bleeding requiring transfusion in no-PA compared to PA group. The rate of surgical site infection (SSI) or postoperative ileus was similar between the two groups. Overall, the most common complication was SSI in both groups. Anastomotic leak occurred in 10 patients of the PA group (9 %) versus 0 in the no-PA group, where 15 out of 32 patients (47 %) had continuity restoration. All leaks were managed by reexploration and reanastomosis. Mortality occurred in 7 cases in PA group and in 8 cases in no-primary anastomosis group (6 versus 25 %) Table 2.

In the PA group, 3 patients died of multiple organ failure (MOF) associated with a sceptic shock of abdominal origin, one caused by an anastomotic leak (14 %). Three patients died of respiratory failure, one caused by pleural effusion, one caused by pulmonary embolism and one caused by bronchoscopic aspiration. One patient died of hemorrhagic shock of colic origin.

In the No-PA group, 4 out of 14 patients died after split stoma (29 %) and 4 out of 18 patients died after two-stage procedure (22 %) before the planned second look. Reasons for postoperative death were multi organ failure (MOF) for 6 patients all caused by a septic shock of abdominal origin. One patient died of postoperative hemorrhagic shock of colic origin and one after ruptured aortic aneurysm.

Mean ICU stay was not different between the two groups while mean of hospital stay was significantly higher in the

no-PA group. More patients were able to go home after discharge in the PA group without transfer to another hospital or to a rehabilitation centre Table 2.

Fourteen patients in the no-PA group had a split stoma and 18 had a two-stage procedure with a planned second look. Median time for planned second look was 48 hours (24–96). These two populations were comparable regarding demographics, co morbidities or surgical indications Table 3.

Five out of 14 patients had an ostomy closure after split stoma within a median of 6 days (4–120). Of those one patient had an ostomy closure during the same hospitalisation, and 4 were readmitted for ostomy closure with a median hospital stay of 16 days (13–39). After ostomy closure, one patient had an anastomotic leak and needed a reoperation and refection of the anastomosis during the same hospitalisation. Four patients died before ostomy closure and 5 were not deemed eligible for another operation for medical reasons.

Six out of 18 patients who underwent a two-stage procedure had an anastomosis performed during the second look except for one patient who needed a complementary colic resection of 5 cm during the second look and anastomosis was performed at third look. One of those 6 patients had a leakage and needed a reoperation and anastomosis refection during the same hospitalisation. Eight patients had a split stoma during the second look. Two patients needed a complementary colic resection of 4 and 10 cm during second look. Four of the 8 patients who had a split stoma after a second

Table 1 Comparison between PA group and no-PA group, Demographic Data

	PA group (n = 116)	No-PA group (n = 32)	P value
Age (range)	62 (15-90)	68 (27-94)	0.004
Sex ratio, (M:F)	67:49	18:14	1.000
Body mass index >25 (Kg/m2)	43 (37 %)	20 (63 %)	0.023
ASA grade III-IV, n (%)	67 (58 %)	29 (91 %)	<0.001
Charlson comorbidity index >3	67 (58 %)	30 (94 %)	<0.001
Comorbidity			
Diabetes, n (%)	20 (17 %)	6 (19 %)	0.798
Cardiopathy, n (%)	28 (24 %)	17 (53 %)	0.002
Tobacco smoking, n (%)	35 (30 %)	12 (38 %)	0.520
Immunosuppression, n (%)	12 (10 %)	10 (31 %)	0.009
Surgical indication			
Mechanical obstruction, n (%)	48 (41 %)	4 (13 %)	0.004
Perforation, n (%)	29 (25 %)	13 (41 %)	0.129
Hemorrhage, n (%)	16 (14 %)	1 (3 %)	0.173
Ischemia, n (%)	14 (12 %)	11 (34 %)	0.006
Other, n (%)	9	3	
Operator			0.551
Junior Consultant, n (%)	57 (49 %)	18 (56 %)	
Senior Consultant, n (%)	59 (51 %)	14 (44 %)	
Surgery time			0.831
Nightshift, n (%)	36 (31 %)	9 (28 %)	
Intraoperative Noradrenalin >10ug/min	36 (30 %)	30 (95 %)	<0.001
Surgical approach			0.202
Open, n (%)	108 (93 %)	32 (100 %)	

Table 2 Comparison between PA group and no-PA group; 30d complications and outcomes

	PA group (n = 116)	No-PA group (n = 32)	P value
30d complications			
overall	72 (62 %)	32 (100 %)	<0.001
III-IV, n (%)	28 (24 %)	28 (88 %)	<0.001
V, n (%)	7 (6 %)	8 (25 %)	0.004
Surgical site infection, n (%)	27 (23 %)	10 (31 %)	0.364
Postoperative ileus, n (%)	19 (16 %)	4 (13 %)	0.784
Need for Transfusion, n (%)	13 (11 %)	12 (38 %)	0.001
Anastomotic leak, n (%)	10 (9 %)	0*	
ICU stay in days (SD)	5 (16)	10 (13)	0.063
LOS in days (SD)	12 (21)	18 (24)	0.163
Discharge home	76 (66 %)	5 (16 %)	<0.001

*15/32 patients had anastomosis

look had an ostomy closure in a third time within a median of 63 days (57–67).

Regarding patients in the No-PA group, more patients had continuity restoration after two-stage procedure compared after split stoma 10 vs. 5, but this numbers were no statistically significant (p = 0.265) Fig. 1.

Discussion

Primary anastomosis was performed in most patients after emergency right colectomy. Due to retrospective data analyse and obvious differences between patients from PA group and from no-PA group are incomparable. Two bailout options were applied in patients at high risk: split stoma confection and two-staged procedure with delayed ostomy or anastomosis. Our results suggest that a two-stage strategy might help to reduce permanent ostomy rate.

In accordance with the current literature[18], primary anastomosis was performed in 80 % of patients in this study Anastomotic leak rate was 9 % which was slightly higher than in the literature (4–6 %) probably because of increased co-morbidities, particularly more cardiac disease (30 % in this present study vs. 15 to 20 % in other studies) and higher ASA score 64 % III-IV vs. 40–50 %)[4, 18, 19]. None of these leaks resulted in death.

As expected, patients in the group with no primary anastomosis were significantly sicker and older. Furthermore, intraoperative risk factors and aetiologies differed significantly. All of these parameters have arguably influenced on surgical decision-making. Unfortunately, due to the retrospective nature of this study, it remains unclear which risk factors influenced surgical strategy most. Of note, the choice of surgical strategy was not influenced by surgeon's experience in our present series as suggested by other reports [4].

Two main factors may probably have influenced the decision-making in the present study, both having a major impact on blood supply of an eventual anastomosis and hence its perceived safety. High intraoperative vasopressor requirements (>10ug/min of noradrenalin/min) and colic ischemia were more common in the no-PA group. In accordance, safety strategies were liberally employed on a case-by-case basis. It would be interesting to analyze the pathway of decision-making but due to emergency and retrospective analysis we could not do that. Interestingly, primary anastomosis was performed with good results even in case of tumour obstruction with proximal bowel dilatation. Surgeon's experience or dayshifts did not play any role on strategy decision or on postoperative complications. Even when bailout procedures were performed and primary anastomosis was avoided, outcomes were disappointing in the high-risk patients group with an overall morbidity of 100 % and a mortality of 25 %. Other groups reported similar results underlining the overwhelming impact of the concomitant metabolic stress

Table 3 Comparison between patient of the no-PA group who underwent split stoma or two stage procedure

	Split stoma (n = 14)	Two stage (n = 18)	P value
Age (range)	68 (27-88)	70 (34-94)	0.912
Sex ratio, (M:F)	7:7	11:7	0.532
Body mass index >25 (Kg/m2)	9 (64 %)	11 (61 %)	0.854
ASA grade			0.400
I-II, n (%)	2 (14 %)	1 (6 %)	
III-IV, n (%)	12 (86 %)	17 (95 %)	
Charlson comorbidity index >3	13 (93 %)	17 (94 %)	0.854
Comorbidity			
Diabetes, n (%)	2 (14 %)	4 (22 %)	0.568
Cardiopathy, n (%)	9 (64 %)	8 (44 %)	0.265
Tobacco smoking, n (%)	5 (36 %)	7 (39 %)	0.854
Immunosuppression, n (%)	4 (29 %)	6 (33 %)	0.773
Surgical indication			
Mechanical obstruction, n (%)	2 (14 %)	2 (11 %)	0.787
Perforation, n (%)	5 (36 %)	8 (44 %)	0.618
Hemorrhage, n (%)	0	1 (6 %)	0.370
Ischemia, n (%)	5 (36 %)	6 (33 %)	0.888
Other, n (%)	2	1	
Operator			0.127
Junior Consultant, n (%)	10 (71 %)	8 (44 %)	
Senior Consultant, n (%)	4 (29 %)	10 (56 %)	
Surgery time			0.960
Nightshift, n (%)	4 (29 %)	5 (28 %)	
Intraoperative Noradrenalin >10ug/min	12 (86 %)	18 (100 %)	0.098

response do to preoperative comorbidities, emergent surgery and hemodynamic instability during anaesthesia [20]. A surgical safety strategy can only aim to obtain local control with low surgical morbidity; avoiding a high-risk anastomosis can certainly play a role in this concept. Further, surgical aggression should be reduced to a minimum in the context of an overshooting systemic inflammatory response; this can be achieved by primary resection, open abdomen and second look once the patient has been stabilized [21]. Nevertheless, outcomes remain dismal and early and aggressive reanimation at the intensive care unit is arguably as decisive with regards to outcomes as surgery[22]. The surgeon's decision seems to be adequate when a primary anastomosis is chosen. Mortality and morbidity rate are low and comparable to series in the literature [1, 23].

One of the most interesting finding of this study was the difference in permanent ostomy rate within the group of 18 patients who had a two-staged procedure. After right colectomy, the surgeon chooses to perform a second-look 2–4 days later either because the patient was deemed to

be unstable to continue the intervention or the surgeon wanted to reassess the viability of the remaining intestine (usually in an ischemic context) before restoring bowel continuity. By applying this strategy more continuity restoration was done compared to the group with primary split soma (10/18 vs. 5/14; $p = 0.265$). The patients in split stoma groups and two-stage procedure do not differ in their co-morbidities, the patients seem to benefit from two-stage procedure. However, this comparison is too small to draw final conclusions, but a two-staged procedure appears to be a valid approach and a bail out option for selected high-risk patients. A two-staged procedure with planed second-look allows a short first surgery ("just" the resection or damage control), minimizes surgical trauma and allows for early intensive care. If the evolution is favourable, some to these patients can still benefit from an anastomosis at planned second or third look. However, a two-staged procedure implies easy access to operating rooms, which could be difficult to achieve in some centres.

This study also shows that junior surgeons more often performed split stoma than two stage procedures. Comparison with senior surgeons was not significant, but a trend can not be denied. Unfortunately, we did not record reasons that drove junior consultants to opt for split stoma.

The present study is limited by its retrospective design. Furthermore, results from a single centre cannot be generalized by principle. However, this audit might help in certain situations with the decision to anastomose or not. It definitely warrants a prospective trial. Only large datasets could help to overcome limitations of heterogeneity and low power.

Conclusions

In conclusion, primary anastomosis was performed in 80 % of patients undergoing emergency right-sided colectomy. In patients considered more fragile (e.g. patients with heart disease, immunocompromised patients, hemodynamically unstable or with ischemic colic lesions) and where the surgeon initially does not anastomose, a two-staged procedure with a second look might facilitate continuity restoration in the long-term.

Abbreviations
ASA: American Society of Anaesthesiologists; ICU: Intensive Care Unit; PA: Primary anastomosis; SSI: Surgical Site Infection.

Competing interests
The authors declare that they have no competing interests.

Authors' contributions
HTF, MH and DH designed the study and wrote the manuscript. HTF and EM were involved in acquisition of data. HTF, EM, DH and MH were involved in statistical analysis and interpretation of the data. DH, MH, and ND participated in the coordination and helped to draft the manuscript. EM, MH, DH and ND were involved in the final corrections. All authors read and approved the final manuscript.

References

1. Kobayashi H, Miyata H, Gotoh M, Baba H, Kimura W, Kitagawa Y, et al. Risk model for right hemicolectomy based on 19,070 Japanese patients in the National Clinical Database. J Gastroenterol. 2014;49(6):1047–55.
2. Lee YM, Law WL, Chu KW, Poon RT. Emergency surgery for obstructing colorectal cancers: a comparison between right-sided and left-sided lesions. J Am Coll Surg. 2001;192(6):719–25.
3. Kingham TP, Pachter HL. Colonic anastomotic leak: risk factors, diagnosis, and treatment. J Am Coll Surg. 2009;208(2):269–78.
4. Leichtle SW, Mouawad NJ, Welch KB, Lampman RM, Cleary RK. Risk factors for anastomotic leakage after colectomy. Dis Colon Rectum. 2012;55(5):569–75.
5. Ruggiero R, Sparavigna L, Docimo G, Gubitosi A, Agresti M, Procaccini E, et al. Post-operative peritonitis due to anastomotic dehiscence after colonic resection. Multicentric experience, retrospective analysis of risk factors and review of the literature. Ann Ital Chir. 2011;82(5):369–75.
6. Klima DA, Brintzenhoff RA, Agee N, Walters A, Heniford BT, Mostafa G. A review of factors that affect mortality following colectomy. J Surg Res. 2012;174(2):192–9.
7. Klein M. Postoperative non-steroidal anti-inflammatory drugs and colorectal anastomotic leakage. NSAIDs and anastomotic leakage. Dan Med J. 2012;59(3):B4420.
8. Ziegler MA, Catto JA, Riggs TW, Gates ER, Grodsky MB, Wasvary HJ. Risk factors for anastomotic leak and mortality in diabetic patients undergoing colectomy: analysis from a statewide surgical quality collaborative. Arch Surg. 2012;147(7):600–5.
9. Breitenstein S, Kraus A, Hahnloser D, Decurtins M, Clavien PA, Demartines N. Emergency left colon resection for acute perforation: primary anastomosis or Hartmann's procedure? A case-matched control study. World J Surg. 2007;31(11):2117–24.
10. Oberkofler CE, Rickenbacher A, Raptis DA, Lehmann K, Villiger P, Buchli C, et al. A multicenter randomized clinical trial of primary anastomosis or Hartmann's procedure for perforated left colonic diverticulitis with purulent or fecal peritonitis. Ann Surg. 2012;256(5):819–26. discussion 26-7.
11. Gainant A. Emergency management of acute colonic cancer obstruction. J Visc Surg. 2012;149(1):e3–e10.
12. Murray JA, Demetriades D, Colson M, Song Z, Velmahos GC, Cornwell 3rd EE, et al. Colonic resection in trauma: colostomy versus anastomosis. J Trauma. 1999;46(2):250–4.
13. Pasternak I, Dietrich M, Woodman R, Metzger U, Wattchow DA, Zingg U. Use of severity classification systems in the surgical decision-making process in emergency laparotomy for perforated diverticulitis. Int J Colorectal Dis. 2010;25(4):463–70.
14. Komen N, Dijk JW, Lalmahomed Z, Klop K, Hop W, Kleinrensink GJ, et al. After-hours colorectal surgery: a risk factor for anastomotic leakage. Int J Colorectal Dis. 2009;24(7):789–95.
15. Zorcolo L, Covotta L, Carlomagno N, Bartolo DC. Toward lowering morbidity, mortality, and stoma formation in emergency colorectal surgery: the role of specialization. Dis Colon Rectum. 2003;46(11):1461–7. discussion 7-8.
16. Golub R, Golub RW, Cantu Jr R, Stein HD. A multivariate analysis of factors contributing to leakage of intestinal anastomoses. J Am Coll Surg. 1997;184(4):364–72.
17. Dindo D, Demartines N, Clavien PA. Classification of surgical complications: a new proposal with evaluation in a cohort of 6336 patients and results of a survey. Ann Surg. 2004;240(2):205–13.
18. Wyrzykowski AD, Feliciano DV, George TA, Tremblay LN, Rozycki GS, Murphy TW, et al. Emergent right hemicolectomies. Am Surg. 2005;71(8):653–6. discussion 6-7.
19. Mealy K, Salman A, Arthur G. Definitive one-stage emergency large bowel surgery. Br J Surg. 1988;75(12):1216–9.
20. Garber A, Hyman N, Osler T. Complications of Hartmann takedown in a decade of preferred primary anastomosis. Am J Surg. 2014;207(1):60–4.
21. Miller PR, Chang MC, Hoth JJ, Holmes JH, Meredith JW. Colonic resection in the setting of damage control laparotomy: is delayed anastomosis safe? Am Surg. 2007;73(6):606–9. discussion 9-10.
22. Godat L, Kobayashi L, Costantini T, Coimbra R. Abdominal damage control surgery and reconstruction: world society of emergency surgery position paper. World journal of emergency surgery : WJES. 2013;8(1):53.
23. Kim J, Mittal R, Konyalian V, King J, Stamos MJ, Kumar RR. Outcome analysis of patients undergoing colorectal resection for emergent and elective indications. Am Surg. 2007;73(10):991–3.

6

The duration of intra-abdominal hypertension strongly predicts outcomes for the critically ill surgical patients

Kyu-Hyouck Kyoung[1] and Suk-Kyung Hong[2*]

Abstract

Introduction: Intra-abdominal hypertension (IAH) is associated with morbidity and mortality in critically ill patients. The present study analyzed the clinical significance of IAH in surgical patients with severe sepsis.

Methods: This was a prospective study carried out in the surgical intensive care unit (SICU). Intra-abdominal pressure (IAP) was measured three times a day via a urinary catheter filled with 25 mL of saline. IAH was defined as an IAP ≥ 12 mmHg, and the peak IAP was recorded as the IAP for the day. Data were analyzed in terms of IAH development and the IAH duration.

Results: Of the 46 patients enrolled in the study, 42 developed IAH while in the SICU. The development of IAH aggravated the clinical outcomes; such as longer SICU stay, requirement of ventilator support, and delayed initiation of enteral feeding (EF). The IAH duration showed a significant correlation with pulmonary, renal, and cardiovascular function, and enteral feeding. The IAH duration was an independent predictor of 60-day mortality (odds ratio: 1.196; $p = 0.014$).

Conclusions: The duration of IAH is a more important prognostic factor than the development of IAH; thus every effort should be made to reduce the IAH duration in critically ill patients.

Trial registration: NCT01784458

Keywords: Severe sepsis, Intra-abdominal hypertension, Intra-abdominal pressure, Enteral feeding, abdominal perfusion pressure

Introduction

Intra-abdominal pressure (IAP) is defined as the steady-state pressure within the abdominal cavity bounded by the abdominal muscles and diaphragm [1]. It is affected by body weight, posture, tension of abdominal muscles, and movement of the diaphragm [2–4]. The World Society of the Abdominal Compartment Syndrome (WSACS) has published a grading system for intra-abdominal hypertension (IAH), with IAH defined as an IAP ≥12 mmHg, and abdominal compartment syndrome as an IAP ≥ 20 mmHg combined with the failure of more than one organ [1, 5]. Ever since then, WSACS have updated consensus definitions and clinical practice guidelines for the patients with IAH [6]. The prevalence of IAH on admission to the intensive care unit (ICU) ranges from 31 to 58.8 % [4, 7, 8], and the incidence increases with the length of ICU stay. Clinical conditions that increase IAP include blood and ascites in the peritoneal cavity, bowel distension and edema [4, 9], high-volume resuscitation and massive transfusion, damage control surgery in traumatic patients, excessive tension after abdominal closure, postoperative ileus, echar in burn patients [10, 11], and hemodilution [12]. IAH causes not only abdominal organ dysfunction by decreasing the abdominal perfusion

* Correspondence: skhong94@amc.seoul.kr
[2]Division of Trauma and Surgical Critical Care, Department of Surgery, Asan Medical Center, University of Ulsan College of Medicine, 388-1 Pungnap-dong, Songpa-gu, Seoul, Republic of Korea
Full list of author information is available at the end of the article

pressure (APP) [13–15] but also cardiopulmonary dysfunction [16], which increases both morbidity and mortality [17].

IAH has been increasingly recognized in the critically ill patients. However, the duration of IAH has not been under consideration. The aim of the present study was to investigate the influence of IAH development and its duration on the clinical course and outcome of critically ill surgical patients with severe sepsis.

Materials and methods
Study design and patients
The study was a prospective observational study in surgical ICU of an academic tertiary care hospital. Patients at least 18 years of age, who admitted for severe sepsis were enrolled within 24 h of admission to the ICU. Patients with urinary tract injury or therapeutic open abdomen were excluded. All subjects provided informed consent. A total of 48 patients admitted to the ICU from March 2009 to October 2009 met the inclusion criteria, of which two were excluded who refused to participate in the study. Overall, 46 patients were enrolled. The study protocols were approved by the Institutional Review Board of Asan Medical Center and registered at http://Clinical Trials.gov under the number NCT01784458.

Definitions
Severe sepsis was defined as a sepsis with a failure of more than one organ due to sepsis, an arterial blood lactate concentration of at least 4 mmol/L, or hypotension (with a systolic blood pressure < 90 mmHg).

Measurements and treatment
IAP was measured using a urinary catheter at the level of the mid-axillary line on the iliac crest with the patient supine. IAP was expressed as mmHg. A 3-lumen urinary catheter was inserted into the bladder. After the urinary drainage lumen was clamped, 25 ml of saline was injected through the irrigation lumen to prevent contamination. IAP was measured three times per day while the patient was in the ICU, with the highest reading recorded as the value for that day. The Acute Physiology and Chronic Health Evaluation (APACHE II) score was recorded every 24 h. Resuscitation was performed according to goal-directed guidelines [18, 19].

Statistical analysis
Statistical analyses were performed using SPSS 21 for windows (SPSS Inc. Chicago, IL). The Chi-square test or Fisher's exact test were used to compare categorical variables and the Mann–Whitney U test was used to compare continuous variables. Correlation analysis was performed using Spearman's rank correlation coefficient. Statistical significance was set at $p < 0.05$.

Results
Baseline characteristics
On admission day, 33 patients (71.7 %) had IAH. Mean IAP was 17.3 ± 5.5 mmHg. During ICU stay, IAH developed in 42 (91.3 %) patients at 1.4 ± 1.0 days after ICU admission. The incidence of IAH was higher in patients with peritonitis [25 (59.5 %) vs. 0 (0 %), $p = 0.037$] and in those who underwent laparotomy [37 (88.1 %) vs. 1 (25 %), $p = 0.013$]. The APACHE II score (22.0 ± 6.1 vs. 14.0 ± 6.2, $p = 0.030$) and total fluid administered ($5,065 \pm 1,814$ ml vs. $2,657 \pm 927$ ml, $p = 0.007$) was significantly high in the IAH group. There were no significant differences in other parameters between IAH group and non-IAH group on admission day to the ICU (Table 1).

Table 1 Baseline characteristics of the study patients upon admission to the intensive care unit

Variable	IAH (n = 42)	Non-IAH (n = 4)	P-value
Age (years)	64.9 ± 12.0	63.8 ± 8.7	0.585
Gender			>0.99
male	32 (76.2)	3 (75.0)	
Female	10 (23.8)	1 (25.0)	
Causes of sepsis			0.037
Peritonitis	25 (59.5)	0	
non- peritonitis	17 (40.5)	4 (100)	
abdominal organ infection	11 (26.2)	3 (75)	
Pneumonia	3 (7.1)	1(25)	
Others	3 (7.1)	0	
Laparotomy			0.013
laparotomy	37 (88.1)	1 (25.0)	
non-laparotomy	5 (11.9)	3 (75.0)	
APACHE II Score	22.0 ± 6.1	14.0 ± 6.2	0.030
Total fluid (mL/day)	5065 ± 1814	2657 ± 927	0.007
Urine output (mL/day)	1615 ± 1148	1243 ± 1011	0.560
RBC transfusion (units)	0.7 ± 1.8	1.3 ± 1.5	0.395
White blood cell ($\times 10^3$/mm^3)	14.4 ± 12.0	9.6 ± 4.7	0.721
Hematocrit (%)	28.4 ± 5.2	27.1 ± 7.3	0.374
Platelet ($\times 10^3$/mm^3)	120.2 ± 119.0	63.0 ± 26.8	0.117
Prothrombin time (%)	45.5 ± 18.9	46.7 ± 15.6	0.638
Total bilirubin (mg/dL)	1.9 ± 1.4	3.8 ± 3.0	0.127
Blood urea nitrogen[1] (mg/dL)	28.2 ± 16.9	34.3 ± 21.5	0.515
Creatinine[1] (mg/dL)	1.6 ± 1.0	1.7 ± 1.0	0.829
Lactate (mmol/L)	3.9 ± 2.4	3.7 ± 1.1	0.836
PaO$_2$/FiO$_2$ Ratio	151.9 ± 69.8	212.5 ± 65.7	0.099

[1]Two patients with chronic renal failure on hemodialysis were excluded from the IAH group

Table 2 Clinical outcomes according to intra-abdominal hypertension

Variable	IAH (n = 42)	Non-IAH (n = 4)	P-value
Mortality			
30-Day mortality	5 (11.9)	0	>0.99
60-Day mortality	13 (31.0)	0	0.313
Length of ICU Stay (days)	17.3 ± 13.2	2.5 ± 2.4	0.002
Length of hospital Stay (days)	42.6 ± 27.6	16.0 ± 2.4	0.003
Mechanical ventilation	38 (90.5)	1 (25.0)	0.009
Duration of ventilatory support (days)	13.1 ± 13.0	1.0 ± 2.0	0.007
Renal replacement therapy[1]	15 (37.5)	0	0.282
Duration of RRT[1] (days)	6.5 ± 10.9	0	0.239
Vasopressor treatment	36 (85.7)	3 (75.0)	0.496
Inotropic treatment	13 (31.0)	0	0.313
Initiation of enteral feeding[2] (days)	8.9 ± 7.5	2.3 ± 1.9	0.019

[1]Two patients with chronic renal failure on hemodialysis were excluded from the IAH group
[2]Two patients in the IAH group (who did not try enteral feeding) were excluded

Clinical outcomes according to intra-abdominal hypertension

The length of ICU stay (17.3 ± 13.2 days vs. 2.5 ± 2.4 days, $p = 0.002$) and length of hospital stay (42.6 ± 27.6 days vs. 16.0 ± 2.4 days, $p = 0.003$) were longer in the IAH group. Patients with the IAH had an increased requirement for mechanical ventilation [38 (90.5 %) vs. 1 (25 %), $p = 0.009$] and duration of ventilatory support (13.1 ± 13.0 day vs. 1.0 ± 2.0 day, $p = 0.007$). Initiation of enteral feeding (EF) was delayed (8.9 ± 7.5 day vs. 2.3 ± 1.9 day, $p = 0.019$) in the IAH group. Renal replacement therapy (RRT) and mortality did not show significant differences (Table 2).

Clinical effect of the duration of intra-abdominal hypertension

The duration of IAH had more impact on outcomes than the development of IAH. Distribution of IAH duration is demonstrated on Fig. 1. There were significant increases in terms of the length of ICU stay (r = 0.860, $p < 0.001$), duration of mechanical ventilation (r = 0.840, $p < 0.001$), duration of RRT (r = 0.603, $p < 0.001$), and initiation of EF (r = 0.330, $p = 0.029$) according to increase of IAH duration (Fig. 2).

Comparison of survivors and non-survivors

There were no significant differences in any of the study variables in terms of 30-day mortality. However, univariate analysis showed that the duration of IAH ($p = 0.001$), the initial APACHE II score ($p = 0.021$), and peritonitis ($p = 0.010$) were significantly associated with 60-day mortality (Table 3). Multivariate logistic regression analysis identified the duration of IAH as an independent predictor of 60 day-mortality (odds ratio: 1.196; 95 % confidence interval: 1.037–1.380; $p = 0.014$) (Table 4).

Discussion

IAP has been measured since the 19th century. Ever since then, its importance has been recognized recently. Since the mid-1990s it was known that IAH could develop without abdominal trauma [20] and numerous studies have measured IAP, examined its clinical outcomes, and classifications.

The prevalence of IAH depends on the patient population. IAH was present in 54.4 % of medical ICU and 65 % of surgical ICU patients [7]. We found a quite high prevalence of IAH (91.3 %) in critically ill surgical patients. The previous study demonstrated that sepsis was the predominant cause of IAH [21], and the population of this study composed of the patients with severe sepsis might make such deviation.

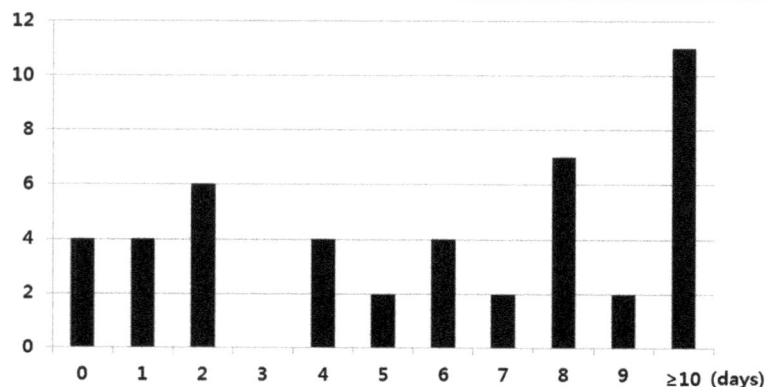

Fig. 1 Distribution of patients by duration of intra-abdominal hypertension

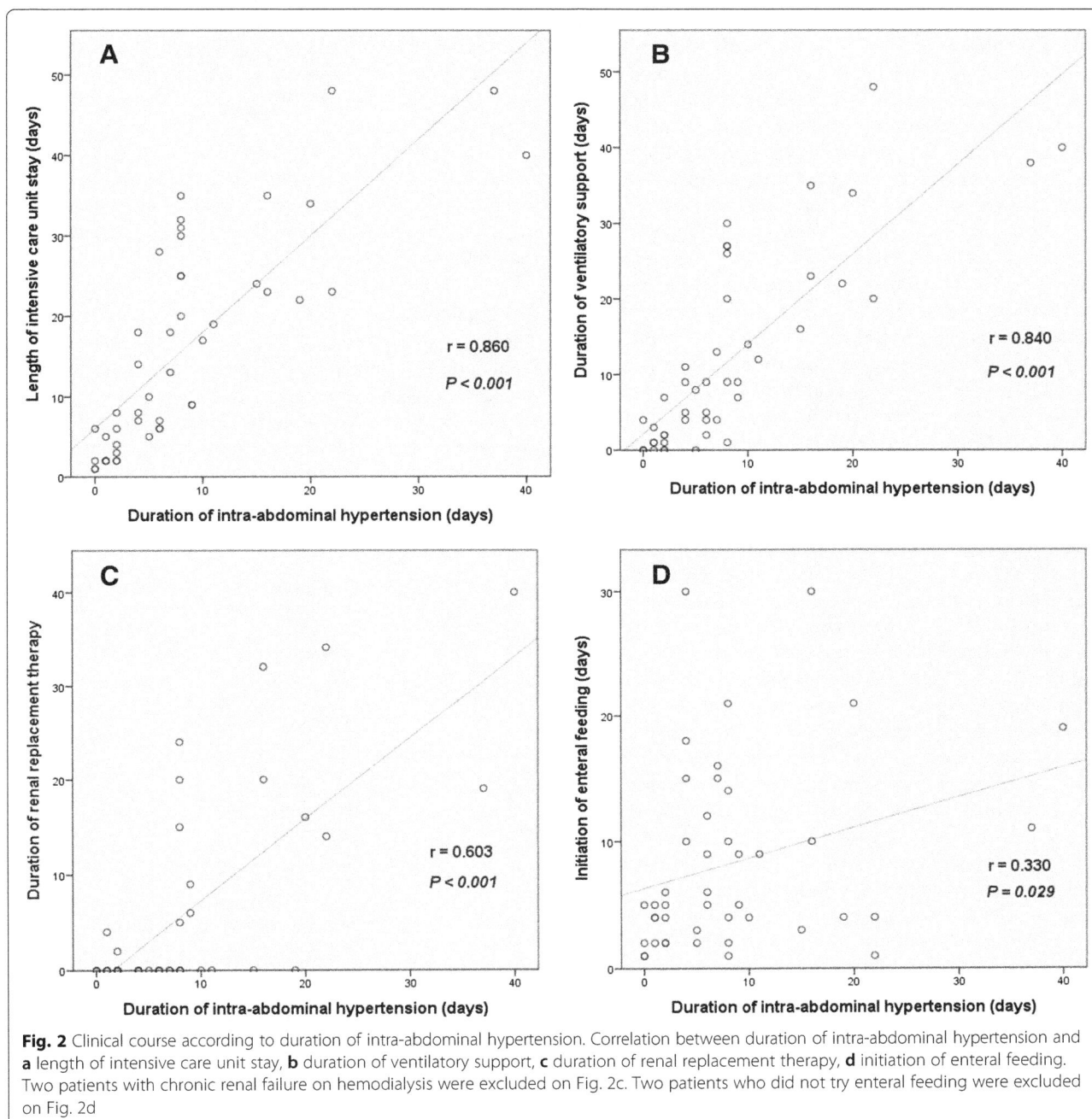

Fig. 2 Clinical course according to duration of intra-abdominal hypertension. Correlation between duration of intra-abdominal hypertension and **a** length of intensive care unit stay, **b** duration of ventilatory support, **c** duration of renal replacement therapy, **d** initiation of enteral feeding. Two patients with chronic renal failure on hemodialysis were excluded on Fig. 2c. Two patients who did not try enteral feeding were excluded on Fig. 2d

Table 3 Univariate analysis on the predictors of 60-Day mortality

Variable	Survivors (n = 33)	Non-survivors (n = 13)	P-value
Age (years)	64.1 ± 12.7	66.5 ± 8.6	0.517
Initial APACHE II Score	19.9 ± 5.9	24.7 ± 6.8	0.021
Peritonitis	14 (42.4)	11 (84.6)	0.010
Development of IAH	29 (87.9)	13 (100)	0.313
Duration of IAH (days)	5.2 ± 4.1	16.3 ± 12.2	0.001

Table 4 Multivariate analysis on predictors of 60-day mortality

Variable	Odds ratio	95 % Confidence interval	P-value
Initial APACHE II Score	1.073	0.917–1.254	0.381
Peritonitis	6.072	0.814–45.278	0.078
Duration of IAH	1.196	1.037–1.380	0.014

This study was to introduce the clinical effects of time-dependence of IAH. The effect off IAH in organ dysfunction involves a myriad of pathologic change. Essentially, the concept of IAH has been established in the area of trauma and experts have been recommended damage control laparotomy and open abdomen to correct physiologic stress in trauma and acute general surgical patients [22]. The main mechanism of organ dysfunction by IAH is suggested as reduction of APP and direct pressure effect on other compartment [17]. Most of previous studies have focused on the effect of IAH. However, the duration of IAH is more important as an outcome prognostic factor than a just presence of IAH. It could be explained that prolonged IAH would accumulate risk for organ failure and worsen the outcomes. This study identified the phenomenon that persistent IAH aggravated organ failure and increased affected mortality independently.

Patients with IAH tend to need more mechanical ventilation and have more difficulty in weaning, both of which represent respiratory organ failure. The transmission of IAH to thorax has a worse impact on the respiratory system. The major reason is a reduction of the functional residual capacity caused by cephalad displacement of the diaphragm in response to unopposed intra-abdominal pressure. In addition, reduction of chest wall compliance cause by IAH is leading to atelectasis [23]. Therefore, patients with IAH need a different ventilator strategy and more specific treatment considering IAH such as positive end-expiratory pressure against IAP [24]. Moreover, persistent IAH can worsen the respiratory mechanics more seriously.

The adverse effects of IAH on abdominal organs have been demonstrated on the basis of renal function in postoperative surgical patients [21, 25]. Acute kidney injury is common consequences of IAH. The detrimental effect of IAH on the kidney is closely related to renal blood flow. IAH lead to significant intrarenal venous congestion and to lower the filtration gradient, which represents the difference between glomerular filtration and proximal tubular pressures [26, 27]. With persistent IAH, not only direct effect of intra-abdominal pressure but also reduction of cardiac output and elevated level of catecholamine, rennin, angiotensin, and inflammatory cytokines may also come into play, further worsening renal function.

Elevated IAP also reduces blood flow to abdominal viscera [28, 29]. Splanchnic ischemia impairs subsequent intestinal barrier function and gastrointestinal motility. Early enteral nutrition is the preferred strategy for feeding the critically ill patients. However, it is not always possible to initiate EN in critically ill patients. Elevated IAP can be a big obstacle to feed early the critically ill patients. In addition, it is very hard to determine the tolerance of enteral feeding in patients with

IAH. Therefore, the results presented herein suggest that IAH and its duration may provide important clues for clinicians to make decisions about whether to proceed with EF. As a result, persistent IAH delays enteral feeding in various reasons.

In addition to IAH development, sustained IAH reduced the chances of recovery and forces patients into a vicious cycle. The results of the present study show that the IAH duration is a more important clinical factor than the development of IAH.

Conclusions

There is a strong relationship 'risk accumulation' between duration of IAH and organ dysfunction. Persistent elevations of IAH are aggravating clinical outcomes including organ failure and mortality. Therefore early recognition and prompt intervention, including surgical intervention if necessary are essential to improve patients' outcomes.

Abbreviations
IAP: Intra-abdominal pressure; WSACS: World Society of the Abdominal Compartment Syndrome; IAH: Intra-abdominal hypertension; ICU: Intensive care unit; APP: Abdominal perfusion pressure; APACHE II: Acute Physiology and Chronic Health Evaluation; EF: Enteral feeding; RRT: Renal replacement therapy; RBC: Red blood cell.

Competing interests
The authors declare that they have no competing interests.

Authors' contributions
KHK participated in the design of the study, data collection and drafted the manuscript. SKH designed the study and supervised study processes, statistical analysis and drafting the manuscript. Both authors read and approved the final manuscript.

Author details
[1]Department of Surgery, Ulsan University Hospital, University of Ulsan College of Medicine, 877 Bangeojinsunhwando-ro, Dong-gu, Ulsan, Republic of Korea. [2]Division of Trauma and Surgical Critical Care, Department of Surgery, Asan Medical Center, University of Ulsan College of Medicine, 388-1 Pungnap-dong, Songpa-gu, Seoul, Republic of Korea.

References
1. Malbrain ML, Cheatham ML, Kirkpatrick A, Sugrue M. Results from the International Conference of Experts on Intra-abdominal Hypertension and Abdominal Compartment Syndrome. I. Definitions. Intensive Care Med. 2006;32:1722–32.
2. Pelosi P, Croci M, Ravagnan I, Cerisara M, Vicardi P, Lissoni A. Respiratory system mechanics in sedated, paralyzed, morbidly obese patients. J Appl Physiol. 1997;82:811–8.
3. Hering R, Wrigge H, Vorwerk R, Brensing KA, Schröder S, Zinserling J. The effects of prone positioning on intra-abdominal pressure and cardiovascular and renal function in patients with acute lung injury. Anesth Analg. 2001;92:1226–31.
4. Malbrain ML, Chiumello D, Pelosi P, Bihari D, Innes R, Ranieri VM. Incidence and prognosis of intra-abdominal hypertension in a mixed population of critically ill patients: a multiple-center epidemiological study. Crit Care Med. 2005;33:315–22.
5. Cheatham ML, Malbrain ML, Kirkpatrick A, Sugrue M. Results from the International Conference of Experts on Intra-abdominal Hypertension and Abdominal Compartment Syndrome. II. Recommendations. Intensive Care Med. 2007;33:951–62.

6. Kirkpatrick AW, Roberts DJ, De Waele J, Jaeschke R, Malbrain ML, De Keulenaer B, et al. Intra-abdominal hypertension and the abdominal compartment syndrome: updated consensus definitions and clinical practice guidelines from the World Society of the Abdominal Compartment Syndrome. Intensive Care Med. 2013;39:1190–206.

7. Vidal MG, Ruiz Weisser J, Gonzalez F, Toro MA, Loudet C. Incidence and clinical effects of intra-abdominal hypertension in critically ill patients. Crit Care Med. 2008;36:1823–31.

8. Malbrain ML, Chiumello D, Pelosi P, Wilmer A. Prevalence of intra-abdominal hypertension in critically ill patients: a multicentre epidemiological study. Intensive Care Med. 2004;30:822–9.

9. Goldman RK, Mullins RJ. Mechanism of acute ascites formation after trauma resuscitation. Arch Surg. 2003;138:773–6.

10. Mahajna A, Mitkal S, Krausz MM. Postoperative gastric dilatation causing abdominal compartment syndrome. World J Emerg Surg. 2008;31:3–7.

11. De Waele JJ, Hoste E, Blot SI, Decruyenaere J, Colardyn F. Intra-abdominal hypertension in patients with severe acute pancreatitis. Crit Care. 2005;9:452–7.

12. Czajkowski M, Dabrowski W. Changes in intra-abdominal pressure during CABG with normovolemic hemodilution. Med Sci Monit. 2006;12:487–92.

13. Diebel LN, Wilson RF, Dulchavsky SA, Saxe J. Effect of increased intra-abdominal pressure on hepatic arterial, portal venous, and hepatic microcirculatory blood flow. J Trauma. 1992;33:279–82.

14. Diebel LN, Dulchavsky SA, Brown WJ. Splanchnic ischemia and bacterial translocation in the abdominal compartment syndrome. J Trauma. 1997;43:852–5.

15. De Laet IE, Ravyts M, Vidts W, Valk J, De Waele JJ. Current insights in intra-abdominal hypertension and abdominal compartment syndrome: open the abdomen and keep it open! Arch Surg. 2008;393:833–47.

16. Ridings PC, Bloomfield GL, Blocher CR, Sugerman HJ. Cardiopulmonary effects of raised intra-abdominal pressure before and after intravascular volume expansion. J Trauma. 1995;39:1071–5.

17. Cheatham ML, White MW, Sagraves SG, Johnson JL, Block EF. Abdominal perfusion pressure: a superior parameter in the assessment of intra-abdominal hypertension. J Trauma. 2000;49:621–6.

18. Rivers E, Nguyen B, Havstad S, Ressler J, Muzzin A. Early goal-directed therapy in the treatment of severe sepsis and septic shock. N Engl J Med. 2001;345:1368–77.

19. Dellinger RP, Carlet JM, Masur H, Gerlach H, Calandra T. Surviving Sepsis Campaign guidelines for management of severe sepsis and septic shock. Crit Care Med. 2004;32:858–73.

20. Greenhalgh DG, Warden GD. The importance of intra-abdominal pressure measurements in burned children. J Trauma. 1994;36:685–90.

21. Sugrue M, Jones F, Deane SA, Bishop G, Bauman A, Hillman K. Intra-abdominal hypertension is an independent cause of postoperative renal impairment. Arch Surg. 1999;134:1082–5.

22. Godat L, Kobayashi L, Costantini T, Coimbra R. Abdominal damage control surgery and reconstruction: world society of emergency surgery position paper. World J Emerg Surg. 2013;17:8–53.

23. Pelosi P, Quintel M, Malbrain ML. Effect of intra-abdominal pressure on respiratory mechanics. Acta Clin Belg Suppl. 2007;1:78–88.

24. Regli A, Chakera J, De Keulenaer BL, Roberts B, Noffsinger B, Singh B, et al. Matching positive end-expiratory pressure to intra-abdominal pressure prevents end-expiratory lung volume decline in a pig model of intra-abdominal hypertension. Crit Care Med. 2012;40:1879–86.

25. Sugrue M, Buist MD, Hourihan F, Deane S, Bauman A, Hillman K. Prospective study of intra-abdominal hypertension and renal function after laparotomy. Br J Surg. 1995;82:235–8.

26. Dalfino L, Tullo L, Donadio I, Malcangi V, Brienza N. Intra-abdominal hypertension and acute renal failure in critically ill patients. Intensive Care Med. 2008;34:707–13.

27. Mohmand H, Goldfarb S. Renal dysfunction associated with intra-abdominal hypertension and the abdominal compartment syndrome. J Am Soc Nephrol. 2011;22:615–21.

28. Gudmundsson FF, Gislason HG, Dicko A, Horn A, Viste A, Grong K, et al. Effects of prolonged increased intra-abdominal pressure on gastrointestinal blood flow in pigs. Surg Endosc. 2001;15:854–60.

29. Correa-Martín L, Castellanos G, García-Lindo M, Díaz-Güemes I, Sánchez-Margallo FM. Tonometry as a predictor of inadequate splanchnic perfusion in an intra-abdominal hypertension animal model. J Surg Res. 2013;184:1028–34.

7

Correlations of perioperative coagulopathy, fluid infusion and blood transfusions with survival prognosis in endovascular aortic repair for ruptured abdominal aortic aneurysm

Yohei Kawatani, Yoshitsugu Nakamura, Hirotsugu Kurobe, Yuji Suda and Takaki Hori[*]

Abstract

Background: Factors associated with survival prognosis among patients who undergo endovascular aortic repair (EVAR) for ruptured abdominal aortic aneurysms (rAAA) have not been sufficiently investigated. In the present study, we examined correlations between perioperative coagulopathy and 24-h and 30-day postoperative survival. Relationships between coagulopathy and the content of blood transfusions, volumes of crystalloid infusion and survival.

Methods: This was a retrospective study of the medical records of all patients who underwent EVAR for rAAA at Chiba-Nishi General Hospital during the period from October 2013 to December 2015. Major coagulopathy was defined using the international normalized ratio or activated partial thromboplastin time (APTT) ratio of at least 1.5, or platelet count less than $50 \times 10/l$. We quantified the amounts of blood transfusions and crystalloid infusions administered from arrival to the hospital to admission to ICU following operations.

Results: Coagulopathy among patients with rAAA was found to progress even after they had presented at the hospital. No statistically significant correlation between preoperative coagulopathy and mortality was found, although a significantly greater degree of postoperative coagulopathy was seen among patients who died both within 24-h and 30 days postoperatively. Among patients with postoperative coagulopathy, lesser quantities of fresh frozen plasma (FFP) compared with red cell concentrate (RCC) were used during the period from hospital arrival to postoperative ICU entry. In both groups of patients who did not survive after 24-h and 30 days, FFP was used less than RCC. Large transfusions of crystalloids administered during the periods from hospital arrival to surgery and from hospital arrival to the end of surgery were associated with postoperative incidence of major coagulopathy, death within 24-h, and death within 30 days.

Conclusion: Coagulopathy progressed during care in the emergency outpatient clinic and operations. Postoperative coagulopathy was associated with poorer outcomes. Smaller FFP/RCC ratios and larger volumes of crystalloid infusion were associated with development of coagulopathy and poorer prognosis of survival.

Trial registration: This study is retrospectively registered in UMIN Clinical Trials Registry (Registration 19 April 2016, registered number is R000025334 UMIN000021978).

Keywords: Ruptured abdominal aortic aneurysm, Endovascular aortic repair, EVAR, Blood transfusion, Crystalloid infusion

* Correspondence: hori@tokushima-cvs.info
Department of Cardiovascular Surgery, Chiba-Nishi General Hospital, 107-1 Kanegasaku, Matsudo-Shi 2702251, Chiba-Ken, Japan

Background

Ruptured abdominal aortic aneurysm (rAAA) is a fatal condition, with mortality rates of 38 to 50 % reported, even in cases where surgery is performed [1–3]. Open repair has generally been the standard operation; however, recent reports have indicated that endovascular aortic repair (EVAR) is equally effective [4]. In a randomized controlled trial, EVAR was found to be not inferior to open repair for treating rAAA [5].

Several studies have found associations between treatment success in open repair of rAAA and factors including advanced age, female sex [6], preoperative kidney failure, chronic obstructive pulmonary disease history [7], and deranged clotting [8]. But, few studies have investigated EVAR for rAAA, and we found limited data examining correlations between perioperative coagulopathy and survival. Furthermore, no data are available concerning preoperative treatment strategies, such as fluid and blood transfusions.

Coagulopathy is thought to be closely linked with rAAA survival [9]. Additionally, an association has been reported between coagulopathy and incidence of abdominal compartment syndrome, a complication of EVAR for rAAA [10]. Therefore, coagulopathy may also be an important factor determining survival prognosis after EVAR.

Similar to rAAA, trauma–induced coagulopathy (TIC) can be detrimental to a patient's overall condition from hemorrhagic shock and is known to worsen prognoses. Moreover, it is known that high doses of crystalloids can further worsen prognoses by contributing to TIC [11]. Early use of blood products is thought to improve prognoses [12]. Among patients undergoing EVAR for rAAA, we expected to find a correlation between coagulopathy incidence and postoperative survival prognosis, the volume and content of blood transfusions, and survival.

We retrospectively investigated associations between preoperative and postoperative coagulopathy in patients who underwent EVAR for rAAA at our hospital and 24-h and 30-day postoperative survival. Additionally, we examined how crystalloid infusion and blood transfusion correlated with coagulopathy incidence. We also examined the relation of crystalloid infusion and blood transfusion with 24-h and 30-day postoperative survival.

Methods

Patient selection

Subjects were all patients who underwent EVAR for rAAA at our hospital during the period from October 2013 to December 2015. Diagnosis of rAAA was made using simple computed tomography (CT) or contrast-enhanced CT. Observation of hematoma led to a diagnosis of rAAA. Patients who underwent emergency surgery for symptomatic abdominal aortic aneurysms were excluded where imaging did not show evidence of rupture.

This was a retrospective observational study. Prior to use of treatment data, consent was obtained in all cases from patients themselves or proxies with permission to make decisions on behalf of patients. The study was approved by a local ethical committee (approval No. TGE 00576-025).

Data collection

Information was gathered from medical, nursing, medication, and emergency medical service records. The results of blood tests performed when patients were admitted to the emergency room were used as the preoperative values, and results from tests performed when patients were admitted to the ICU after surgery were used as the postoperative values. Major coagulopathy was defined by an activated partial thrombin time ratio (APTT) greater than 1.5, by a prothrombin time and international normalized ratio (PT-INR) greater than 1.5, or by a platelet count less than $50 \times 10/l$. To investigate the content of blood products used, we calculated RCC/FFP ratios and differences (RCC-FFP) based on the volumes of blood products used during the period from hospital arrival to ICU entry just after surgery.

Three treatment outcomes were observed: intraoperative death, 24-h postoperative survival, or 30-day postoperative survival.

Pre- and intraoperative management

Decisions to administer fluid and blood transfusions, and about which compositions should be used, were made by the physicians in charge of outpatient care from hospital arrival to the start of surgery. In the period after patients entered the operating room, during surgery, and until the patients arrived in the ICU these decisions were made by anesthesiologists.

In principle, surgeries commenced under local anesthesia and general anesthesia was introduced after preparation for use of an aortic occlusion balloon. General anesthesia was administered before any incisions were made if the anesthesiologist and surgeon agreed this could be done safely.

Surgeries began without the use of heparin; however, heparin was administered in cases where it was possible to insert a balloon to occlude the aorta in order to ensure that activated clotting time was at least 200 s. Protamine was used to reverse the effects of heparin at the end of the operation, administered at a dose equivalent quantity. Following the end of the operation, all patients were transferred to the ICU while sedated and connected to an artificial respiratory device.

Statistical analysis

For continuous variables, means and standard deviations were calculated. Categorical variables were presented as n (percentage of total [%]). The Mann-Whitney test was used for analysis of continuous variables, whilst categorical variables were compared using the chi-square test. Differences were considered statistically significant at a p-value of <0.05.

All statistical analyses were performed on a personal computer using the statistical software package SPSS for Mac (Version 22; SPSS Inc., Chicago, IL, USA).

Results

Treatment outcome

Forty-seven patients presenting with rAAA in our hospital were enrolled in the study. One patient was considered unfit for surgery. Of the 46 patients who went to theater, 25 underwent EVAR and thus were included in our analyses.

With regard to treatment outcomes, no patients died in the operating theater, whilst three died due to abdominal compartment syndrome (ACS) within 24-h postsurgery, and an additional two died between 24-h and 30 days postsurgery. One of these two patients died due to respiratory failure and one of cancer.

Comparison of preoperative and postoperative examination values

Data from the 25 subjects before and after surgery were compared using paired t-tests. Statistically significant changes were seen in APTT and PT-INR, which increased, and platelet counts, which decreased. No patients presented with major coagulopathy prior to surgery, although nine patients experienced major coagulopathy afterward (Table 1).

Coagulopathy, fluid infusion, and blood transfusion

Patients who presented major coagulopathy after surgery received larger total fluid transfusions from hospital arrival to the end of surgery. More patients in the nonsurvival groups for both 24-h and 30-day survival received fluid transfusions of 1.5 L (Table 2).

The values for RCC/FFP ratio and RCC-FFP were significantly larger in the group that exhibited major coagulopathy than in the group that did not.

Table 1 Comparison of the preoperative and postoperative coagulation profiles in all participants

	Preoperative	Postoperative	p
APTT (second)	27.8 +/- 5.2	47.3 +/- 30.1	0.002
PT-INR	1.2 +/- 0.2	1.4 +/- 0.2	<0.001
PLT counts (10^4/μL)	16.3 +/- 5.2	9.9 +/- 4.7	<0.001
Major coagulopathy (n)	0	9	<0.001

APTT activated partial thromboplastin time ratio, PT-INR prothrombin time and international normalized ratio, PLT platelet

Table 2 Survival and coagulation profiles

	Survival	Non-survival	p
24-h survival			
n	22	3	
Preoperative APTT (second)	27.0 +/- 4.3	33.6 +/- 8.4	0.21
Postoperative APTT (second)	38.9 +/- 8.7	108.7 +/- 63.4	0.006
APTT change (second)	11.9 +/- 9.2	75.0 +/- 58.9	0.006
Preoperative PT-INR	1.2 +/- 0.16	1.2 +/- 0.2	0.802
Postoperative PT-INR	1.3 +/- 0.20	1.5 +/- 0.28	0.295
PT-INR change	0.16 +/- 0.17	0.33 +/- 0.33	0.503
Preoperative platelet counts (10^4/μL)	16.1 +/- 5.4	17.3 +/- 3.0	0.616
Postoperative platelet counts (10^4/μL)	10.2 +/- 5.0	7.7 +/- 1.9	0.558
Platelet count change (10^4/μL)	5.9 +/- 6.2	9.5 +/- 5.2	0.452
Preoperative major coagulopathy (n)	0 (0 %)	0 (0 %)	NS
Postoperative major coagulopathy (n)	6 (27 %)	3 (100 %)	0.037
NS: not significant			
30-day survival			
n	20	5	
Preoperative APTT (second)	26.8 +/- 4.3	32 +/- 7.0	0.119
Postoperative APTT (second)	38.1 +/- 7.9	95.7 +/- 57.9	0.002
APTT change (second)	11.3 +/- 8.9	62.7 +/- 54.1	0.002
Preoperative PT-INR	1.2 +/- 0.16	1.23 +/- 0.19	0.0767
Postoperative PT-INR	1.4 +/- 0.2	1.5 +/- 0.2	0.148
PT-INR change	0.16 +/- 0.18	0.30 +/- 0.28	0.436
Preoperative platelet counts (10^4/μL)	16.2 +/-5.54	16.8 +/- 2.7	0.767
Postoperative platelet counts (10^4/μL)	10.4 +/- 5.0	7.2 +/- 1.9	0.299
Platelet count change (10^4/μL)	−5.7 +/-6.3	−9.6 +/- 4.0	0.335
Preoperative major coagulopathy (n)	0 (0 %)	0 (0 %)	NS
Postoperative major coagulopathy (n)	5 (25 %)	4 (80 %)	0.01

APTT activated partial thromboplastin time ratio, PT-INR prothrombin time and international normalized ratio, PLT platelet

Coagulopathy and survival

Postoperative APTT was significantly longer in the 24-h and 30-day non-survival groups in comparison with the respective survival groups (Table 3).

A significantly greater number of patients in the 24-h non-survival group exhibited major coagulopathy postoperatively compared with the survival group. Similarly, there more instances of major coagulopathy were observed in the 30-day non-survival group than in the survival group.

Fluid and blood transfusions and survival

Values for RCC/FFP ratios and RCC-FFP were significantly larger in both the 24-h and 30-day non-survival groups compared with the respective survival groups

Table 3 Postoperative major coagulopathy and blood and fluid transfusions

	Postoperative major coagulopathy		
	Non-presented	Presented	p
RCC (units)	5.63 +/- 5.3	13.6 +/- 7.0	0.004
FFP (units)	5.75 +/- 6.4	6.2 +/- 7.5	0.743
PC (units)	5.6 +/- 11.5	4.4 +/- 8.8	0.57
RCC/FFP ratio	1.1 +/- 0.23	2.00 +/- 0.73	0.015
RCC - FFP (units)	2.3 +/- 3.5	7.9 +/- 4.3	0.001
Preoperative crystalloid volume (mL)	750 +/- 408	1589 +/- 1071	0.022
Total crystalloid volume (mL)	2214 +/- 893	3572 +/- 1391	0.014
Total crystalloids >1.5 L (n)	4 (25 %)	5 (56 %)	0.137

RCC red cell concentrate, FFP fresh frozen plasma, PC platelet concentrate

(Table 4). Patients with RCC/FFP ratios greater than 1.5 had higher risks of mortality.

Larger quantities of crystalloids were used in the both the 24-h and 30-day non-survival groups compared with the respective survival groups.

Discussion

For all subjects, values for postoperative APTT and PT-INR were significantly longer than preoperative values.

Table 4 Survival and blood and fluid transfusions

	Survival	Non-survival	p
24-h survival			
RCC (units)	7.3 +/- 5.3	17.7 +/- 7.8	0.035
FFP (units)	3.6 +/- 4.2	12.0 +/- 6.9	0.02
PC (units)	5.7 +/- 12.9	13.3 +/- 11.5	0.271
RCC/FFP ratio	1.3 +/- 0.6	1.6 +/- 0.8	0.014
RCC/FFP >1.5 L (n)	2 (9 %)	3 (100 %)	0.018
RCC - FFP (units)	4.5 +/- 4.7	5.7 +/- 5.7	0.006
Preoperative crystalloid volume (mL)	877 +/- 615	2333 +/- 1041	0.01
Total crystalloid volume (mL)	2386 +/- 912	5083 +/-803	0.028
Total crystalloid >1.5 L (n)	5 (23 %)	3 (100 %)	0.037
30-day survival			
RCC (units)	6.9 +/- 5.6	15.8 +/- 7.4	0.017
FFP (units)	3.4 +/- 4.2	10.0 +/- 6.9	0.116
PC (units)	5.7 +/- 12.9	10.0 +/- 11.5	0.96
RCC/FFP ratio	1.1 +/- 0.6	1.8 +/- 0.8	0.001
RCC/FFP > 1.5 L (n)	1 (5 %)	4 (70 %)	0.03
RCC - FFP (units)	3.5+/-4.7	5.8+/-4.6	0.03
Preoperative crystalloid volume (mL)	847 +/- 615	2125 +/- 946	0.003
Total crystalloid volume (mL)	2341 +/- 9.6	4550 +/- 1252	0.012
Crystalloids >1.5 L (n)	5 (25 %)	4 (80 %)	0.01

RCC red cell concentrate, FFP fresh frozen plasma, PC platelet concentrate

While there were no instances of major coagulopathy preoperatively, the condition was observed in nine patients postoperatively.

At both 24-h and 30 days postoperation, there were no significant differences in preoperative APTT, PT-INR, or major coagulopathy between the survival groups and non-survival groups. These results concur with findings from a previous study that examined factors related to survival after open repair for rAAA and found no correlation between preoperative coagulopathy and mortality [13].

Conversely, our findings show that postoperative APTT was significantly longer in the non-survival groups than in the survival groups at both 24 h and 30 days. Furthermore, APTT increased by a significantly larger proportion between pre- and postsurgery in the non-survival groups at both 24 h and 30 days.

There were more instances of postoperative major coagulopathy in the non-survival groups than in the survival groups at both 24 h and 30 days. In a previous study of patients who underwent open repair for rAAA, prolonged PT and prolonged APTT at postoperative ICU entry were associated with poorer prognoses [14]. The same appears to be true for patients treated with EVAR.

In the present study, a tendency for coagulopathy to progress during the period from hospital arrival to the end of surgery was observed among all cases, with patients who exhibited greater progression also exhibiting higher mortality risks. Efforts to control the progression of coagulopathy after hospital arrival could help to improve survival prognoses.

ACS is a serious condition that can occur after EVAR for rAAA and negatively affects survival [15]. Its mortality rate is nearly 100 % without treatment and is still high (30–60 %) with appropriate treatment [16]. ACS is thought to be caused by massive retroperitoneal hematoma and diffuse visceral edema and is diagnosed when the abdominal pressure exceeds 20 mmHg in combination with endo-organ dysfunction. Early recognition and surgical decompression of ACS is essential [17]. Coagulopathy is reportedly a risk factor for ACS [12]. In fact, all the patients who died within 24 h in the present study experienced ACS and exhibited postoperative major coagulopathy. Routine measurement of intraabdominal pressure is useful for detecting ACS. Especially in patients with coagulopathy after EVAR for rAAA, intraabdominal pressure should be monitored carefully. Additionally, we believe that maintaining clotting function by FFP blood trans fusion and limitation of crystalloid use can prevent ACS development.

In a report on trauma treatment by Veena et al. [18], greater administered quantities of crystalloids were associated with coagulopathy progression, cellular distension, heart complications, and elevated abdominal compartment pressure. In addition, incidence of ACS has been linked to large fluid transfusions [19].

In the present study, quantities of crystalloids administered were significantly higher among patients with major coagulopathy. Furthermore, quantities of crystalloids used were significantly higher in the non-survival groups at both 24-h and 30 days. Crystalloid transfusion is associated with coagulopathy onset in rAAA patients who undergo EVAR and is thought to have a negative effect on prognosis. In a study of trauma patients, cases that received large quantities of crystalloids in initial transfusions reportedly required larger blood transfusions [20]. It is possible that limiting use of crystalloids can prevent postoperative coagulopathy and can make better the prognosis of survival.

In the present study, values for both RCC/FFP ratio and RCC-FFP were larger among patients with postoperative major coagulopathy. Previously, a prospective study of patients who underwent open surgery for rAAA found that aggressive FFP and PLT administration significantly inhibited the prolongation of postoperative APTT [21].

In this study, the relatively lesser use of FFP compared with RCC appears to be associated with major coagulopathy.

Studies investigating blood transfusion composition and survival prognosis in trauma patients have indicated that an appropriate target for RCC/FFP ratios is between 3 and 4 [22]. However, a study conducted by the military found that maintaining an RCC/FFP ratio close to 1 led to increased survival rates [23]. A retrospective investigation of RCC/FFP ratios in trauma patients reported a link between a 1:1 RCC/FFP ratio and positive prognoses [24]. Furthermore, the PROPPR randomized clinical trial, which divided trauma patients into an RCC:FFP:PC = 1:1:1 group and an RCC:FFP:PC = 2:1:1 group, found that the former group achieved hemostasis and experienced less exsanguination in 24 h, although no significant differences in mortality between the two groups were observed [25]. Most of the above results suggest that quantities of FFP equal to those of RCC can be useful for improving the survival prognoses of patients with rAAA receiving EVAR by maintaining a coagulation profile and achieving hemostasis.

Our hospital does not have a protocol for blood transfusion in rAAA patients. The physician in charge determines the content of transfusions based on test results. Mean transfusion quantities were RCC 10.0 +/- 5.70 units and FFP 4.4 +/- 3.3 units, representing a RCC/FFP ratio greater than 1. On the basis of results from the present and previous studies, it appears that basing decisions for how much FFP to administer on test results may not keep up with the patient's progression. For rAAA patients undergoing EVAR who require blood transfusions, coagulopathy may be controlled and survival prognosis improved by following a transfusion protocol that uses a 1:1 RCC/FFP ratio and administers FFP early.

Conclusion

Coagulopathy progressed during care in the emergency outpatient clinic and the operations, and postoperative coagulopathy was associated with poorer outcomes. We suggest that smaller FFP/RCC ratios and larger volumes of crystalloid infusions potentially contributed to coagulopathy and ACS development, and poor survival prognosis. Limitations of this study include the small sample number and its retrospective design, and further investigation is needed.

Abbreviations

ACS, abdominal compartment syndrome; APTT, activated partial thrombin time ratio; EVAR, endovascular aortic repair; FFP, fresh frozen plasma; ICU, intensive care unit; PC, platelet concentrate; PT-INR, prothrombin time international normalized ratio; RCC, red cell concentrated.

Acknowledgement
None.

Funding
None.

Authors' contribution

YK and TH conducted the study and drafted manuscript. YK, YN, HK, YS and TH contributed to the operative and postoperative care and discussion during patient care and preparing the manuscript. All the authors have approved the final text.

Authors' information
None.

Competing interests
The authors declare that they have no competing interests.

References

1. Bown MJ, Sutton AJ, Bell PR, Sayers RD. A meta-analysis of 50 years of ruptured abdominal aortic aneurysm repair. Br J Surg. 2002;89:714–30.
2. Heller JA, Weinberg A, Arons R, Krishnasastry KV, Lyon RT, Deitch JS, et al. Two decades of abdominal aortic aneurysm repair: have we made any progress? J Vas Surg. 2000;32:1091–100.
3. Egorova N, Giacovelli J, Greco G, Gelijns A, Kent CK, McKinsey JF. National outcomes for the treatment of ruptured abdominal aortic aneurysm: comparison of open versus endovascular repairs. J Vasc Surg. 2008;48:1092–100.
4. Antoniou GA, Georgiadis GS, Antoniou SA, Pavlidis P, Maras D, Sfyroeras GS, et al. Endovascular repair for ruptured abdominal aortic aneurysm confers an early survival benefit over open repair. J Vasc Surg. 2013;58:1091–105.
5. IMPROVE Trial Investigators. Endovascular strategy or open repair for ruptured abdominal aortic aneurysm: one-year outcomes from the IMPROVE randomized trial. Eur Heart J. 2015;36:2061–9.
6. Dueck AD, Kucey DS, Johnston KW, Alter D, Laupacis A. Survival after ruptured abdominal aortic aneurysm: effect of patient, surgeon, and hospital factors. J Vasc Surg. 2004;39:1261–7.

7. Ouriel K, Geary K, Green RM, Fiore W, Geary JE, DeWeese JA. Factors determining survival after ruptured aortic aneurysm: the hospital, the surgeon, and the patient. J Vasc Surg. 1990;11:493–6.
8. Davies MJ, Murphy WG, Murie JA, Elton RA, Bell K, Gillon JG, et al. Ruptured aortic aneurysm: the decision not to operate. Br J Surg. 1993;80:974–6.
9. Tambyraja AL, Murie JA, Chalmers RT. Prediction of outcome after abdominal aortic aneurysm rupture. J Vasc Surg. 2008;47:222–30.
10. Mehta M, Darling 3rd RC, Roddy SP, Fecteau S, Ozsvath KJ, Kreienberg PB, et al. Factors associated with abdominal compartment syndrome complicating endovascular repair of ruptured abdominal aortic aneurysms. J Vasc Surg. 2005; 42:1047–51.
11. Ley EJ, Clond MA, Srour MK, Barnajian M, Mirocha J, Margulies DR, et al. Emergency department crystalloid resuscitation of 1.5 L or more is associated with increased mortality in elderly and nonelderly trauma patients. J Trauma. 2011;70:398–400.
12. Ball CG. Damage control resuscitation: history, theory and technique. Can J Surg. 2014;57:55–60.
13. Reed MJ, Burfield LC. Initial emergency department coagulation profile does not predict survival in ruptured abdominal aortic aneurysm. Eur J Emerg Med. 2013;20:397–401.
14. Gierek D, Cyzowski T, Kaczmarska A, Janowska-Rodak A, Budziarz B, Koczur T. Perioperative prognostic factors in patients with ruptured abdominal aortic aneurysms treated in the intensive care unit. Anaesthesiol Intensive Ther. 2013;45:25–9.
15. Mehta M, Darling 3rd RC, Roddy SP. Factors associated with abdominal compartment syndrome complicating endovascular repair of reuptured abdominal aortic aneurysms. J Vasc Surg. 2005;42(6):1047–51.
16. Ersryd S, Djavani-Gidulund K, Wanhainen A. Abdominal compartment syndrome after surgery for abdominal aortic aneurysm: A Nation wide population based study. Eur J Vasc Endovasc Surg. 2016. doi:10.1016/j.ejvs.2016.03.011.
17. Kirkpatrick AW, Roberts DJ, De Waele J. Intra-abdominal hypertension and the abdominal compartment syndrome: updated consensus definitions and clinical practice guidelines from the World Society of the Abdominal Compartment Syndrome. Intensive Care Med. 2013;39(7):1190–206.
18. Chatrath V, Khetarpal R, Ahuja J. Fluid management in patients with trauma: Restrictive versus liberal approach. J Anaesthesiol Clin Pharmacol. 2015;31:308–16.
19. Kwan I, Bunn F, Roberts I, WHO Pre-Hospital Trauma Care Steering Committee. Timing and volume of fluid administration for patients with bleeding. Cochrane Database Syst Rev. 2003;3, CD002245.
20. Wang H, Robinson RD, Phillips JL, Kirk AJ, Duane TM, Umejiego J, et al. Benefits of Initial Limited Crystalloid Resuscitation in Severely Injured Trauma Patients at Emergency Department. J Clin Med Res. 2015;7:947–55.
21. Johansson PI, Stensballe J, Rosenberg I, Hilsløv TL, Jørgensen L, Secher NH. Proactive administration of platelets and plasma for patients with a ruptured abdominal aortic aneurysm: evaluating a change in transfusion practice. Transfusion. 2007;47:593–8.
22. Tu JV, Austin PC, Johnston KW. The influence of surgical specialty training on the outcomes of elective abdominal aortic aneurysm surgery. J Vasc Surg. 2001;33:447–52.
23. Spinella PC, Perkins JG, Grathwohl KW, Beekley AC, Niles SE, McLaughlin DF, et al. Effect of plasma and red blood cell transfusions on survival in patients with combat related traumatic injuries. J Trauma. 2008;64:S69–78.
24. Zehtabchi S, Nishijima DK. Impact of transfusion of fresh-frozen plasma and packed red blood cells in a 1:1 ratio on survival of emergency department patients with severe trauma. Acad Emerg Med. 2009;16:371–8.
25. Holcomb JB, Tilley BC, Baraniuk S, Fox EE, Wade CE, Podbielski JM, et al. Transfusion of plasma, platelets, and red blood cells in a 1:1:1 vs a 1:1:2 ratio and mortality in patients with severe trauma: the PROPPR randomized clinical trial. JAMA. 2015;313:471–82.

8

Which cause of diffuse peritonitis is the deadliest in the tropics? A retrospective analysis of 305 cases from the South-West Region of Cameroon

Alain Chichom-Mefire*, Tabe Alain Fon and Marcelin Ngowe-Ngowe

Abstract

Background: Acute diffuse peritonitis is a common surgical emergency worldwide and a major contributor to non-trauma related death toll. Its causes vary widely and are correlated with mortality. Community acquired peritonitis seems to play a major role and is frequently related to hollow viscus perforation. Data on the outcome of peritonitis in the tropics are scarce. The aim of this study is to analyze the impact of tropic latitude causes of diffuse peritonitis on morbidity and mortality.

Methods: We retrospectively reviewed the records of 305 patients operated on for a diffuse peritonitis in two regional hospitals in the South-West Region of Cameroon over a 7 years period. The contributions of various causes of peritonitis to morbidity and mortality were analyzed.

Results: The diagnosis of diffuse peritonitis was suggested on clinical ground only in more than 93 % of cases. The most common causes of diffuse peritonitis included peptic ulcer perforation ($n = 69$), complications of acute appendicitis ($n = 53$) and spontaneous perforations of the terminal ileum ($n = 43$). A total of 142 complications were recorded in 96 patients (31.5 % complication rate). The most common complications included wound dehiscence, sepsis, prolonged paralytic ileus and multi-organ failure. Patients with typhoid perforation of the terminal ileum carried a significantly higher risk of developing a complication ($p = 0.002$). The overall mortality rate was 15.1 %. The most common cause of death was septic shock. Differential analysis of mortality of various causes of peritonitis indicated that the highest contributors to death toll were typhoid perforation of terminal ileum (34.7 % of deaths), post-operative peritonitis (19.5 %) and peptic ulcer perforation (15.2 %).

Conclusion: The diagnosis of diffuse peritonitis can still rely on clinical assessment alone in the absence of sophisticated imaging tools. Peptic ulcer and typhoid perforations are still major contributors to death toll. Patients presenting with these conditions require specific attention and prevention policies must be reinforced.

Keywords: Diffuse peritonitis, Morbidity, Mortality, Menheim Peritonitis index, Hollow viscus perforation, Septic shock

Background

Pathological conditions requiring surgery contribute significantly to the global disease burden [1]. It is well established that injuries contribute more than 70 % of death toll in the emergency departments of low and middle-income countries (LMICs) [2]. However,

* Correspondence: chichomefire@gmail.com
Department of Surgery, Faculty of Health Sciences, University of Buea and Regional Hospital Limbe, P.O. Box 25526, Yaoundé, Cameroon

non-trauma related conditions are still responsible for a high number of in-hospital deaths and require specific attention, especially in the tropics [2–4].

Acute generalized peritonitis is a common surgical emergency worldwide and has been reported as one of the major contributors to non-trauma deaths in the emergency department despite improvements in diagnosis, surgical treatment and intensive care support [4–6]. The causes of generalized peritonitis vary widely from one setting to another and seem to be correlated to mortality [3, 7, 8]. It is known that community acquired peritonitis represent the vast majority of cases and is largely related to bowel perforation [3, 9]. This latter cause of peritonitis seems to carry the highest mortality rate (10 to 32 %) [7, 9–12]. Analysis of the contribution of various forms of perforative peritonitis to morbidity and mortality indicate that while results of treatment of peritonitis secondary to peptic ulcer perforation seem to have improved over the past decades [13–15], other frequent causes in the tropics such as typhoid fever related perforation of the small bowel still carry a heavy morbidity and mortality rates [4, 16–18].

Some factors influencing outcome of peritonitis which have been studied and reported so far include age, co-morbidities, severity of sepsis, delay before initiation of treatment and immune suppression [3, 6, 8]. Early prognostic evaluation of patients with acute generalized peritonitis is desirable to select patients with a higher risk of adverse event who may be eligible for a more aggressive treatment. Various approaches to anticipate the outcome by grading the severity of peritonitis have been proposed. They generally rely on scoring systems such as APACHE II and the Mannheim Peritonitis Index (MPI).

Data on the burden and outcome of peritonitis in sub-Saharan Africa are very scarce and few studies have attempted a differential analysis of various causes of diffuse peritonitis. As a consequence, surgeons performing in these areas of the world generally lack management guidelines which are adapted to their local conditions characterized by absence of health insurance, poor technical background and limited access to intensive care unit.

The aim of this study is to identify the most common causes of diffuse peritonitis in the tropical latitudes and their relative contribution to morbidity and to death toll. The ultimate goal is to help surgeons identify cases which are likely to require a more aggressive therapy and rationalize the decision to refer patients towards a center with an intensive care unit. We hypothesized that peritonitis secondary to peptic ulcer perforation was the highest contributor to death toll in the tropics.

Methods
Study design and setting
This observational retrospective analysis covered a period of 7 years (from January 01st 2007 to December 31st 2013) in the two regional hospitals of the Fako division in the South-West Region of Cameroon. These level III institutions are located in the cities of Limbe and Buea respectively and are easily accessible from most tributary health institutions thanks to the acceptable road network of the Fako division. They have a total admission capacity of 326 beds. The total catchment population is estimated at 527,000 people. These two institutions are organized in a similar model with an emergency department where all urgent cases are initially admitted. Cases requiring surgery are transferred to corresponding surgical wards with a cumulated admission capacity of 58 beds managed by four surgeons during the study period. Surgical interventions are carried out in one of the two operative rooms of each institution. They both possess a laboratory and an imaging department where most basic work-up can be performed. Computerized tomography, bacterial culture and intensive care units are available in none of the institutions. Cases requiring more specialized investigations or intensive care can however be referred to the city of Douala located about 70 km from both cities where two large central hospitals possessing all the services are available and functional.

Study population and procedure
We included in this study all patients operated on for an intra-abdominal sepsis for which a final diagnosis of diffuse peritonitis was made. Diffuse peritonitis was defined as any intra-abdominal infection extending beyond the transverse mesocolon. The exclusion criteria were the following:

- All patients with a localized peritonitis.
- All patients with a primary peritonitis defined as diffuse peritonitis with no identifiable source of infection during surgical exploration.
- All patients with suspected peritonitis for whom a laparotomy was not performed.
- All patients whose file did not contain follow-up data.

Data source included admission registers of the emergency department, patient's admission files, post-operative note registers and report books of the surgical wards. For each patient included, we recorded on a pre-designed data collection form data regarding patient's characteristics, clinical and para-clinical characteristics of the peritonitis, findings of the surgical exploration, follow-up data and final outcome. Sepsis, septic shock and multiorgan failure were defined according to the American College of Chest Physicians/Society of Critical Care Medicine Consensus Conference Committee of 1991 as modified in 2001 [19, 20]. Only adverse events occurring during the same admission were considered.

The characteristics of the peritonitis were classified according to the MPI which has been extensively used to predict the outcome of various forms of peritonitis [6, 21, 22]. The severity of complications was graded according to the Clavien-Dindo classification [23, 24].

Statistical analysis

All data were entered in an excel database (Excel 2007, Microsoft corporation®) and later one converted into an Epi-info 7 for the purpose of statistical analysis. Pairwise comparisons were done using Epi-info Statalc function. Spontaneous comparisons were done using STATA 10.

Ethical consideration

The procedures of this study respected the Helsinki declaration and were in conformity with the laws of the republic of Cameroon about research on human subjects. An ethical approval was obtained from the Institutional Review Board of the University of Buea.

Reporting

The STROBE guidelines were used in reporting this study [25].

Results

Patient's characteristics

A total of 378 patients were admitted in these two institutions with the post-operative diagnosis of acute diffuse peritonitis over the study period.

These included 230 patients from Buea Regional Hospital and 148 patients from Limbe Regional hospital. A total of 73 patients were excluded for the following reasons:

- Thirty four records had incomplete data. These included four patients with a presumptive diagnosis of peritonitis who died before a laparotomy could be performed.
- For the remaining 39 files, analysis of the operative notes indicated that no cause was identified for the peritonitis during surgical exploration and they were classified as primary peritonitis.

A total of 305 files could finally be analyzed, 201 (65.9 %) from Buea Regional Hospital and 104 (34.1 %) from Limbe Regional Hospital.

Our sample included 168 males and 137 females, giving a sex-ratio of 1.23/1. The ages of our patients ranged from 3 to 82 years with a mean of 30.6 ± 16.0 years. As shown on Fig. 1, a total of 269 patients (88.2 %) were aged 50 years or below.

Characteristics of the peritonitis

As shown in Table 1, the most common clinical findings were diffuse abdominal pain (100 %), abnormal temperature (83 %) and signs of peritoneal irritation (tenderness, rebound tenderness, guarding, rigidity: 91 %). A total of 138 patients (45 %) presented with signs of sepsis on admission. The delay between onset

of symptoms and admission ranged from 16 h to 9 days with a mean of 3.62 days.

Most patients (80 %) for whom a leucocyte count was requested and had a leucocytosis above 12.000/ml.

The diagnosis of acute generalized peritonitis was suspected on clinical ground in all cases and the most common confirmatory tool was ultrasound used in 238 (78 %) cases. The cause of peritonitis was suspected pre-operatively based on the combination of clinical and ultrasonographical findings in 246 (81 %) of cases. An erect chest X-ray was requested and performed in 231 (75.7 %) patients and revealed a pneumoperitoneum in 37 % of cases, all with a final diagnosis of either peptic ulcer or small bowel perforation.

All patients with a suspicion of diffuse peritonitis had an antibiotic regimen started in the emergency department. As shown on Fig. 2, most patients (79 %) received a combination of ceftriaxone and metronidazole with or without gentamicine.

Table 2 indicates all the causes of diffuse peritonitis as reported by the surgical exploration. According to this table, the five most common causes included peptic ulcer perforation ($n = 69$), complications of acute appendicitis ($n = 53$), post-operative peritonitis ($n = 44$), typhoid related perforation of the terminal ileum ($n = 43$) and abdominal injuries (38). As Table 3 shows, the age distribution of these five most common causes of diffuse peritonitis indicates that almost 75 % of cases of typhoid perforation of small bowel occurred before the age of 20. Also, 26 of the 44 cases of post-operative diffuse peritonitis (59 %) were consecutive to the septic complications of illegal abortion, performed by a health care provider out of the hospital in most cases.

When assessing the severity of the peritonitis, the MPI ranged from 6 to 34 points with a mean of 19.88 ± 9.68. We divided our patients in three groups: those with a MPI of <15, those with MPI ranging from 16 to 25 and those with MPI >26. As shown on Fig. 3, 60 (19.7 %) patients had a MPI > 26.

Analysis of post-operative notes indicated that source control was successful in 286 patients (93.8 %). All cases of peptic ulcer perforation were located on the proximal duodenum, except for three cases of gastric ulcers. The most frequent treatment modality for cases of peptic ulcer perforation was suture with omentum patch after Graham applied in 92.8 % of patients. Three patients (4.34 %), all from Limbe Regional hospital had a bilateral trunkal vagotomy performed as definitive treatment of the peptic ulcer disease. All typhoid related perforations of the small bowel were located in the last 100 cm of the ileum. Simple suturing of the ileal perforation was the most frequently used treatment modality applied in 31 (74.4 %) of patients.

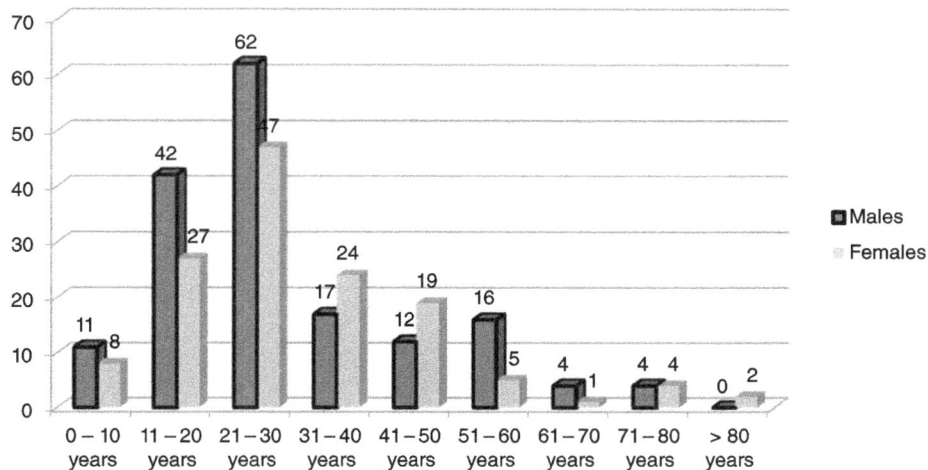

Fig. 1 Age and sex distribution of cases of diffuse peritonitis in Limbe and Buea Regional Hospitals

Outcome

The outcome data are shown in Table 4-6. A total of 142 complications were recorded in 96 patients (31.5 % complication rate). The most common complications recorded included wound dehiscence, sepsis, prolonged paralytic ileus and multi-organ failure. The most common combination was the association of signs of septic shock with paralytic ileus. According to the Clavien-Dindo classification, as shown in Fig. 4, when excluding those who died (classified as Clavien-Dindo V), the majority of patients developed a Grade I complication. A total of 100 of these complications occurred in 84 of the 247 patients whose laparotomy was performed for one of the five most

Table 1 Clinical and para-clinical characterisitics of diffuse community acquired peritonitis in Limbe and Buea Regioanl Hospitals

Clinical and para-clinical findings	Number	Percentage
Abdominal pain	305	100
Nausea/vomiting	128	42
Diarrhea/constipation	214	70.1
Fever or hypothermia	253	83
Tachycardia	219	71.8
Tachypnoea	133	43.6
Abdominal distention	198	64.7
Signs of peritoneal irritation	277	90.8
Signs of shock	138	45.1
Leucocyte count >12.000	138/196	80.4
Leucocyte count < 4000	32/196	16.3
Pneumoperitoneum	86/231	37.22
Air fluid levels	82/231	35.5
Suggestive ultrasound findings	156/238	96.9

common causes of diffuse peritonitis listed above (34 % complication rate). According to Table 7, septic shock and multi-organ failure were very frequent complications in patients with typhoid perforation of the ileum. Patients with MPI of 16 or more carried a significantly higher risk of developing a complication ($P < 0.0001$). Differential analysis indicates that patients with typhoid perforation of the terminal ileum carried a significantly higher risk of developing a complication ($p = 0.002$).

A total of 46 patients were reported death during the course of management, giving an overall mortality rate of 15.1 %. The most common cause of death was septic shock. Those who died each developed a mean of 1.43 complications. Two patients died in the operative room, both with a severe pre-operative sepsis. Differential analysis of mortality of various causes of peritonitis indicated that the highest contributors to death toll were perforation of terminal ileum (34.7 % of deaths), post-operative peritonitis (19.5 %) and peptic ulcer perforation (15.2 %). As shown on Table 4, perforation of sigmoid colon, perforation of the terminal ileum and post-operative peritonitis carried a significantly higher relative risk of death.

Discussion

This study is one of the few conducted in the LMICs, that includes a large sample size and analyzes complications and fatality rates for various causes of diffuse peritonitis.. It is a contribution to the advocacy in favour of global surgery as outlined by the Lancet commission for Global surgery and its objectives for the year 2030 and by the World Health Assembly's resolutions on the need to reduce the global burden of surgical conditions potentially correctable by surgery, especially in Low and middle income countries [26, 27].

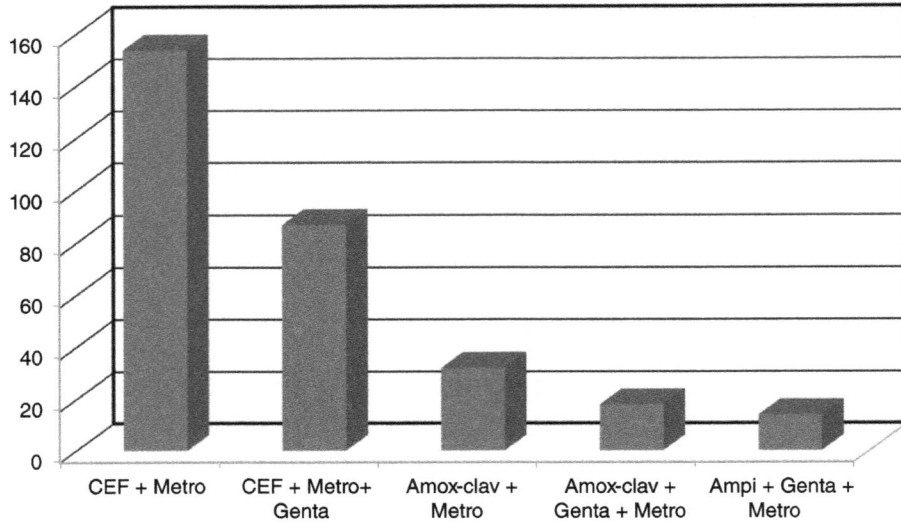

Fig. 2 The various antibiotic regimens proposed to patients with diffuse community acquired peritonitis in Limbe and Buea. CEF + Metro: combination of ceftriaxone and metronidazole. CEF + Metro + Genta: combination of ceftriaxone, metronidazole and gentamicine. Amox-clav + Metro: combination of amoxicillin-clavulanic acid and metronidazole. Amox-clav + Metro + genta: combination of amoxicillin-clavulanic acid, metronidazole and gentamicine. Ampi + Genta + Metro: combination of Ampicillin,Gentamicine and Metronidazole

Our study suggests that spontaneous perforation of small bowel, usually typhoid fever related is a substantial problem especially in paediatric populations. Also, peptic ulcer perforation is still a major concern in these areas of the world. Septic complications of illegal abortions also require a specific attention. Large proportion of patients with diffuse peritonitis still present to the hospital with unacceptable delays and this probably accounts for the high incidence of sepsis and high MPI scores at the time of diagnosis with the consequences that it entails in terms of outcome. In settings with limited technical background, the diagnosis of this common clinical entity can still rely largely on clinical arguments. Patients operated on for diffuse peritonitis are likely to develop wound dehiscence, sepsis, prolonged paralytic ileus or multi-organ failure. These complications often occur in

Table 2 Relative frequency and sex distribution of causes of diffuse community acquired peritonitis in Limbe and Buea Regional hospitals

Cause	Males	Females	Total	Percentage
Peptic Ulcer Perforation	49	20	69	22.6
Spontaneous perforation of terminal ileum	19	24	43	14.1
Complications of acute appendicitis	34	19	53	17.4
Splenic Abscess	4	2	6	2
Tubo-Ovarian Abscess	0	7	7	2.3
Acute cholecystitis	1	7	8	2.6
Incarcerated hernia	8	0	8	2.6
Intestinal obstruction	4	9	13	4.3
Intussusception	3	0	3	1
Volvulus of sigmoid colon	8	1	9	3
Infection of haemoperitoneum	0	2	2	0.6
Rupture of liver abscess	1	1	2	0.6
Hospital-acquired	10	34	44	14.4
Blunt abdominal injury	21	6	27	8.9
Penetrating abdominal injury	6	5	11	3.6
Total	168	137	305	100

Table 3 Age distribution of the five most common causes of diffuse community acquired peritonitis in Limbe and Buea

Age group	Peptic ulcer perforation	Perforation of terminal ileum	Complications of appendicitis	Hospital-acquired	Abdominal injuries	Total
0–10 years	0	11	3	0	6	20
11–20 years	14	21	14	12	13	74
21–30 years	27	5	22	22	11	87
31–40 years	15	3	10	7	4	39
41–50 years	7	1	3	3	1	15
51–60 years	4	1	1	0	2	8
61–70 years	0	1	0	0	1	2
71–80 years	1	0	0	0	0	1
>80 years	1	0	0	0	0	1
Total	69	43	53	44	38	247

combination especially in those with typhoid related small bowel perforation, and can be deadly in more than 15 % of cases. The highest contributors to death toll are all cases of peritonitis originating from bowel perforations, especially those related to complications of typhoid fever which is endemic in the region.

This study brings to light once more the crucial problem of filing and conservation of data in LMICs with nearly 10 % of patients excluded for incomplete data. However, higher rates of patients with incomplete files have been reported in similar settings [2]. Also, it is questionable how the findings of this study can be compared to those from other centers where all the facilities for diagnosis and management are available. In particular, the absence of equipment for the laparoscopic approach is likely to influence the outcome. It has been reported that this approach could be proposed to as much as 27 % of patients [5] with a supposedly better outcome. Our choice to limit this study to diffuse peritonitis is inspired by the

fact that this form of peritonitis is by far the most frequent with a higher death toll [3–5].

While multiple reports indicate that diffuse peritonitis, especially when related to bowel perforation seem to affect young patients with a predominance of male sex [4, 8, 17, 28, 29], major differences in causes between LMICs and developed countries have been reported. In general, patients from LMICs tend to suffer perforations of the proximal gut while does in the western countries are more often affected with perforations of the large intestine [30]. The five most common causes of secondary peritonitis described in our study have been reported in numerous studies in similar settings [7, 9, 12, 29, 31, 32]. Peptic ulcer perforation is still a frequent complication and affects the duodenum in the large majority of cases [7, 9, 33, 34]. Typhoid related perforation of the ileum appears to be a major problem in paediatric populations together with appendicular peritonitis [35–37]. Involvement of the biliary tract is rare as opposed to findings of western countries [5]. Health care induced

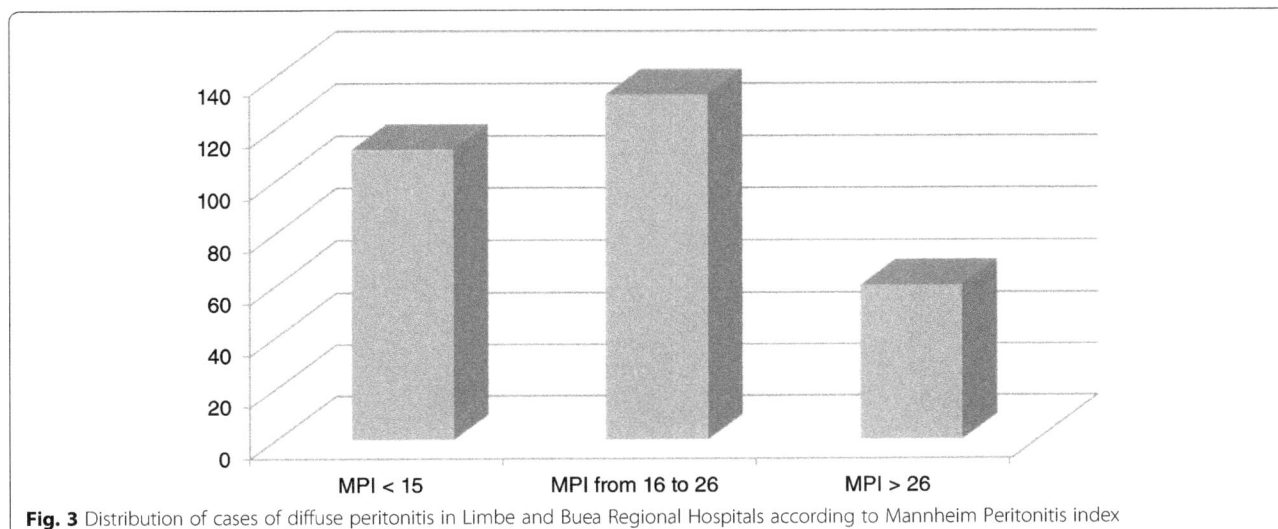

Fig. 3 Distribution of cases of diffuse peritonitis in Limbe and Buea Regional Hospitals according to Mannheim Peritonitis index

Table 4 outcome of the management of diffuse peritonitis in Limbe and Buea Regional Hospitals

Complications recorded

Type of complication	Number recorded	Percentage
Sepsis	28	9.2
Respiratory infection	6	2
Multi-organ failure	17	5.6
Wound dehiscence	36	11.8
Prolonged paralytic ileus	23	7.5
Post-operative peritonitis	12	4
Post-operative fistula	4	1.3
Residual/recurrent abscess	16	5.2

peritonitis represents a smaller fraction but tend to be more severe [4, 38].

Late presentation is a major concern in many areas of the world and delays as long as 13 days have been reported [11, 16, 17]. The absence of modern diagnostic tools in settings with limited technical background cannot be considered a major problem as diffused peritonitis can generally be diagnosed or at least suspected on purely clinical grounds in more than 97 % of cases [8, 39].

The choice of antibiotics seem to rely to a large extend on the fact that *E. coli* has been identified as the most frequent causative agent [8, 40]. Its sensitivity pattern validates our choice of antibiotics combination which elements are very widely used [40, 41], although some studies have reported other germs with a different sensitivity pattern [42]. The replacement of 3rd generation cephalosporin by ampicillin in the protocol has been proved to be a valid cost-effective regimen, especially if combined with gentamicin [43]. The use of chloramphenicol must be advocated in cases of perforation of terminal ileum suspected to be of typhoid origin [29]. Tertiary peritonitis is frequently polymicrobial and a strategy to tackle fungal infection needs to be considered [3, 38].

Although numerous scoring systems have been proposed to assess the severity of peritonitis, MPI has been largely recognized as a valid and reliable predictor of outcome [6, 8, 21, 44]. This simple, purely clinical assessment tool is particularly adapted to settings with limited access to para-clinical work-up tools and can be extensively used with accuracy comparable to other validated tools such as the various version of the APACHE scoring system [5, 10].

There is strong evidence that the management of diffuse peritonitis should still rely on three fundamental principles: (1) Elimination of the source of infection; (2) reduction of bacterial contamination of the peritoneal

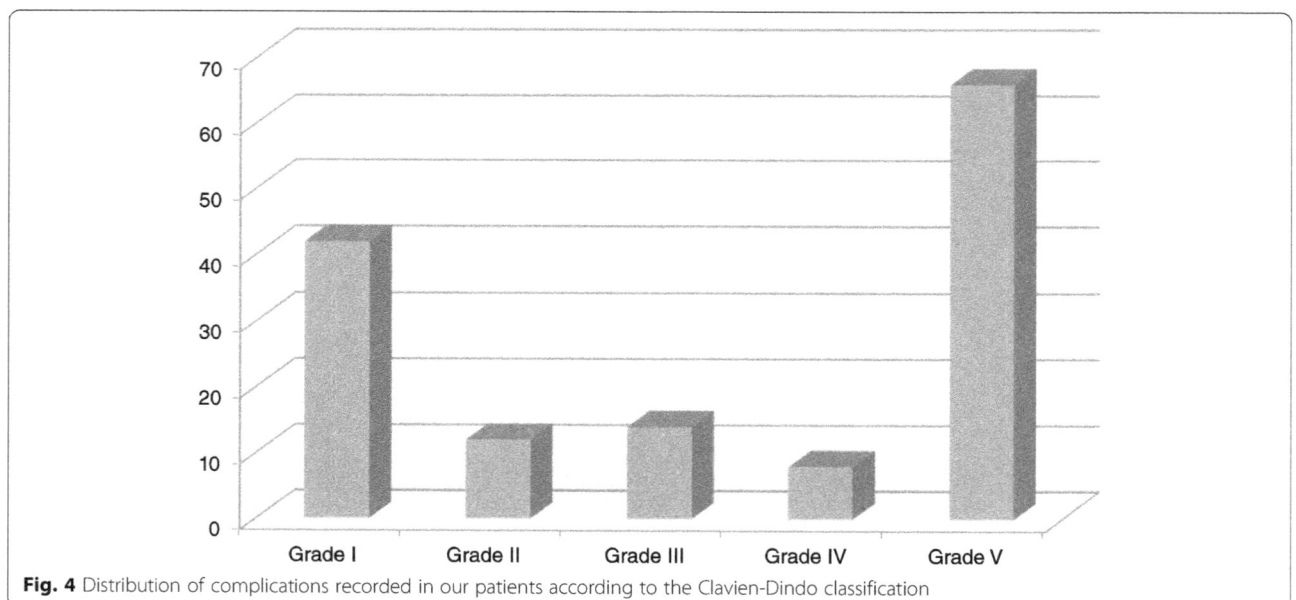

Fig. 4 Distribution of complications recorded in our patients according to the Clavien-Dindo classification

Table 5 Outcome of the management of diffuse peritonitis in Limbe and Buea Regional Hospitals

Complication rates for the five most common causes of diffuse peritonitis

Cause of peritonitis	Number with complications	Complication rate	Risk ratio (RR)	95 % CI	Fisher's P-value
Peptic ulcer perforation	18	25.4 %	0.77	0.50, 1.19	0.25
Perforation of ileum	25	58.1 %	1.77	1.30, 2.41	0.002
Acute appendicitis	13	24.5 %	0.74	0.45, 1.23	0.26
Post-operative	14	31.8 %	0.97	0.61, 1.54	1.00
Abdominal injury	12	31.6 %	0.96	0.58, 1.58	1.00

cavity; and (3) prevention of persistent or recurrent intra-abdominal infection [4]. Concerning the suppression of the cause, the source of peritonitis can usually be controlled in almost 90 % of cases [4, 28, 45]. Generally it appears that surgeon seem to be generally reluctant using the laparoscopic approach [5]. It has been proven that the results of this approach are equivalent to those of open surgery [13]. In peptic ulcer perforations, the surgical definitive treatment of the peptic ulcer disease is rarely proposed and procedures such has suture and omentoplasty after Graham is generally considered sufficient on the condition that the medical treatment be proposed post-operatively [3, 46]. This approach has the advantage of shortening the operation time and

improving the outcome, especially in patients with sepsis. In fact, the results of treatment of all bowel perforation seem to favour simple suturing rather that resections and anatomosis, especially in typhoid related perforations of the small bowel [3, 16, 46–48]. The need to protect the suture or anastomosis with a loop ileostomy has been discussed [36]. The prevention of persistent intra-abdominal infection currently opposes two strategies: on-demand re-laparotomy and systematic planned relaparotomies. Current literature seem to favour the on-demand approach in terms of length of hospitalization and intensive care unit stay [3, 49–51].

Morbidity and mortality rates are extremely variable and do not seem to be superior in settings with a limited technical background [4, 8, 9, 18, 28, 29, 39, 45, 52], even in tertiary peritonitis [38]. The mortality rate reported in our study is unacceptably high. This is probably a direct consequence of some of the local conditions of surgical practice such as the scarcity of surgeons, the lack of appropriate diagnosis and management tools and the socio-economic conditions characterized by the total absence of social security even for such critical and potentially deadly conditions. Also, they are no clear standards and guidelines for the management of surgical emergencies which are adapted our settings. However, this heavy mortality rate is not exceptional. It is comparable to what have been reported in other regions and countries with similar settings [43, 46]. Even in some western countries, overall complication rates as high as 41 % have been reported [39, 45].

Table 6 Outcome of the management of diffuse peritonitis in Limbe and Buea Regional Hospitals

Analysis of mortality rate

Cause of peritonitis	Number of deaths	Mortality rate	Contribution to death toll	Risk ratio (RR)	95 % CI	Fisher's P-value
Peptic Ulcer Perforation	7	10.1 %	15.2 %	0.67	0.32, 1.43	0.34
Spontaneous perforation of terminal ileum	16	37.2 %	34.7 %	2.47	1.54, 3.95	0.001
Complications of acute appendicitis	4	7.6 %	8.7 %	0.50	0.19, 1.33	0.20
Splenic Abscess	0	0	0	0	Undefined	0.60
Tubo-Ovarian Abscess	0	0	0	0	Undefined	0.60
Acute cholecystitis	0	0	0	0	Undefined	0.61
Incarcerated hernia	1	12.5 %	2.2 %	0.83	0.13, 5.29	1.00
Intestinal obstruction	2	15.4 %	4.4 %	1.02	0.28, 3.75	1.00
Intussusception	0	0	0	0	Undefined	1.00
Perforation of sigmoid colon	4	44.4 %	8.7 %	2.95	1.35, 6.41	0.04
Infection of haemoperitoneum	0	0	0	0	Undefined	1.00
Rupture of liver abscess	0	0	0	0	Undefined	1.00
Post-operative	9	20.5 %	19.5 %	1.36	0.71, 2.57	0.38
Abdominal injury	3	7.9 %	6.6 %	0.52	0.17, 1.60	0.33
Total	46	15.1 %	100 %	Ref.	-	-

Table 7 Complications recorded in patients operated for the five most common causes of peritonitis in Limbe and Buea regional Hospitals

Cause Complication	Peptic ulcer perforation	Perforation of terminal ileum	Complications of appendicitis	Post-operative	Abdominal injuries	Total
Septic shock	4	10	2	4	1	21
Respiratory infection	3	1	0	0	1	5
Multi-organ failure	3	5	2	2	0	12
Surgical site infection	1	3	6	0	1	11
Wound dehiscence	4	5	1	0	1	11
Prolonged paralytic ileus	4	6	1	2	2	15
Post-operative peritonitis	2	1	2	4	1	10
Post-operative fistula	0	2	0	0	0	2
Residual abscess	2	3	2	3	3	13
Total	23	36	16	15	10	100

In differential analysis of relative contributors to death toll, our study clearly points complications of typhoid fever as a major problem. Over the past two decades, the trend of mortality of this type of peritonitis has been on the decline [16, 53, 54]. Such reduction can only be achieved by early recognition and diagnosis, timely surgical intervention, appropriate antibiotics and surgical technique and peri-operative care which all play a key role in reducing mortality in typhoid intestinal perforation [53]. Also, policies on typhoid vaccine and public health education may help to reduce morbidity and mortality due to this endemic disease [55].

Some factors have been reported as related to the morbidity of diffuse peritonitis. One of these factors is the delay before intervention which is considered by many as an important key [2, 4, 6, 17, 56, 57]. Other factors include the source of peritonitis with a higher complication rate for bowel perforations [4, 52, 58] and MPI [21, 22, 56]. The ability to suppress the source of infection also seems to play an important role [58].

The types of complications recorded in our study are generally the rule, especially in low-income settings [29, 31, 37, 59, 60]. Adesunkanmi et al. recorded 58 % of wound dehiscence in a neighbouring country [29].

Despite all the recent advances in the medical management of peptic ulcer disease, its contribution to the death toll of diffuse peritonitis is still unacceptably high and can be predicted with special scoring systems [14, 15, 34, 61]. It has been reported that the number of deaths attributable to peptic ulcer perforation is seven times the one of acute appendicitis [13]. Although the outcome of management of typhoid related perforation of small bowel seems to have improved over the recent years, it is still frequently reported as a major contributor to mortality rates [1, 18, 47]. Recognized mortality factors include age, origin of sepsis, MPI greater than 26 and multi-organ failure [6, 8, 21, 44, 58, 62]. Demmel et al. reported more than 50 % of sepsis related deaths [21].

Conclusion

Diffuse peritonitis is still a major life-threatening condition in LMICs. The diagnosis can reasonably still rely to a very large extend on a meticulous clinical assessment rather than sophisticated tools such as CT scan. In all cases, the clinical assessment must lead to the estimation of severity based on simple but reliable grading systems such as the MPI. Peritonitis originating from the perforation of a hollow viscus deserves special attention. The morbidity and mortality rates of diffuse peritonitis in the Fako are unacceptable high and health authorities need to consider the need for financing the management of such life-threatening surgical conditions as it is the main way to mprove their outcome. Some specific situations require special attention based on public health intervention. These include typhoid ileal perforation for which prevention and early detection are desirable, especially in children. Once the peritonitis has occurred, the adjustment of antibiotic regimen to match the special sensitivity pattern of Salmonella typhi will likely improve overall outcome. The same approach is applicable to complications of peptic ulcer perforation for which the reinforcement of the identification and management of patients suffering from this medical condition before perforation occurs would be beneficial.

For the prevention of persistent abdominal sepsis, surgeons in low-income setting can safely apply the on demand re-laparotomy approach which is likely to be cost-effective.

Competing interests
The authors declare that they have no competing interest.

Authors' contributions

CM contributed in designing the study, writing the protocole, analyzing the data, conceiving, writing and reviewing the final paper. FA contributed in designing the study, writing the protocole, collecting and analyzing the data and reviewing the final version of the paper. NN contributed in designing the study, analyzing the data, drafting and revising the final paper. All authors read and approved the final manuscript.

Acknowledgement

The authors wish to acknowledge the contribution of Dr Julius Atashili[†], M.D. and PhD, senior epidemiologist of blessed memory who contributed to the statistical analysis of the data and kindly accepted to review the final version of the article.

References

1. Stewart B, Khanduri P, McCord C, Ohene-Yeboah M, Uranues S, Vega Rivera F, Mock C. Global disease burden of conditions requiring emergency surgery. Br J Surg. 2014;101(1):e9–e22. doi:10.1002/bjs.9329.
2. Ofoegbu CK, Odi T, Ogundipe O, Taiwo J, Solagberu BA. Epidemiology of non-trauma surgical deaths. West Afr J Med. 2005;24(4):321–4.
3. Sartelli M, Viale P, Catena F, Ansaloni L, Moore E, Malangoni M, Moore FA, Velmahos G, Coimbra R, Ivatury R, Peitzman A, Koike K, Leppaniemi A, Biffl W, Burlew CC, Balogh ZJ, Boffard K, Bendinelli C, Gupta S, Kluger Y, Agresta F, Di Saverio S, Wani I, Escalona A, Ordonez C, Fraga GP, Junior GA, Bala M, Cui Y, Marwah S, Sakakushev B, Kong V, Naidoo N, Ahmed A, Abbas A, Guercioni G, Vettoretto N, Díaz-Nieto R, Gerych I, Tranà C, Faro MP, Yuan KC, Kok KY, Mefire AC, Lee JG, Hong SK, Ghnnam W, Siribumrungwong B, Sato N, Murata K, Irahara T, Coccolini F, Segovia Lohse HA, Verni A, Shoko T. 2013 WSES guidelines for management of intra-abdominal infections. World J Emerg Surg. 2013;8(1):3.
4. Sartelli M, Catena F, Ansaloni L, Coccolini F, Corbella D, Moore EE, Malangoni M, Velmahos G, Coimbra R, Koike K, Leppaniemi A, Biffl W, Balogh Z, Bendinelli C, Gupta S, Kluger Y, Agresta F, Di Saverio S, Tugnoli G, Jovine E, Ordonez CA, Whelan JF, Fraga GP, Gomes CA, Pereira GA, Yuan KC, Bala M, Peev MP, Ben-Ishay O, Cui Y, Marwah S, Zachariah S, Wani I, Rangarajan M, Sakakushev B, Kong V, Ahmed A, Abbas A, Gonsaga RA, Guercioni G, Vettoretto N, Poiasina E, Díaz-Nieto R, Massalou D, Skrovina M, Gerych I, Augustin G, Kenig J, Khokha V, Tranà C, Kok KY, Mefire AC, Lee JG, Hong SK, Lohse HA, Ghnnam W, Verni A, Lohsiriwat V, Siribumrungwong B, El Zalabany T, Tavares A, Baiocchi G, Das K, Jarry J, Zida M, Sato N, Murata K, Shoko T, Irahara T, Hamedelneel AO, Naidoo N, Adesunkanmi AR, Kobe Y, Ishii W, Oka K, Izawa Y, Hamid H, Khan I, Attri A, Sharma R, Sanjuan J, Badiel M, Barnabé R. Complicated intra-abdominal infections worldwide: the definitive data of the CIAOW Study. World J Emerg Surg. 2014;9:37
5. Gauzit R, Péan Y, Barth X, Mistretta F, Lalaude O, Top Study Team. Epidemiology, management, and prognosis of secondary non-postoperative peritonitis: a French prospective observational multicenter study. Surg Infect (Larchmt). 2009;10(2):119–27.
6. Scapellato S, Parrinello V, Sciuto GS, Castorina G, Buffone A, Cirino E. Valuation on prognostic factors about secondary acute peritonitis: review of 255 cases. Ann Ital Chir. 2004;75(2):241–5. discussion 246.
7. Bali RS, Verma S, Agarwal PN, Singh R, Talwar N. Perforation peritonitis and the developing world. ISRN Surg. 2014;105492. doi:10.1155/2014/105492.
8. Agrawal CS, Niranjan M, Adhikary S, Karki BS, Pandey R, Chalise PR. Quality assurance in the management of peritonitis: a prospective study. Nepal Med Coll J. 2009;11(2):83–7.
9. Agarwal N, Saha S, Srivastava A, Chumber S, Dhar A, Garg S. Peritonitis: 10 years' experience in a single surgical unit. Trop Gastroenterol. 2007;28(3):117–20.
10. Ahuja A, Pal R. Prognostic scoring indicator in evaluation of clinical outcome in intestinal perforations. J Clin Diagn Res. 2013;7(9):1953–5.
11. Chakma SM, Singh RL, Parmekar MV, Singh KH, Kapa B, Sharatchandra KH, Longkumer AT, Rudrappa S. Spectrum of perforation peritonitis. J Clin Diagn Res. 2013;7(11):2518–20.
12. Jhobta RS, Attri AK, Kaushik R, Sharma R, Jhobta A. Spectrum of perforation peritonitis in India–review of 504 consecutive cases. World J Emerg Surg. 2006;1:26.
13. Søreide K, Thorsen K, Søreide JA. Strategies to improve the outcome of emergency surgery for perforated peptic ulcer. Br J Surg. 2014;101(1):e51–64.
14. Arici C, Mesci A, Dincer D, Dinckan A, Colak T. Analysis of risk factors predicting (affecting) mortality and morbidity of peptic ulcer perforations. Int Surg. 2007;92(3):147–54.
15. Møller MH, Engebjerg MC, Adamsen S, Bendix J, Thomsen RW. The Peptic Ulcer Perforation (PULP) score: a predictor of mortality following peptic ulcer perforation. A cohort study. Acta Anaesthesiol Scand. 2012;56(5):655–62.
16. Ugochukwu AI, Amu OC, Nzegwu MA. Ileal perforation due to typhoid fever - review of operative management and outcome in an urban centre in Nigeria. Int J Surg. 2013;11(3):218–22.
17. Sanogo ZZ, Camara M, Doumbia MM, Soumaré L, Koumaré S, Keïta S, Koïta AK, Ouattara MA, Togo S, Yéna S, Sangaré D. Digestive tract perforations at Point G Teaching Hospital in Bamako. Mali Mali Med. 2012;27(1):19–22.
18. Nuhu A, Dahwa S, Hamza A. Operative management of typhoid ileal perforation in children. Afr J Paediatr Surg. 2010;7(1):9–13.
19. Levy MM, Fink MP, Marshall JC, Abraham E, Angus D, Cook D, Cohen J, Opal SM, Vincent JL, Ramsay G. SCCM/ESICM/ACCP/ATS/SIS. 2001 SCCM/ESICM/ACCP/ATS/SIS International Sepsis Definitions Conference. Crit Care Med. 2003;31(4):1250–6.
20. Bone RC, Balk RA, Cerra FB, Dellinger RP, Fein AM, Knaus WA, Schein RM, Sibbald WJ. Definitions for sepsis and organ failure and guidelines for the use of innovative therapies in sepsis. The ACCP/SCCM Consensus Conference Committee. American College of Chest Physicians/Society of Critical Care Medicine. Chest. 1992;101(6):1644–55.
21. Demmel N, Maag K, Osterholzer G. The value of clinical parameters for determining the prognosis of peritonitis–validation of the Mannheim Peritonitis Index. Langenbecks Arch Chir. 1994;379(3):152–8.
22. Tan KK, Bang SL, Sim R. Surgery for small bowel perforation in an Asian population: predictors of morbidity and mortality. J Gastrointest Surg. 2010;14(3):493–9.
23. Clavien PA, Barkun J, de Oliveira ML, Vauthey JN, Dindo D, Schulick RD, de Santibañes E, Pekolj J, Slankamenac K, Bassi C, Graf R, Vonlanthen R, Padbury R, Cameron JL, Makuuchi M. The Clavien-Dindo classification of surgical complications: five-year experience. Ann Surg. 2009;250(2):187–96.
24. Mentula PJ, Leppäniemi AK. Applicability of the Clavien-Dindo classification to emergency surgical procedures: a retrospective cohort study on 444 consecutive patients. Patient Saf Surg. 2014;8:31.
25. von Elm E, Altman DG, Egger M, et al. STROBE Initiative. The Strengthening the Reporting of Observational Studies in Epidemiology (STROBE) Statement: guidelines for reporting observational studies. Int J Surg. 2014;12(12):1495–9.
26. Meara JG, Leather AJ, Hagander L, Alkire BC, Alonso N, Ameh EA, et al. Global Surgery 2030: evidence and solutions for achieving health, welfare, and economic development. Lancet. 2015;386(9993):569–624.
27. Debas HT, Donkor P, Gawande A, Jamison DT, Kruk ME, Mock CN, editors. Essential Surgery: Disease Control Priorities, Third Edition (Volume 1). Washington (DC): The International Bank for Reconstruction and Development / The World Bank; 2015.
28. Stănescu D, Mihalache D, Irimescu O, Buciu A, Nistor A. Treatment of acute peritonitis. Results in County Hospital Suceava with 317 cases. Rev Med Chir Soc Med Nat Iasi. 2010;114(2):372–5.
29. Adesunkanmi AR, Badmus TA. Pattern of antibiotic therapy and clinical outcome in acute generalized peritonitis in semi-urban and rural Nigerians. Chemotherapy. 2006;52(2):69–72.
30. Sharma L, Gupta S, Soin AS, Sikora S, Kapoor V. Generalized peritonitis in India–the tropical spectrum. Jpn J Surg. 1991;21(3):272–7.
31. Dieng M, Ndiaye A, Ka O, Konaté I, Dia A, Touré CT. Etiology and therapeutic aspects of generalized acute peritonitis of digestive origin. A survey of 207 cases operated in five years. Mali Med. 2006;21(4):47–51.
32. Ohene-Yeboah M. Causes of acute peritonitis in 1188 consecutive adult patients in Ghana. Trop Doct. 2005;35(2):84–5.
33. Afridi SP, Malik F, Ur-Rahman S, Shamim S, Samo KA. Spectrum of perforation peritonitis in Pakistan: 300 cases Eastern experience. World J Emerg Surg. 2008;3:31.
34. Ohene-Yeboah M, Togbe B. Perforated gastric and duodenal ulcers in an urban African population. West Afr J Med. 2006;25(3):205–11.

35. Osifo OD, Ogiemwonyi SO. Peritonitis in children: our experience in Benin City, Nigeria. Surg Infect (Larchmt). 2011;12(2):127–30.

36. Khalid S, Burhanulhuq, Bhatti AA. Non-traumatic spontaneous ileal perforation: experience with 125 cases. J Ayub Med Coll AbbOttabad. 2014;26(4):526–9.

37. Oheneh-Yeboah M. Postoperative complications after surgery for typhoid ileal perforation in adults in Kumasi. West Afr J Med. 2007;26(1):32–6.

38. Panhofer P, Izay B, Riedl M, Ferenc V, Ploder M, Jakesz R, Götzinger P.. Age, microbiology and prognostic scores help to differentiate between secondary and tertiary peritonitis. Langenbecks Arch Surg. 2009;394(2):265–71.

39. Memon AA, Siddiqui FG, Abro AH, Agha AH, Lubna S, Memon AS. An audit of secondary peritonitis at a tertiary care university hospital of Sindh, Pakistan. World J Emerg Surg. 2012;7:6.

40. Mouaffak Y, Boutbaoucht M, Soraa N, Chabaa L, Salama T, Oulad Saiad M, Younous S. Bacteriology of community-acquired peritonitis in children treated in the university hospital of Marrakech. Ann Fr Anesth Reanim. 2013;32(1):60–2.

41. Mittelkötter U, Endter F, Reith HB, Thielemann H, Schmitz R, Ihle P, Kullmann KH. Prospective comparative observational study on the antibiotic treatment of secondary peritonitis in Germany – efficacy and cost analysis. Chirurg. 2003;74(12):1134–42.

42. Montravers P, Lepape A, Dubreuil L, Gauzit R, Pean Y, Benchimol D, Dupont H. Clinical and microbiological profiles of community-acquired and nosocomial intra-abdominal infections: results of the French prospective, observational EBIIA study. J Antimicrob Chemother. 2009;63(4):785–94.

43. Ramakrishnaiah VP, Chandrakasan C, Dharanipragadha K, Sistla S, Krishnamachari S. Community acquired secondary bacterial peritonitis in a tertiary hospital of South India: an audit with special reference to peritoneal fluid culture. Trop Gastroenterol. 2012;33(4):275–81.

44. Qureshi AM, Zafar A, Saeed K, Quddus A. Predictive power of Mannheim Peritonitis Index. J Coll Physicians Surg Pak. 2005;15(11):693–6.

45. Seiler CA, Brügger L, Forssmann U, Baer HU, Büchler MW. Conservative surgical treatment of diffuse peritonitis. Surgery. 2000;127(2):178–84.

46. Nuhu A, Kassama Y. Experience with acute perforated duodenal ulcer in a West African population. Niger J Med. 2008;17(4):403–6.

47. Saxe JM, Cropsey R. Is operative management effective in treatment of perforated typhoid? Am J Surg. 2005;189(3):342–4.

48. Caronna R, Boukari AK, Zaongo D, Hessou T, Gayito RC, Ahononga C, Adeniran S, Priuli G. Comparative analysis of primary repair vs resection and anastomosis, with laparostomy, in management of typhoid intestinal perforation: results of a rural hospital in northwestern Benin. BMC Gastroenterol. 2013;13:102.

49. Chichom Mefire A, Tchounzou R, Masso Misse P, Pisoh C, Pagbe JJ, Essomba A, Takongmo S, Malonga EE. Analysis of operative indications and outcomes in 238 re-operations after abdominal surgery in an economically disadvantaged setting. J Chir (Paris). 2009;146(4):387–91.

50. Van Ruler O, Mahler CW, Boer KR, Reuland EA, Gooszen HG, Opmeer BC, de Graaf PW, Lamme B, Gerhards MF, Steller EP, van Till JW, de Borgie CJ, Gouma DJ, Reitsma JB. Boermeester MA: comparison of on-demand vs planned relaparotomy strategy in patients with severe peritonitis: a randomized trial. JAMA. 2007;298:865–72.

51. Rakić M, Popović D, Rakić M, Druzijanić N, Lojpur M, Hall BA, Williams BA, Sprung J. Comparison of on-demand vs planned relaparotomy for treatment of severe intra-abdominal infections. Croat Med J. 2005;46(6):957–63.

52. Ngowe Ngowe M, Toure A, Mouafo Tambo FF, Chichom A, Tchounzou R, Ako-Egbe L, Sosso M. Prevalence and risk factors associated with post-operative infections in the Limbe Regional Hospital of Cameroon. The open Surgery Journal. 2014;8:1–8.

53. Anupama PK, Ashok AC, Rudresh HK, Srikantaiah HC, Girish KS, Suhas KR. Mortality in Typhoid Intestinal Perforation-A Declining Trend. J Clin Diagn Res. 2013;7(9):1946–8.

54. Mogasale V, Desai SN, Mogasale VV, Park JK, Ochiai RL. Wierzba TF Case fatality rate and length of hospital stay among patients with typhoid intestinal perforation in developing countries: a systematic literature review. PLoS One. 2014;9(4):e93784.

55. Qamar FN, Azmatullah A, Bhutta ZA. Challenges in measuring complications and death due to invasive Salmonella infections. Vaccine. 2015;33 Suppl 3:C16–20.

56. Gedik E, Girgin S, Taçyildiz IH, Akgün Y. Risk factors affecting morbidity in typhoid enteric perforation. Langenbecks Arch Surg. 2008;393(6):973–7.

57. Chichom Mefire A, Weledji PE, Verla VS, Lidwine NM. Diagnostic and therapeutic challenges of isolated small bowel perforations after blunt abdominal injury in low income settings: analysis of twenty three new cases. Injury. 2014;45(1):141–5.

58. Wacha H, Hau T, Dittmer R, Ohmann C. Risk factors associated with intraabdominal infections: a prospective multicenter study. Peritonitis Study Group. Langenbecks Arch Surg. 1999;384(1):24–32.

59. Riché FC, Dray X, Laisné MJ, Matéo J, Raskine L, Sanson-Le Pors MJ, Payen D, Valleur P, Cholley BP. Factors associated with septic shock and mortality in generalized peritonitis: comparison between community-acquired and postoperative peritonitis. Crit Care. 2009;13(3):R99. doi:10.1186/cc7931.

60. Bielecki K, Kamiński P, Klukowski M. Large bowel perforation: morbidity and mortality. Tech Coloprocto. 2002;6(3):177–82.

61. Lohsiriwat V, Prapasrivorakul S, Lohsiriwat D. Perforated peptic ulcer: clinical presentation, surgical outcomes, and the accuracy of the Boey scoring system in predicting postoperative morbidity and mortality. World J Surg. 2009;33(1):80–5.

62. Hernández-Palazón J, Fuentes-García D, Burguillos-López S, Domenech-Asensi P, Sansano-Sánchez TV, Acosta-Villegas F. Analysis of organ failure and mortality in sepsis due to secondary peritonitis. Med Intensiva. 2013;37(7):461–7.

9

Patterns and management of degloving injuries: a single national level 1 trauma center experience

Suhail Hakim[1], Khalid Ahmed[1], Ayman El-Menyar[2,3]* (iD), Gaby Jabbour[1], Ruben Peralta[1], Syed Nabir[4],
Ahammed Mekkodathil[2], Husham Abdelrahman[1], Ammar Al-Hassani[1] and Hassan Al-Thani[1]

Abstract

Background: Degloving soft tissue injuries (DSTIs) are serious surgical conditions. We aimed to evaluate the pattern, management and outcome of DSTIs in a single institute.

Methods: A retrospective analysis was performed for patients admitted with DSTIs from 2011to 2013. Presentation, management and outcomes were analyzed according to the type of DSTI.

Results: Of 178 DSTI patients, 91 % were males with a mean age of 30.5 ± 12.8. Three-quarter of cases was due to traffic–related injuries. Eighty percent of open DSTI cases were identified. Primary debridement and closure (62.9 %) was the frequent intervention used. Intermediate closed drainage under ultrasound guidance was performed in 7 patients; however, recurrence occurred in 4 patients who underwent closed serial drainage for recollection and ended with a proper debridement with or without vacuum assisted closure (VAC). Closed DSTIs were mainly seen in the lower extremity and back region and initially treated with conservative management as compared to open DSTIs. Infection and skin necrosis were reported in 9 cases only. Open DSTIs were more likely involving head and neck region and being treated by primary debridement/suturing and serial debridement/washout with or without VAC. All-cause DSTI mortality was 9 % that was higher in the closed DSTIs (19.4 vs 6.3 %; $p = 0.01$).

Conclusion: The incidence of DSTIs is 4 % among trauma admissions over 3 years, with a greater predilection to males and young population. DSTIs are mostly underestimated particularly in the closed type that are usually missed at the initial presentation and associated with poor outcomes. Treatment guidelines are not well established and therefore further studies are warranted.

Keywords: Degloving, Soft tissue injury, Debridement, Management, Trauma

Abbreviations: CT scanning, Computerized Tomography; DSTI, Degloving soft tissue injuries; MVC, Motor vehicle crash; VAC, Vacuum assisted closure

Background

Degloving soft-tissue injuries (DSTIs) are often serious surgical conditions characterized by avulsions or detachment of the skin and subcutaneous tissue from the underlying muscle and fascia secondary to a sudden shearing force applied to the skin surface [1]. DSTIs are more commonly observed in males due to disproportionately higher burden of traumatic injuries [2]. Although it may occur anywhere in the body, the main sites of DSTIs are lower extremities, trunk, scalp and face with a variable amount of skin and soft tissue loss [3–5]. DSTIs could be categorized as either closed/internal or open/external lesions [6]. Delayed diagnosis and treatment of these injuries often result in full-thickness necrosis due to jeopardized blood supply to the avulsed skin flap [7]. Moreover, patients with severe DSTI could develop infection or even necrotizing fasciitis due to mismanagement leading to high morbidity and mortality [6].

* Correspondence: aymanco65@yahoo.com
[2]Clinical Research, Trauma Surgery Section, Hamad General Hospital, Doha, Qatar
[3]Clinical Medicine, Weill Cornell Medical College, Doha, Qatar
Full list of author information is available at the end of the article

DSTIs are mostly underestimated lesions due to lack of clinical diagnostic and prognostic indicators and well established treatment guidelines. In addition, the marked variability in the type, magnitude and severity of DSTI makes it difficult to set a standard management and to predict outcomes. In closed or internal degloving injury the shearing forces create a cavity which subsequently gets filled with hematoma and liquefied fat [8]. Such closed internal degloving lesions usually develop over the greater trochanter and are known as Morel-Lavallee lesions [9].

The DSTI treatment varies considerably from close observation to active interventions such as early primary definitive skin closure, superior skin cover, early return of function and secondary procedures, if needed [5]. However, distinction between viable and nonviable tissues may be difficult during early wound management in both types of injuries [6]. Since, every injury is unique with variety of lesions; it is difficult to develop an appropriate decision-making algorithm for treatment and therefore, the outcome of DSTI often remains underestimated. Interestingly, there is a paucity of information on DSTI from our region in the Arab Middle East. In this study, we retrospectively reviewed the frequency, pattern, management and outcome of DSTIs from a single institute over a 3-year period in Qatar.

Methods

Data were acquired retrospectively for all DSTI patients identified from the trauma registry database who were admitted to the section of trauma surgery at Hamad general hospital (HGH) between January 2011 and November 2013. HGH is the only Level 1 trauma center facility in Qatar which admits and treats all traumatic injury patients. DSTIs are defined as avulsion of soft tissue, in which an extensive portion of skin and subcutaneous tissue is detached from the underlying fascia and muscles [6]. We mainly diagnosed DSTI by clinical assessment, ultrasound and CT scanning. DSTI are classified as either open or closed. In an open DSTI, the skin is torn off the body though it may still be attached as a flap. Closed DSTI are soft tissue injuries with disintegration of the underlying layers in which the subcutaneous tissue is torn away from the underlying fascia, creating a cavity filled with hematoma and liquefied fat (i.e., Morel-Lavallée lesion). We excluded patients in whom the skin is completely detached as these are considered open wounds rather than DSTIs. Patients with open wounds are more likely to require some form of advanced soft tissue coverage. On arrival, all patients underwent thorough clinical assessment and resuscitation according to Advanced TRAUMA Life Support (ATLS) guidelines. Collected data included age, gender, mechanism of injury, injury severity score (ISS), type of degloving injury (open and closed), anatomical

location (head, neck, back, limbs, abdomen and perineum), associated injuries, comorbidities, laboratory findings, blood transfusion and management [primary debridement/suturing; initial conservative treatment; serial debridement and washout with or without vacuum assisted closure (VAC)]. The term (early) vs (late) was used based on the initial treatment after the initial assessment. Complications (infection, skin necrosis and flap necrosis), discharge disposition (plastic surgery or rehabilitation), length of stay and mortality were also reported. Baseline demographic characteristics, mechanism of injury, site of injury, associated injury, management, and outcomes were also compared according to open and closed type of DSTIs.

Statistical analysis

Data were expressed as proportions, medians, or mean ± standard deviation (SD), as appropriate. Differences in categorical variables between respective comparison groups were analyzed using Chi-Square test or Fisher exact (observed cell values less than 5) test for categorical variables. The continuous variables were analyzed using student's t-test. Two-tailed p values < 0.05 were considered to be significant. Multivariate analysis was performed to look for ISS whether it has a prognostic role or not in both types of DSTIs. Data analysis was carried out using the Statistical Package for Social Sciences version 18 (SPSS Inc. Chicago, Illinois, USA).

Results

A total of 178 patients with DSTIs were included in this study who was admitted to the Section of Trauma Surgery during three years period. The mean age of patients was 30.5 ± 12.8 years, and the majority were males (91 %) and expatriates (83.3 %). Demographics, clinical presentation, laboratory findings and type of DSTI are presented in Table 1. Motor vehicle crash (MVC) was the leading mechanism of injury (54.5 %) followed by falls from height (12.9 %) and pedestrian injuries (12.4 %). Lower extremity (40.4 %), head (23.0 %), upper extremity (19.1 %) and pelvis (16.9 %) were the most frequent associated injuries. Co-morbidities included diabetes (3.4 %) and hypertension (1.7 %). The median myoglobin level was 846 with a range from 21 to 6698 ng/ml. A higher proportion of cases sustained open/external type (79.8 %) DSTI followed by closed/internal type (20.2 %). The most frequent anatomic site of DSTI was lower extremity (44 %) followed by head/neck (37.3 %) and back (13.5 %) region (Fig. 1).

Table 2 shows the laboratory results, management, complications and outcome according to the type of degloving injury. Figures 2 and 3 show examples of open and closed degloving injuries.

The blood transfusion was needed primarily for associated injuries, rather than the degloving injury per se.

Table 1 Demographics and patient characteristics by type of degloving injury

	Overall (n = 178)	Open (n = 142)	Close (n = 36)	P
Age; years (mean ± SD)	30.5 ± 12.8	30.2 ± 13.1	31.9 ± 11.9	0.51
Males	162 (91 %)	129 (91.5)	33 (91.7)	0.97
Nationality				
Qatari	28 (16.7 %)	25 (18.3)	3 (9.7)	0.08 for all
Non-nationals	140 (83.3 %)	112 (81.7)	28 (90.3)	
Mechanism of Injury				0.63 for all
Motor vehicle crashes	97 (54.5 %)	80 (56.3)	17 (47.2)	
Fall from height	23 (12.9 %)	16 (11.3)	7 (19.4)	
Pedestrian injuries	22 (12.4 %)	16 (11.3)	6 (16.7)	
Fall of heavy objects	16 (9.0 %)	13 (9.2)	3 (8.3)	
Others	20 (11.2)	17 (12 %)	3 (8 %)	
Associated injuries				
Head	41 (23 %)	36 (25.4)	5 (13.9)	0.15
Lower extremity	72 (40.4 %)	58 (40.8)	14 (38.9)	0.83
Upper extremity	34 (19 %)	28 (19.7)	6 (16.7)	0.67
Pelvic fracture	30 (17 %)	19 (13.4)	11 (30.6)	0.01
Spinal	25 (14.2 %)	21 (15.0)	4 (11.1)	0.55
Solid organ injury	14 (7.9 %)	9 (6.3)	5 (13.9)	0.13
Facial	14 (8 %)	14 (9.9)	0.0	0.05
Chest	10 (5.7 %)	7 (5.0)	3 (8.3)	0.44
Bowel	6 (3.4 %)	3 (2.1)	3 (8.3)	0.09
Injury severity score (mean ± SD)	13.80 ± 10.9	13.11 ± 10.2	16.5 ± 13.04	0.09
Degloving injury size[a] (n = 37)	90 (18–1080)[b]	75 (18–741)	380 (36–1080)	0.003
Anatomic site of DSTI[c]				
Head/Neck	66 (37.3 %)	65 (46.1)	1 (2.8)	0.001
Lower extremity	78 (44 %)	55 (39.0)	23 (63.9)	0.007
Upper extremity	13 (7.4 %)	12 (8.6)	1 (2.9)	0.24
Back	24 (13.5 %)	12 (8.5)	12 (33.3)	0.001
Perineum	8 (4.6 %)	6 (4.3)	2 (5.7)	0.72
Abdomen	6 (3.6 %)	4 (2.8)	2 (5.6 %)	0.41

[a]CT volume in cc, [b]data present as median and range, [c]there are overlapped sites

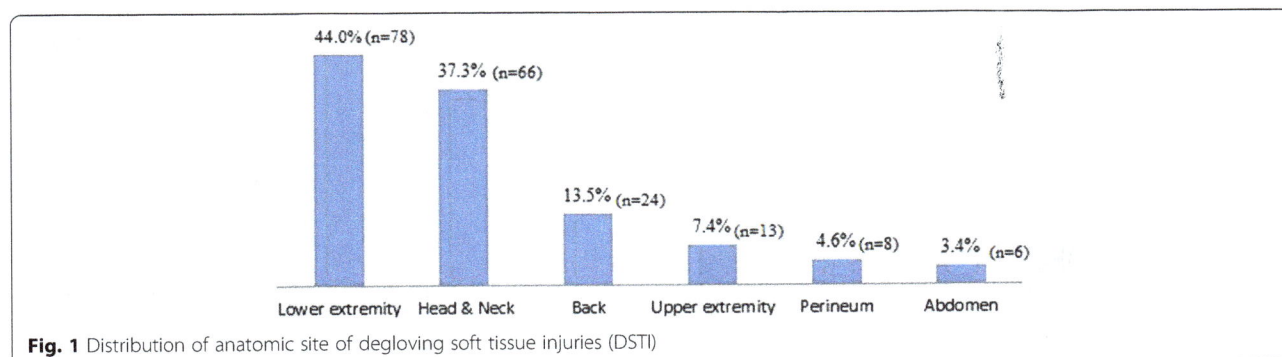

Fig. 1 Distribution of anatomic site of degloving soft tissue injuries (DSTI)

Table 2 Management, complications and outcome by type of degloving injury

	Overall (n = 178)	Open (n = 142)	Close (n = 36)	P
Laboratory results				
Myoglobin	1190 ± 1179[b]	1076 ± 1125	1636 ± 1293	0.02
Blood Urea Nitrogen	4.8 ± 1.6[b]	4.6 ± 1.4	5.5 ± 2	0.004
Serum Creatinine	86.6 ± 37.3[b]	81.6 ± 31	107 ± 52	0.01
White blood cells	17.6 ± 7.7[b]	18 ± 8	16 ± 7	0.09
Platelets	250.8 ± 86.5[b]	258 ± 86	224 ± 84	0.04
Hemoglobin	12.9 ± 2.6[b]	13 ± 2.5	12.6 ± 3	0.42
INR	1.2 ± 0.3[b]	1.19 ± 0.3	1.19 ± 0.2	0.92
Serum Lactate	3.9 ± 2.4[b]	4.05 ± 2.6	3.31 ± 1.9	0.72
Treatment of degloving Injury				
Packed RBC units	3 (1–25)[a]	2 (1–20)	6 (1–25)	0.03
Fresh Frozen Plasma units	6 (2–24)[a]	5.5 (2–24)	6 (4–13)	0.46
Platelets units	9 (1–28)[a]	10 (1–28)	5 (1–11)	0.19
Primary Debridement/suturing	112 (62.9 %)	105 (73.9 %)	7 (19.4 %)	0.001
Initial conservative	28 (15.7 %)	0 (0.0 %)	28 (77.8 %)	0.001
Serial debridement[b]	34 (19.1 %)	33 (23.2 %)	1 (2.8 %)	0.003
Late flap	22 (12.3 %)	21 (14.8 %)	1 (2.8 %)	0.05
Disposition				
Plastic surgery	26 (14.6 %)	23 (16.4 %)	3 (8.3 %)	0.22
Rehabilitation	7 (3.9 %)	7 (4.9 %)	0 (0.0 %)	0.17
Hospital length of stay; days	10 (1–393)[a]	11 (1–393)	6 (1–365)	0.11
Complications				
Skin Infection	7 (3.9 %)	6 (4.3 %)	1 (2.8 %)	0.68
Skin necrosis	2 (1.1 %)	2 (1.4 %)	0 (0.0 %)	0.47
Mortality	16 (9.0 %)	9 (6.3 %)	7 (19.4 %)	0.01

[a]Median and range, [b]Serial debridement and washout (with or without vacuum assisted closure)

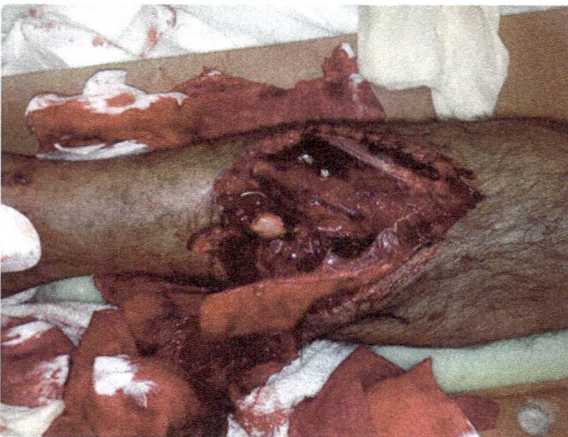

Fig. 2 Open degloving with flap and underlying bony injury

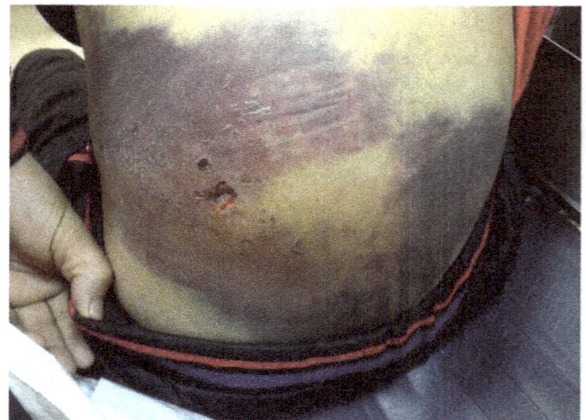

Fig. 3 Closed degloving with frank bruising but intact skin

Primary debridement and closure (62.9 %) was the main intervention for DSTI cases followed by serial debridement and washout with or without VAC (19.1 %). Intermediate closed drainage was done under ultrasound guidance for 7 cases out of which recurrence observed in four cases that had to undergo closed serial drainage for recollection. The definitive treatment for these patients was finally a proper debridement with or without VAC. One patient had undergone serial drainage over a period of three months before final resolution. Initial conservative management was adopted in 28 (15.7 %) patients. Late flap (i.e., serial debridement that eventually required rotational skin flap to close the defect) coverage was needed in 22 (12.3 %) cases. In those who underwent serial debridement some of them required closure by secondary suturing and others left to heal by secondary intention. Complications such as infection and skin necrosis were observed in 3.9 % and 1.1 % cases, respectively. Plastic surgical referral was sought for 26 (14.6 %) patients. The median hospital length of stay was 10 (1–393) days.

There were no differences between the two groups with respect to age, gender, mechanism of injuries and associated injuries. However, the frequency of pelvic fracture was significantly higher in the closed group (30.6 % vs. 13.4 %; $p = 0.01$) as compared to open DSTI. Regarding the anatomic site, DSTI at the lower extremity (63.9 % vs. 39 %, $p = 0.007$) and back (33.3 % vs. 8.5 %, $p = 0.001$) region were significantly higher in closed group compared to open group. In contrast, head (scalp) and neck region were mainly affected in the open group of degloving injuries (46.1 % vs. 2.8 %, $p = 0.001$) than closed group.

In comparison to closed DSTI, patients in open group were more likely to be treated by primary debridement/suturing (73.9 % vs. 19.4 %, $p = 0.001$) and serial debridement and washout with or without VAC (23.2 % vs. 2.8 %, $p = 0.003$). On the other hand, the frequency of initial conservative management (77.8 % vs. 0 %, $p = 0.001$) was higher in patients with closed group when compared to open DSTI. There was no significant difference in terms of complications or discharge dispositions between the two groups. The overall mortality was 9.0 % ($n = 16$) and around half ($n = 7$) of them died within the first 24 h of admission due to severe associated injuries. Moreover, the mortality rate was significantly higher in the closed group (19.4 % vs. 6.3 %, $p = 0.01$) as compared to open DSTI group. The mean ISS was greater in the closed DSTI in comparison to the opened type of DSTI (16.5 ± 13.04 vs 13.11 ± 10.2; $p = 0.09$). Multivariate analysis showed that ISS is a predictor of mortality in closed DSTI (Odd ratio 1.2; 95 % confidence interval 1.06-1.35; $p = 0.004$), however, this effect on mortality was not observed in the opened type of DSTI (Odd ratio 1.07; 95 % confidence interval 0.99-1.45; $p = 0.07$).

Discussion

This is a unique study from the Arab Middle Eastern region which provides an insight on the frequency, patterns, management and outcome of DSTIs among trauma patients in Qatar. This is a large single-institution study which enrolled 178 patients as compared to earlier descriptive studies [10–12]. Our study shows that the incidence of DSTI is around 4 % with a greater predilection to males and young patients. Three quarter of the cases is traffic-related injuries. It has significant implications for the treatment and final outcome of our trauma patients. Most of the current literature on DSTI is mainly based on specific anatomic regions and are usually drived from case series or case reports. An earlier study from South Africa reviewed 16 cases with closed degloving injuries treated during one-year period [10]. Another study from Pakistan demonstrated the pattern of degloving injuries in 50 cases; of which majority sustained open type of degloving injuries [11]. Consistent with small number of cases, Milcheski et al. [12] reported 21 patients with degloving injuries from Brazil. In the present study, majority of the DSTI patients were young males which reflect the disproportionately higher burden of road traffic injuries in Qatar. Our findings are consistent with previous reports, which also documented a higher involvement of young males (88 %) in road traffic injuries [13].

DSTIs are often associated with severe concomitant injuries and massive blood loss [6].

Early diagnosis of DSTI remains challenging as the initial clinical evaluation could not predict avulsion of underlying soft tissue particularly in the closed DSTI [14]. On the other hand, prompt recognition of these injuries are crucial as treatment may be time consuming and such delay may increase the risk of infection or progression to necrotizing fasciitis. Severity of DSTI mainly depends on the mechanism of injury, comorbidities (particularly Diabetes mellitus), concomitant injuries, anatomic site and type (open or closed) of DSTI [6]. Our study showed MVC to be the most common cause of DSTI with frequent involvement of lower limb and head/neck regions. Consistent with our findings, several studies have demonstrated a higher association of lower limb DSTI and MVC [10, 12]. Similarly, Khan et al. [11] reported that higher frequency of young males (74 %) had degloving injuries of the lower limb. The present study also showed greater frequency of open DSTI which mainly affect head (scalp) and neck region. Although, less frequent closed DSTI were mainly associated with lower extremity and back. Contrarily, an earlier study reported greater involvement of open type (94 %) in patients with degloving injuries of the lower limb [11]. The present analysis showed that ISS was greater in the closed DSTI in comparison to the opened type, moreover ISS was found as a predictor of mortality only in the closed type of DSTIs.

Diagnosis of DSTI can be made by clinical assessment of fluctuant area as well as using imaging modalities such as ultrasonography, computed tomography (Fig. 4) and magnetic resonance imaging (MRI) [14]. Open DSTI is clinically self-evident condition that usually presented as a soft tissue loss of variable extent together with avulsed skin, subcutaneous tissue flaps from the underlying deep tissues which is the hallmark of physical finding together with overlying abrasion, ecchymosis or skin wound [9]. However, the diagnosis of closed DSTI is usually difficult and can be missed on the initial clinical evaluation and require radiological investigation for accurate diagnosis. Closed degloving injury with suspected Morel-Lavallée lesions (Fig. 4) could be diagnosed by CT scan, however, evaluation using MRI is more informative [15]. As ultrasound typically shows these lesions as anechoic or hypoechoic, with or without echogenic foci or even fluid/fluid levels. Therefore, for such cases MRI is the modality of choice which clearly determines the relationship of the collection with the underlying fascia [9, 14].

Direct injury to the cutaneous layers may result in necrosis of the skin overlying the degloved area. It can also occur on a delayed basis secondary to swelling of the degloved cavity, resulting in ischemia of the overlying skin [16]. To prevent potential complications such as, secondary infection and necrosis, early diagnosis and

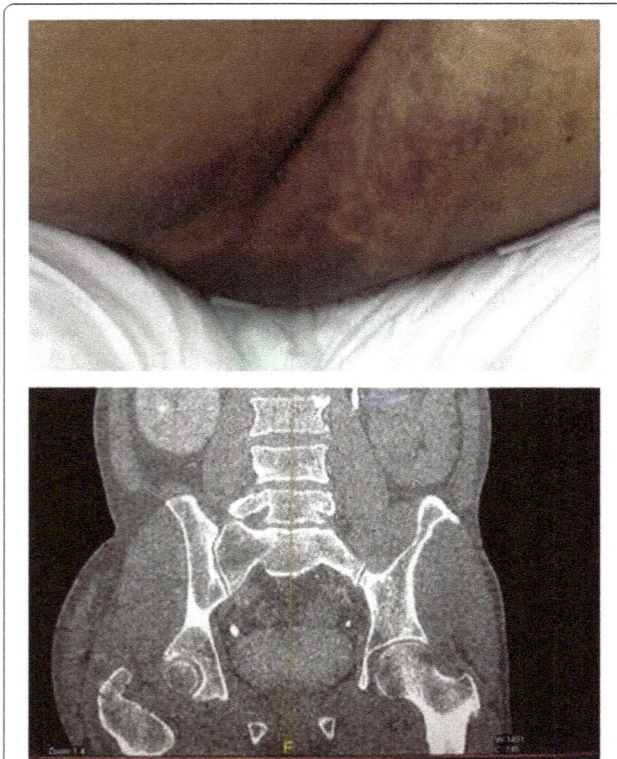

Fig. 4 Morel Lavallee lesion (common site) and Coronal CT view of the lesion

intervention are needed. In our series, skin necrosis was developed only in two cases with open DSTI and was not evident in the closed type of injuries. Although, skin necrosis was commonly considered as a complication of closed degloving injury, it was not observed in any of the patients in our series.

The primary management approach for DSTI ranges from optimal preservation of individual structure to early primary definitive skin cover, superior skin cover, early return of function and secondary procedures, if required [5]. Particularly, various modalities for the treatment of open DSTI include simple debridement with repair to more complex procedures like flaps, skin grafts, free tissue transfer, replantation or revascularization depending on the site, extent, severity and availability of the treatment. In our series, nearly 74 % of the cases with the open type and 20 % of the closed type of DSTI underwent primary debridement and closure. Plastic surgery consultation was sought in 26 (23 open and 3 closed) DSTIs cases due to wound complexity which necessitated a complex wound management including flap coverage and skin reconstruction.

Vacuum-assisted closure is an advanced management therapy often used to cover open degloving wounds of the lower-limb [17–19]. Utility of this device to develop the wound bed for grafting gained wide applicability which is directly applied to the wound to promote granulation tissue formation and skin grafting [18]. The present study showed that thirty four patients who needed serial debridement and washout due to re-accumulation were benefitted with an early wound closure from VAC therapy.

Management of closed DSTI is more challenging due to lack of evidence-based guidelines, these injuries are either treated by non-operative therapy or percutaneous and operative techniques. In our study, majority of patients with closed DSTI (78 %) underwent conservative treatment. Hak et al [9] performed open debridement of the Morel-Lavallée lesion with the incision placed close to the middle of the degloved area with thorough exploration for possible loculations. However, due to high incidence of complications such as re-accumulation of hematoma, wound breakdown and infection, the authors left the wound open post debridement [9]. A retrospective study by Nickerson et al [20] reported various treatment options for Morel-Lavallée lesions or closed DSTI such as compression wraps or observation, percutaneous aspiration or operative management with incision/drainage and formal debridement of skin and soft tissues. The authors observed that aspiration of more than 50 mL of fluid from Morel-Lavallée lesions was more frequent among lesions that recurred (83 %) as compared to those that resolved (33 %). Therefore, it has been recommend that aspiration of more than 50 mL of fluid from a Morel-Lavallée lesion should prompt operative intervention [20]. However, data of Morel-Lavallée lesions were not documented in the present series. Although, we did not quantify the initial drained amount of fluid in simple drainages, recurrent collection was observed in patients with initial copious drainage. Such patients should undergo repeated drainages and ultimately required proper debridement. The mortality rate was higher in closed type of degloving injuries. Notably, severe associated injuries such as traumatic brain injury and pelvic fracture were predominant in fatal cases which in fact were the contributing factors for increased mortality in closed DSTI. In addition, severe associated injuries may also lead to increased hospital length of stay.

The retrospective nature of the present study is one limitation. Detailed intervention and management of specific anatomical injuries were not well elaborated and the exact volume and the amount of fluid in the degloving injuries were available only for 37 cases based on computed tomography findings. Moreover, despite 11 cases with pelvic fracture had closed DSTI, Morel-Lavallée lesions were not documented which could be due to delayed diagnosis secondary to possible inconsistent clinical presentation. Lastly, this study lacks the exact details of the radiological investigation particularly for closed DSTI as the initial diagnose was primarily based on the clinical assessment. The tissue viability of the open/closed degloving injury, which is supposed to be a key factor relating to morbidity, mortality and ultimate result, was lacking in the available registry data and need further prospective work to be addressed. The time frame of management was not given in the database.

Conclusions

Diagnosis of degloving injury is a challenge as initially the emphasis concentrates on the most urgent life and limb threatening issues. Also the fact that some of these injuries are initially subtle and tend to deteriorate over time to become obvious as swelling or skin changes and for that some lesions can be missed and diagnosed at late stage. Although modern imaging like CT and MRI can pick these injuries early, they are not asked for that particular indication and it is commonly observed that the radiologic report of these images underestimate or not properly comment on these injuries which are considered as less important incidental injuries of the subcutaneous tissue and unless we change our stand and start to think of it ahead, document and communicate proactively with the radiologist and multidisciplinary treating teams; the same challenges won't be fixed. Early diagnosis and on-time management of degloving injury depend on a high index of suspicion, clear protocols and guidelines on the approaches of management, standardized diagnostic criteria, and more reliance on clinical

guidance of imaging technology. Current evidence support the use of MRI to diagnose, characterize and guide treatment and follow up, whereas ultrasound tends to be useful at later stage and or for follow up.

The incidence of DSTI is around 4 % with greater predilection to males and young patients in our series. Three quarter of the cases is traffic-related injuries. DSTI injuries are mostly underestimated lesions, with higher association of morbidity and mortality, if mismanaged. Open DSTI are more likely to be associated with head and scalp region whereas closed type are evident in lower extremity injuries and pelvic fractures. A high index of suspicion is crucial for the diagnosis and management of closed DSTI as it needs a multidisciplinary tailored approach. Moreover, the lower incidence of skin complication could probably attribute to the early interventions. To provide appropriate care for these patients, early tissue restoration and effective rehabilitation are crucial. Still, the treatment guidelines for DSTI are not well established; so further studies are needed to resolve controversial issues for DSTI grading and optimal diagnostic and treatment approaches guided by evidence-based practice.

Acknowledgement
The authors thank the entire registry database team in the Trauma Surgery Section, SICU and TICU staff, Hamad General Hospital, Doha, Qatar. All authors have declared no conflict of interest, no financial issues to disclose and no funding was received for this study. All authors contributed to the creation of and approved the manuscript.
This study was presented in part at 17th Congress of the European Society for Trauma and Emergency Surgery in Austria, Vienna from April 24 – 26, 2016.

Authors' contributions
SH was involved in study design, data acquisition, writing manuscript and review, KA: data acquisition, interpretation and drafting manuscript; GJ: data acquisition, interpretation and drafting manuscript; AE: study design, data analysis and interpretation, drafting and critical review of manuscript; RP: data interpretation, drafting and review of manuscript; SN: data acquisition, data interpretation, and review manuscript; AM: study design, data interpretation, and manuscript drafting; HA data analysis and interpretation, drafting and manuscript review; AA: data interpretation, drafting and review of manuscript and HA study design, data interpretation and critical review. Data availability: anonymous data will be available after getting permission according to the medical research center (MRC) policy at HMC, Qatar; research@hamad.qa. All authors read and approved the final manuscript.

Competing interests
The authors declare that they have no competing interests.

Author details
[1]Trauma Surgery Section, Hamad General Hospital, Doha, Qatar. [2]Clinical Research, Trauma Surgery Section, Hamad General Hospital, Doha, Qatar. [3]Clinical Medicine, Weill Cornell Medical College, Doha, Qatar. [4]Department of Radiology, Hamad General Hospital, Doha, Qatar.

References
1.   Morris M, Schreiber MA, Ham B. Novel Management of Closed Degloving Injuries. J Trauma Inj Inf Crit Care. 2009;67:E121–3.
2.   Mello DF, Assef JC, Soldá SC, Helene Jr A. Degloving injuries of trunk and limbs: comparison of outcomes of early versus delayed assessment by the plastic surgery team. Rev Col Bras Cir. 2015;42:143–8. doi:10.1590/0100-69912015003003.
3.   Wójcicki P, Wojtkiewicz W, Drozdowski P. Severe lower extremities degloving injuries-medical problems and treatment results. Pol Przegl Chir. 2011;83:276–82.
4.   Antoniou D, Kyriakidis A, Zaharopoulos A, Moskoklaidis S. Degloving Injury. Eur J Trauma. 2005;31:593–6.
5.   Krishnamoorthy R, Karthikeyan G. Degloving injuries of the hand. Indian J Plast Surg. 2011;44:227–36.
6.   Latifi R, El-Hennawy H, El-Menyar A, et al. The therapeutic challenges of degloving soft-tissue injuries. J Emerg Trauma Shock. 2014;7:228–32.
7.   Yan H, Gao W, Li Z, et al. The management of degloving injury of lower extremities: technical refinement and classification. J Trauma. 2013;74:604–10.
8.   Gummalla KM, George M, Dutta R. Morel-Lavallee lesion: case report of a rare extensive degloving soft tissue injury. Ulus Travma Acil Cerrahi Derg. 2014;20:63–5. doi:10.5505/tjtes.2014.88403.
9.   Hak DJ, Olson SA, Matta JM. Diagnosis and management of closed internal degloving injuries associated with pelvic and acetabular fractures: the Morel-Lavallée lesion. J Trauma. 1997;42:1046–51.
10. Hudson DA, Knottenbelt JD, Krige JE. Closed degloving injuries: results following conservative surgery. Plast Reconstr Surg. 1992;89:853–5.
11. Khan AT, Tahmeedullah O. Degloving injuries of the lower limb. J Coll Physicians Surg Pak. 2004;14:416–8.
12. Milcheski DA, Ferreira MC, Nakamoto HA, Tuma Jr P, Gemperli R. Degloving injuries of lower extremity–proposal of a treatment protocol. Rev Col Bras Cir. 2010;37:199–203.
13. El-Menyar A, Consunji R, Asim M, et al. Underutilization Of Occupant Restraint Systems In Motor Vehicle Injury Crashes: A Quantitative Analysis From Qatar. Traffic Inj Prev. 2015;13:1–9 [Epub ahead of print].
14. Latifi R. The Diagnostic and Therapeutic Challenges of Degloving Soft-Tissue Injuries. SOJ Surgery. 2013;1(1):01. Retrieved from http://www.symbiosis onlinepublishing.com/surgery/surgery01.php. Accessed 21 July 2016.
15. Gilbert BC, Bui-Mansfield LT, Dejong S. MRI of a Morel-Lavellée lesion. AJR Am J Roentgenol. 2004;182:1347–8.
16. Kottmeier SA, Wilson SC, Born CT, Hanks GA, Innacone WM, DeLong WG. Surgical management of soft tissue lesions associated with pelvic ring injury. Clin Orthop Relat Res. 1996;329:446–53.
17. Meara JG, Guo L, Smith JD, Pribaz JJ, Breuing KH, Orgill DP. Vacuum-assisted closure in the treatment of degloving injuries. Ann Plast Surg. 1999;42:589–94.
18. Wong LK, Nesbit RD, Turner LA, Sargent LA. Management of a circumferential lower extremity degloving injury with the use of vacuum-assisted closure. South Med J. 2006;99:628–30.
19. Dini M, Quercioli F, Mori A, Romano GF, Lee AQ, Agostini T. Vacuum-assisted closure, dermal regeneration template and degloved cryopreserved skin as useful tools in subtotal degloving of the lower limb. Injury. 2012;43:957–9.
20. Nickerson TP, Zielinski MD, Jenkins DH, Schiller HJ. The Mayo Clinic experience with Morel-Lavallée lesions: establishment of a practice management guideline. J Trauma Acute Care Surg. 2014;76:493–7.

10

The limitations of using risk factors to screen for blunt cerebrovascular injuries

Lewis E. Jacobson[1]*, Mary Ziemba-Davis[2] and Argenis J. Herrera[1]

Abstract

Introduction: Blunt cerebrovascular injury (BCVI) is reported to occur in 1–2 % of blunt trauma patients. Clinical and radiologic risk factors for BCVI have been described to help identify patients that require screening for these injuries. However, recent studies have suggested that BCVI frequently occurs even in the absence of these risk factors. The purpose of this study was to determine the incidence of BCVI in blunt trauma patients without risk factors and whether these patients could be identified by a more liberal CTA screening protocol.

Methods: We conducted a retrospective cohort study of all blunt trauma patients seen between November 2010 and May 2014. In May 2012, a clinical practice guideline for CTA screening for BCVI was implemented. The records of all patients with BCVI were reviewed for the presence of risk factors for BCVI previously described in the literature.

Results: During the 43 month study period, 6,602 blunt trauma patients were evaluated, 2,374 prior to, and 4,228 after implementation of the clinical practice guideline. Nineteen percent of all blunt trauma patients underwent CTA of the neck after protocol implementation compared to only 1.5 % prior to protocol implementation ($p = 0.001$). As a result, a 5-fold increase in the identification of BCVI was observed ($p = 0.00003$). Thirty-seven percent of patients with BCVI identified with the enhanced CT screening protocol had none of the signs, symptoms, or risk factors usually associated with these injuries.

Conclusions: Our findings demonstrate that reliance on clinical or radiologic risk factors alone as indications for screening for BCVI is inadequate. We recommend routine CTA screening for BCVI in all patients who have sustained a mechanism of injury sufficient to warrant either a CT of the cervical spine or a CTA of the chest.

Keywords: Blunt cerebrovascular injury, Carotid artery injury, Vertebral artery injury, Blunt trauma, Computer tomography, CT angiography, CTA screening, Risk factors for BCVI, Signs/symptoms of BCVI, Stroke

Introduction

Although previously thought to be rare, blunt cerebrovascular injury (BCVI) is now reported to occur in 1–2 % of blunt trauma patients [1–3]. Early recognition of these injuries is crucial as the stroke rate in untreated patients with BCVI is reported to be 20–60 % [4–9]. The majority of these strokes occur following a latent, asymptomatic time interval that can vary from hours to weeks [7, 10]. Initiation of treatment with antiplatelet agents or anticoagulation therapy during this asymptomatic period appears to reduce the stroke rate to below 1 % [7, 11, 12].

Screening criteria and optimal imaging modalities to identify patients with BCVI have been vigorously debated over the last 15 years. The groups in Denver [13] and Memphis [1] have identified an extensive list of clinical and radiologic risk factors that warrant diagnostic imaging and these studies have formed the basis of practice management guidelines published by the Western Trauma Association (WTA) in 2009 [13] and the Eastern Association for the Surgery of Trauma (EAST) in 2010 [1]. Despite these extensive lists of risk factors, several groups using whole body multi-slice screening computed tomography (CT) in multiple blunt trauma patients have recognized

* Correspondence: lejacobs@stvincent.org
[1]Department of Surgery, St. Vincent Indianapolis Hospital, 2001 West 86th Street, Indianapolis, IN 46260, USA
Full list of author information is available at the end of the article

that as many as 30 % of patients with BCVI have none of these risks factors [14]. In most of these patients, the first sign of an undetected BCVI will be a completed stroke.

Because of our concern that using risk factors alone might fail to identify a significant proportion of patients with BCVI, our group initiated a protocol of routine CT angiography (CTA) of the neck in any blunt trauma patient who was already undergoing CT of the cervical spine (C-spine) and/or CTA of the chest to screen for these injuries. The purpose of this study was to determine the incidence of BCVI in blunt trauma patients in the absence of any of the widely accepted risk factors currently included in published practice management guidelines and whether these patients could be identified by a more liberal CTA screening.

Methods

St. Vincent Indianapolis Hospital is a 566 bed American College of Surgeons-verified Level II trauma center located in Indianapolis, Indiana. It serves as the receiving trauma center for the 22 hospital St. Vincent Health system within the state and has a fleet of five helicopters to facilitate scene and inter-facility transports. In May of 2012, we initiated a clinical practice guideline for screening of blunt trauma patients for BCVI. All patients evaluated by the trauma service with a mechanism or injury significant enough to warrant a CT of the C-spine and/or a CTA of the chest underwent a CTA of the neck. Patients transferred from outside hospitals who had already undergone CT of the C-spine and/or CTA of the chest were not mandated to undergo routine screening for BCVI due to the increased risk of a second dose of contrast within 24 hours and the additional radiation exposure to the neck. Similarly, emergency department physicians, who evaluated many of the low mechanism/low risk patients initially, were not bound by the routine CTA of the neck screening guideline. In these patients, CTA of the neck was obtained at the discretion of the attending trauma surgeon based on mechanism of injury, signs or symptoms of BCVI, or the presence of known risk factors for BCVI. In these cases, the study was performed immediately. Prior to initiation of the protocol, CTA screening for BCVI was based on the clinical judgment of the trauma surgeon on call guided by the WTA and EAST guidelines available at that time.

Imaging Protocol

All trauma studies were performed on one of two 64 slice CT scanners, the GE 750 HD or the GE LightSpeed VCT (GE Healthcare, Waukesha, WI). The sequence of the exams and the timing of the contrast injections were optimized to minimize both the radiation and the contrast load delivered to the patient. All trauma patients were positioned supine, head first, with their arms down at their sides. CT scans of the head and face, when indicated, were performed first without IV contrast. Patients then underwent CTA of the neck and CT of the C-spine, acquired during a single run, followed by CTA of the chest (arterial phase) and CT of the abdomen and pelvis (venous phase).

For the CTA of the neck, contrast injection was performed using 60 mL of iohexol 350 at 4 mL per second, followed by 20 mL of 0.9 % sodium chloride. Once contrast was seen entering the aortic arch, scanning was initiated. Images were acquired at 0.625 mm slice thickness and at 0.625 mm intervals (0.625 mm × 0.625 mm). Sagittal images were reformatted at 2 mm × 2 mm and both coronal and sagittal reformats were done in Maximal Intensity Projection (MIP) mode at 10 mm × 2.5 mm.

Images for the CT of the C-spine were obtained during scanning for the CTA of the neck at 0.625 mm × 0.625 mm. Reformats were then done manually with coronal and sagittal images in bone window at 2 mm × 2 mm, sagittal images in standard window at 2 mm × 2 mm and angled axial reformats in bone and standard window at 2.5 mm × 2.5 mm.

For the CTA of the chest, 90 ml of iohexol 350 was used, at an injection rate of 4 mL per second, followed by 20 mL of 0.9 % sodium chloride. Arterial phase images were acquired at 0.625 mm × 0.625 mm. Coronal and sagittal reformats were done at 3 mm × 2 mm as well as coronal and sagittal images in MIP mode at 5 mm × 3 mm.

CT of the abdomen and pelvis (venous phase) was then automatically done 50 seconds after the start of the CTA chest (arterial phase) and images were acquired at 1.25 mm × 0.75 mm with coronal and sagittal reformats at 3 mm × 2 mm.

Treatment Protocol

All CTA studies of the neck done during the day were read by an attending neuroradiologist. At night an experienced in-house attending CT radiologist provided a preliminary reading and any positive or equivocal studies were reviewed the next morning by the attending neuroradiologist.

Patients with CTA findings suggestive of a BCVI were seen by an attending neurosurgeon or vascular surgeon and complex or equivocal studies were reviewed by an interventional neuroradiologist. Additional imaging with magnetic resonance angiography or repeat CTA was occasionally performed to help differentiate injuries from atherosclerotic disease. Treatment was initiated at the discretion of the attending neurosurgeon or vascular surgeon. Patients with a CTA reading equivocal for BCVI who were not felt to have injuries by the neurosurgeon or vascular surgeon, and for whom no treatment was initiated, were considered to be false positive studies and were excluded.

Patient Population

This retrospective cohort study was reviewed and approved by our organization's Institutional Review Board. The trauma registry was used to identify all blunt trauma patients seen at our trauma center between November 1, 2010 and May 31, 2014. Our trauma registry is compliant with the National Trauma Data Standard™ developed by the American College of Surgeons Committee on Trauma for inclusion in the National Trauma Data Bank™. Subjects were divided into two groups based on whether they were seen prior to (pre-protocol) or after (post-protocol) implementation of our routine CTA screening guideline for BCVI which was initiated on May 1, 2012.

Data collection from the registry included age, sex, mechanism of injury, Glasgow Coma Scale (GCS) score [15] in the emergency department (ED), Abbreviated Injury Scale (AIS08) scores [16], Injury Severity Score (ISS) [17], ICD-9 diagnosis codes, whether the patient underwent CTA of the neck, and mortality prior to discharge. All CTA of the neck reports were reviewed individually by the primary author and all studies with findings suggestive of BCVI were identified and the BCVI graded based on the grading scale proposed by Biffl [18]. If a patient had more than one CTA of the neck done, only the initial study was included.

The medical records of all the patients with positive studies were then reviewed for the presence of any of the signs/symptoms or risk factors for BCVI outlined in the new Denver Health Medical Center BCVI screening guideline described by Burlew [11] (Table 1).

Statistical Analysis

Minitab 17 (State College, PA) was used for statistical analyses. Proportions and means with ranges were used to summarize and compare patient demographics and the prevalence of CTA screening and BCVI in pre- and post-protocol groups. Pearson's Chi-Square test for independence (χ^2) and Student's t test were used to assess differences by study group. Probability (p) values associated with Fisher's exact test are reported for 2×2 χ^2 tables. Yates correction for continuity was used if expected frequencies were less than 5 in 2×2 χ^2 tables. Binary Logistic Regression was used to calculate the odds of BCVI based on GCS and ISS (mild, moderate, and severe).

Results

During the 43 month study period, 6,602 patients who had sustained blunt trauma were identified, 2,374 prior to implementation of the routine CTA of the neck guideline (pre-protocol) and 4,228 after implementation (post-protocol). Patient demographics are provided in Table 2.

Of the 2,374 pre-protocol patients only 35 (1.5 %) underwent CTA of the neck to evaluate for BCVI whereas post-protocol 802 (19 %) were screened. Pre-protocol

Table 1 New Denver Health Medical Center BCVI screening criteria [11] and prevalence in post-protocol sample

Screening criteria	Prevalence in post-protocol sample
Signs/symptoms of BCVI	
Potential arterial hemorrhage from neck/nose/mouth	0
Cervical bruit in patients < 50 years old	0
Expanding cervical hematoma	1
Focal neurologic deficit (TIA, hemiparesis, vertebrobasilar symptoms, Horner's Syndrome)	1
Neurologic deficit inconsistent with head CT scan findings	0
Stroke on CT or MRI	4
Risk factors for BCVI	
High-energy transfer mechanism associated with:	
Displaced mid-face fracture (LeForte II or III)	1
Mandible fracture	3
Complex skull fracture/basilar skull fracture/occipital condyle fracture	5
Closed head injury with diffuse axonal injury and GCS <6	7
Cervical subluxation or ligamentous injury, transverse foramen fracture, any body fracture, any fracture C1–C3	18
Near hanging with anoxic brain injury	1
Clothesline type injury or seat belt abrasion with significant swelling, pain, or altered mental status	0
Traumatic brain injury with thoracic injuries	7
Scalp degloving	3
Thoracic vascular injuries	3
Blunt cardiac rupture	0

there were 5 patients with BCVI identified for an incidence of 0.2 % (Table 3). Post-protocol, 46 patients with BCVI were identified for an overall incidence of 1.1 % in all blunt trauma patients. However, in patients who underwent CTA of the neck, the incidence was 5.7 % (46/802).

In all, 61 BCVIs were identified in 51 patients. There were 30 common or internal carotid artery injuries and 31 vertebral artery injuries. Forty-two patients had one BCVI, eight patients had 2 injuries and one patient had 3 injuries. The grading of these injuries is outlined in Table 4.

Compared to non-BCVI patients, those with BCVI had significantly greater mechanism of injury as indicated by higher incidences of motor vehicle crashes (54.9 % vs 23.5 %, $p = 0.001$), motorcycle crashes (7.8 % vs 6.7 %, $p = 0.016$), pedestrians hit by car (13.7 % vs 4.3 %, $p = 0.006$), and hangings/strangulations (2 % vs 0.1 %, $p = 0.045$) and lower incidences of falls (21.6 % vs 52.4 %, $p = 0.001$). BCVI patients were also a more severely injured group as indicated by lower initial GCS scores (10.5 vs. 14.1, $p = 0.001$), higher ISS (23.2 vs. 8.4, $p = 0.001$), and higher

Table 2 Demographic characteristics of study populations

	Pre-Protocol		Post-Protocol			No BCVI		BCVI		
	n	%	n	%	p	n	%	n	%	p
Patients	2374	36.0	4228	64.0		6551	99.2	51	0.8	
Male	1258	53.0	2330	55.1	0.100	3539	54.3	29	57.0	0.7787
Mortality	74	3.1	136	3.2	0.884	202	3.1	8	15.7	0.001
	Mean	**Range**	**Mean**	**Range**	**p**	**Mean**	**Range**	**Mean**	**Range**	**p**
Age (years)	54.6	15 to 100	54.6	14 to 100	0.974	54.6	14 to 100	54.0	16 to 89	0.800
GCS in ED	14.1	3 to 15	14.1	3 to 15	0.711	14.1	3 to 15	10.5	3 to 15	0.001
ISS	8.2	1 to 75	8.6	1 to 75	0.052	8.4	1 to 75	23.2	4 to 75	0.001

GCS = Glasgow Coma Scale; ISS = Injury Severity Score

mortality (15.7 % vs. 3.1 %, $p = 0.001$) (Table 2). As shown in Table 5, the likelihood of BCVI increased with decreasing GCS score in the ED ($p < 0.005$) and increasing ISS ($p < 0.005$). BCVI was 3.5 times more likely in patients with moderate compared to mild GCS scores, and 7.9 times more likely in patients with moderate compared to mild ISS. These odds ratios were 2.6 and 4.8 respectively, as scores increased from moderate to severe. Patients with severe GCS scores and ISS were 9.4 and 38.3 times more likely to have a BCVI than patients with mild scores.

Treatment of patients with BCVI was tailored to the severity of the BCVI and the patient's other injuries. Thirty-five patients were treated with antiplatelet agents, 5 with systemic anticoagulation, and 4 with a combination of both. Seven patients received no treatment either because they were too critical or because they died before treatment could be initiated.

Of the 46 post-protocol patients with BCVI, 29 (63 %) had at least one of the signs/symptoms or risk factors outlined in the new Denver Health Medical Center BCVI screening guideline [11] (Table 1). Seventeen patients had a single sign/symptom or risk factor, seven patients had 2, two patients had 3, two patients had 4, and one patient had 6 of the new Denver screening criteria. Cervical spine injury (n = 18) was the most common risk factor, followed by closed head injury with diffuse axonal injury and GCS <6 (n = 7) and traumatic brain injury with thoracic injury (n = 7). Finally, 17 (37 %) of the 46 post-protocol patients with BCVI had no identifiable signs/symptoms or risk factors outlined in the new Denver screening guidelines.

Discussion

In 2012, we initiated a protocol of routine CTA of the neck in any blunt trauma patient who was already undergoing CT of the C-spine and/or CTA of the chest. The purpose of this study was to determine whether identification of patients with BCVI was improved by this CT screening protocol. Pre-protocol only 1.5 % of blunt trauma patients underwent CTA of the neck to screen for BCVI, while post-protocol 19 % were screened ($p = 0.001$), representing a 13-fold increase in CTA screening (Fig. 1). As a result, a 5-fold increase in the incidence of BCVI was identified in our patient population (5/2,374 patients, 0.2 % vs 46/4,228 patients, 1.1 %; $p = 0.001$). This apparent increase in the incidence of BCVI is almost certainly the result of more intensive screening rather than a true increase in incidence. In all likelihood, these injuries were being missed prior to the implementation of our BCVI screening guideline.

Thirty-seven percent of BCVI patients identified with this enhanced CT screening protocol had none of the clinical or radiologic risk factors listed in the expanded Denver screening guidelines [11]. It therefore seems clear that reliance on risk factors alone as the indication for BCVI screening is likely to result in missed injuries and potentially avoidable strokes.

Blunt cerebrovascular injuries are thought to result from a combination of stretch induced disruption of the layers of the vessel wall and direct injury caused by

Table 3 CTA screening and identification of BCVI by study group

	Pre-Protocol		Post-Protocol		
	n	%	n	%	p
All patients	2374	36.0	4228	64.0	
CTA of the neck	35	1.5	802	19.0	0.001
BCVI	5	0.2	46	1.1	0.00003

Table 4 Grading of BCVIs [18]

Grade	Definition	n	%
I	Luminal irregularity or dissection with <25 % luminal narrowing	34	55.7
II	Dissection or intramural hematoma with ≥25 % luminal narrowing	7	11.5
III	Pseudoaneurysm	6	9.8
IV	Occlusion	14	23.0
V	Transection with free extravasation	0	0.0
	Total	61	100.0

Table 5 Prevalence and likelihood of BCVI based on GCS score and ISS

	No BCVI		BCVI		Likelihood of BCVI based on GCS/ISS	Odds ratio [95 % CI]	χ^2	p
	n	%	n	%				
GCS in ED								
Mild	4655	99.4	27	0.6	Moderate vs. Mild	3.5 [1.2:10.2]	38.3	<0.005
Moderate	195	98.0	4	2.0	Severe vs. Moderate	2.6 [0.9:8.0]		
Severe	295	94.9	16	5.1	Severe vs. Mild	9.4 [5.0:17.5]		
ISS								
Mild	4679	99.8	9	0.2	Moderate vs. Mild	7.9 [3.6:17.1]	88.1	<0.005
Moderate	1513	98.5	23	1.5	Severe vs. Moderate	4.8 [2.6:9.0]		
Severe	258	93.1	19	6.9	Severe vs. Mild	38.3 [17.2:85.5]		

GCS = Glasgow Coma Scale Score: Mild 14–15, Moderate 8–13, Severe < 8
ISS = Injury Severity Score: Mild 1–9, Moderate 10–25, Severe > 25

fractures of the transverse foramina of the cervical vertebrae [2]. Identification of these lesions and treatment with anticoagulation or antiplatelet agents is recognized to be crucial to prevent embolization or propagation of thrombus into the distal cerebral vessels.

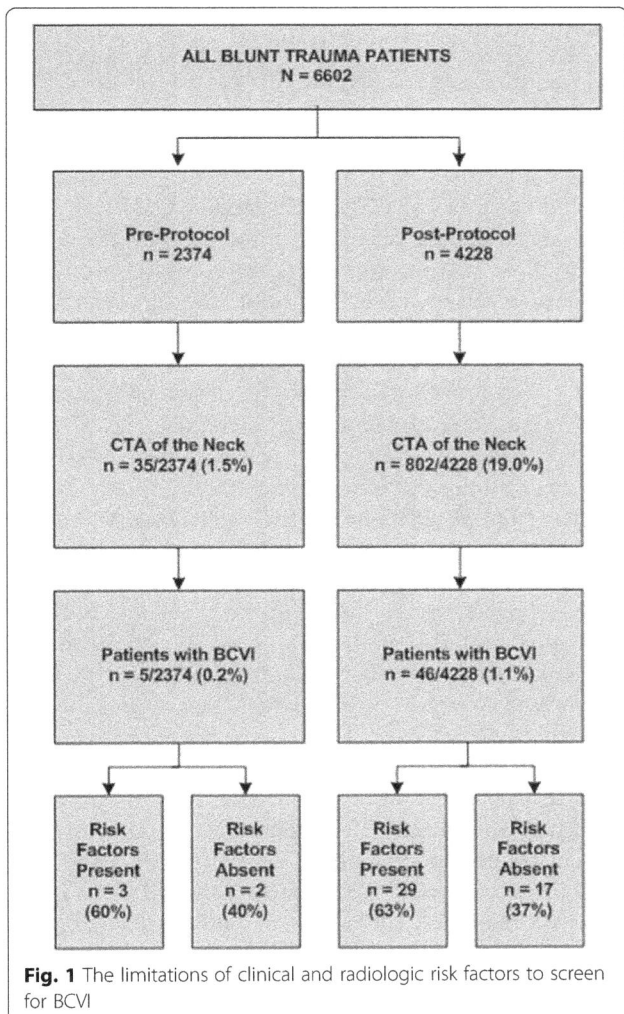

Fig. 1 The limitations of clinical and radiologic risk factors to screen for BCVI

Until relatively recently, blunt cerebrovascular injury was thought to be a rare entity. In 1990, Davis et al. [19] reported on a series of 15,935 blunt trauma patients admitted over a 5 year period in San Diego County and identified 14 patients with blunt carotid injuries for a detected incidence of 0.08 %. Consistent with the standard of care at that time, all injuries were diagnosed by angiography and the majority (11/14, 79 %) only after symptoms or CT findings of completed stroke. Over the next 20 years, however, several crucial observations significantly altered the management and prognosis of these lesions.

Firstly, anticoagulation was shown to improve neurologic outcomes in patients with strokes related to BCVI [2, 5, 6, 9, 11, 19, 20]. In addition, early anticoagulation or antiplatelet therapy has been shown to decrease stroke rate in asymptomatic patients with BCVI from as high as 60 % to less than 1 % [7, 11, 12, 21]. Full anticoagulation is frequently contraindicated in blunt trauma patients due to associated injuries. A recent Cochrane review [22], however, failed to demonstrate a difference in efficacy between anticoagulation and aspirin and concluded that aspirin was as effective as anticoagulation, but with a lower risk of hemorrhage. This would support early initiation of effective therapy in the form of aspirin, even in high risk trauma patients.

Secondly, it has been widely recognized that the vast majority of BCVIs are asymptomatic at the time of presentation and that neurologic symptoms only develop after some variable time interval. This latent, asymptomatic period prior to development of stroke can vary from minutes to years but most commonly lasts from 10 to 72 hours following injury [2, 4, 6–8, 11, 18, 23–26]. Although patients may occasionally present with symptoms of transient ischemic attack, in most the first symptom will be a completed ischemic stroke. It is therefore crucial to identify BCVI during this latent period and to initiate treatment before irreversible neurologic injury occurs.

This recognition led to the third important discovery that has reduced the morbidity and mortality of these lesions, namely the identification of risk factors in blunt trauma patients that warrant screening for BCVI prior to the development of neurologic sequelae. By the late 1990's it was clear that there was an unrecognized epidemic of BCVI [20]. In a meta-analysis done by Franz et al. [2] the incidence range was 0.45–1.63 % in studies using 16-slice or greater CTA. At the high end, this is 20 times higher than the incidence in Davis' study in 1990 [19] of 0.08 %. Recognizing that most of these injuries are asymptomatic at the time of presentation, the groups in Denver [11, 13, 21] and Memphis [1, 27–29] have, over the last decade, elucidated an extensive list of clinical and radiologic risk factors that warrant screening for BCVI. Publication of practice management guidelines by the WTA in 2009 [13] and EAST in 2010 [1] led to widespread adoption of these screening criteria for BCVI. However, despite subsequent broadening of the list of risk factors, it has been recognized that at least 20–30 % of patients with BCVI have none of the risk factors for screening outlined in these organizational guidelines or other published research [9, 14, 28].

In a study by Emmett et al. [28], most patients with significant blunt trauma who warranted a head, C-spine, or face CT to evaluate for potential injury underwent CTA of the neck at the time of their initial trauma evaluation. They found that this routine screening with CTA identified that 16 % of their patients with BCVI had none of the conventional risk factors for screening. Further confirmation of the lack of sensitivity of these widely used risk factors as screening criteria for BCVI has been published by the group from Baltimore [9, 14]. Since 2004 they have used a whole-body, multi-detector CT screening protocol for blunt trauma patients clinically judged to be at high risk for significant injury. In a study published in 2014 they found that 30 % of patients diagnosed with BCVI using this technique had none of the radiologic or clinical risk factors previously described for BCVI screening [14]. They concluded that the use of currently available risk factors to identify patients for screening would lead to missed injury and stroke and that more liberalized screening for BCVI during initial whole-body CT imaging based on mechanism alone is warranted.

Based on our analysis of the literature, we had come to a similar conclusion, even prior to publication of the Baltimore study [14], and initiated a guideline for routine CTA of the neck in patients undergoing CT of the C-spine and/ or CTA of the chest. This conclusion is now supported by the finding in this study that 37 % of patients with BCVI had none of these widely accepted risk factors.

Although 4-vessel digital subtraction angiography (DSA) had long been considered the gold standard for the diagnosis of BCVI, most trauma surgeons do not currently consider it to be the preferred method for screening patients for these injuries. The technique is invasive, expensive, labor intensive, and continues to have a small but measurable potential for complications, including stroke [2, 29]. In addition, it may not be available outside of high volume trauma centers and tertiary care hospitals [9, 14]. CTA, in comparison, is widely available, non-invasive, rapid and cost effective and can be used to detect other injuries in the neck with a single imaging series. Although earlier studies cautioned against use of CTA to identify BCVI due to inadequate sensitivity, more recent data from studies using multi-slice CT scanners have demonstrated improved sensitivity allowing recommendation of its use for screening [29–31]. Moreover, based on a recent survey, the use of CTA of the neck seems to be widespread, with 93 % of 137 trauma surgeons reporting CTA as their preferred method of imaging for the diagnosis of BCVI [32].

There are several limitations to this study. The intent of our screening protocol was to order a CTA of the neck in any patient with sufficient mechanism or clinical suspicion of injury to warrant imaging with CT of the C-spine and/ or CTA of the chest. However, only 19 % of post-protocol blunt trauma patients underwent CTA of the neck. This resulted from several factors. A significant number of low mechanism and low risk patients were not felt to warrant either CT of the C-spine or CTA of the chest and therefore did not undergo CTA of the neck. In addition, CTA of the neck was not mandated in the absence of risk factors in those patients who had already undergone CT of the C-spine and/or CTA of the chest, either prior to transfer from an outside hospital or prior to consultation by the trauma service. Nevertheless, institution of this guideline resulted in a 13-fold increase in the number of CTAs of the neck obtained and a 5-fold increase in the percentage of patients in whom BCVI was identified. Given the high risk of undiagnosed and untreated BCVI reported in the literature, identification of these additional injuries by a liberal screening guideline, and subsequent treatment, almost certainly reduced the number of strokes in these patients. Furthermore, although the incidence of BCVI in all post-protocol patients was 1.1 %, the incidence in the 19 % of patients who were screened with CTA of the neck was 5.7 %. It is likely that more intensive screening would yield an even higher incidence of BCVI. For instance, approximately 40 % of our patients were transferred from outside hospitals and most of them had undergone CT imaging prior to transfer and were therefore not mandated to undergo CTA of the neck in the absence of risk factors. Based on our results we plan to recommend our clinical practice guideline for BCVI screening to the 22 hospitals in our system as well as other referring hospitals, and to implement it within our emergency department physician group for patients seen prior to consultation by the trauma service.

The optimal strategy for identification of BCVI continues to evolve. CTA now appears to be widely accepted as the screening study of choice and given its low risk, ubiquitous availability and reasonable cost in comparison to angiography, it could even be considered the new gold standard. Currently available screening guidelines fail to identify more than a third of patients with BCVI and should therefore no longer be considered adequate by themselves for this purpose. In patients undergoing CT of the C-spine and/or CTA of the chest, a dedicated CTA of the neck can be obtained with no increase in radiation exposure and minimal increase in the amount of contrast administered. In addition, this technique of routine, simultaneous CTA of the neck in moderate and high risk blunt trauma patients obviates the need for a return trip to the CT scanner and additional radiation and contrast in patients who have risk factors identified on initial imaging. This allows the earliest possible identification of these potentially devastating injuries and initiation of simple, low risk treatment (such as aspirin) which appears to reduce the stroke rate to less than 1 % [5, 11, 21, 22]. Based on the findings of this study we would recommend routine CTA of the neck in all patients who have sustained a mechanism of injury sufficient to warrant either a CT of the C-spine or a CTA of the chest. This should minimize the risk of missing occult BCVI in patients with these injuries who have none of the clinical or radiologic risk factors identified in currently available clinical screening guidelines.

Competing interests
The authors declare that they have no competing interests.

Authors' contributions
LEJ conceived of the study and participated in its design and protocol development; reviewed the medical records of all BCVI patients for the presence of signs, symptoms, and risk factors for BCVI; participated in data interpretation; and was involved in the preparation and critical review of the manuscript. MZD participated in study design and protocol development; oversaw data compilation, management, and verification; analyzed the data; and was involved in the preparation of the manuscript. AJH participated in study design and protocol development and reviewed medical records of BCVI patients. All authors read and approved the final manuscript.

Acknowledgements
This research received no grant from any funding agency in the public, commercial or not-for-profit sectors. The authors thank Melinda Dillow, BSW (St. Vincent Trauma Center) for data management and supplemental medical chart review. We also thank Kathy J. Cookman, BS, CSTR, CAISS (KJ Trauma Consulting, LLC) and Marissa Byrd (St. Vincent Trauma Center) for trauma registry data extraction, and Sharon Woodland, BSBA (St. Vincent Trauma Center) for support in the preparation of the manuscript.

Author details
[1]Department of Surgery, St. Vincent Indianapolis Hospital, 2001 West 86th Street, Indianapolis, IN 46260, USA. [2]St. Vincent Neuroscience Institute, 8333 Naab Road, Indianapolis, IN 46260, USA.

References
1. Bromberg WJ, Collier BC, Diebel LN, Dwyer KM, Holevar MR, Jacobs DG, et al. Blunt cerebrovascular injury practice management guidelines: the Eastern Association for the Surgery of Trauma. J Trauma. 2010;68(2):471–7.
2. Franz RW, Willette PA, Wood MJ, Wright ML, Hartman JF. A systematic review and meta-analysis of diagnostic screening criteria for blunt cerebrovascular injuries. J Am Coll Surg. 2012;214(3):313–27.
3. Harrigan MR, Falola MI, Shannon CN, Westrick AC, Walters BC. Incidence and trends in the diagnosis of traumatic extracranial cerebrovascular injury in the nationwide inpatient sample database, 2003–2010. J Neurotrauma. 2014;31(11):1056–62.
4. Biffl WL, Ray Jr CE, Moore EE, Franciose RJ, Aly S, Heyrosa MG, et al. Treatment-related outcomes from blunt cerebrovascular injuries: importance of routine follow-up arteriography. Ann Surg. 2002;235(5):699–706.
5. Burlew CC, Biffl WL. Imaging for blunt carotid and vertebral artery injuries. Surg Clin North Am. 2011;91(1):217–31.
6. Cogbill TH, Moore EE, Meissner M, Fischer RP, Hoyt DB, Morris JA, et al. The spectrum of blunt injury to the carotid artery: a multicenter perspective. J Trauma. 1994;37(3):473–9.
7. Cothren CC, Biffl WL, Moore EE, Kashuk JL, Johnson JL. Treatment for blunt cerebrovascular injuries: equivalence of anticoagulation and antiplatelet agents. Arch Surg. 2009;144(7):685–90.
8. Liang T, McLaughlin PD, Louis L, Nicolaou S. Review of multidetector computed tomography angiography as a screening modality in the assessment of blunt vascular neck injuries. Can Assoc Radiol J. 2013;64(2):130–9.
9. Stein DM, Boswell S, Sliker CW, Lui FY, Scalea TM. Blunt cerebrovascular injuries: does treatment always matter? J Trauma Acute Care Surg. 2009;66(1):132–44.
10. Ahmad HA, Gerraty RP, Davis SM, Cameron PA. Cervicocerebral artery dissections. J Accid Emerg Med. 1999;16(6):3.
11. Burlew CC, Biffl WL, Moore EE, Barnett CC, Johnson JL, Bensard DD. Blunt cerebrovascular injuries: redefining screening criteria in the era of noninvasive diagnosis. J Trauma Acute Care Surg. 2012;72(2):330–7.
12. Cothren CC, Moore EE, Ray Jr CE, Ciesla DJ, Johnson JL, Moore JB, et al. Screening for blunt cerebrovascular injuries is cost-effective. Am J Surg. 2005;190(6):845–9.
13. Biffl WL, Cothren CC, Moore EE, Kozar R, Cocanour C, Davis JW, et al. Western Trauma Association critical decisions in trauma: screening for and treatment of blunt cerebrovascular injuries. J Trauma. 2009;67(6):1150–3.
14. Bruns BR, Tesoriero R, Kufera J, Sliker C, Laser A, Scalea TM, et al. Blunt cerebrovascular injury screening guidelines: what are we willing to miss? J Trauma Acute Care Surg. 2014;76(3):691–5.
15. Teasdale G, Jennett B. Assessment of coma and impaired consciousness. A practical scale. Lancet. 1974;13(2):81–4.
16. Gennarelli TA, Wodzin E. The Abbreviated Injury Scale 2005 - Update 2008. Association for the Advancement of Automotive Medicine. 2008.
17. Baker SP, O'Neill B, Haddon Jr W, Long WB. The injury severity score: a method for describing patients with multiple injuries and evaluating emergency care. J Trauma. 1974;14(3):187–96.
18. Biffl WL, Moore EE, Offner PJ, Brega KE, Franciose RJ, Burch JM. Blunt carotid arterial injuries: implications of a new grading scale. J Trauma. 1999;47(5):845–53.
19. Davis JW, Holbrook TL, Hoyt DB, Mackersie RC, Field Jr TO, Shackford SR. Blunt carotid artery dissection: incidence, associated injuries, screening, and treatment. J Trauma. 1990;30(12):1514–7.
20. Biffl WL, Moore EE, Ryu RK, Offner PJ, Novak Z, Coldwell DM, et al. The unrecognized epidemic of blunt carotid arterial injuries: early diagnosis improves neurologic outcome. Ann Surg. 1998;228(4):462–70.
21. Burlew CC, Biffl WL, Moore EE, Pieracci FM, Beauchamp KM, Stovall R, et al. Endovascular stenting is rarely necessary for the management of blunt cerebrovascular injuries. J Am Coll Surg. 2014;218(5):1012–7.
22. Lyrer P, Engelter S. Antithrombotic drugs for carotid artery dissection. Cochrane Database of Systematic Reviews (Art No: CD000255). 2010(10).
23. Burlew CC, Biffl WL. Blunt cerebrovascular trauma. Curr Opin Crit Care. 2010;16(6):587–95.
24. Cothren CC, Moore EE, Biffl WL, Ciesla DJ, Ray Jr CE, Johnson JL, et al. Anticoagulation is the gold standard therapy for blunt carotid injuries to reduce stroke rate. Arch Surg. 2004;139(5):540–6.

25. Krajewski LP, Hertzer NR. Blunt carotid artery trauma: report of two cases and review of the literature. Ann Surg. 1980;191(3):341–6.
26. Mokri B, Piepgras DG, Houser OW. Traumatic dissections of the extracranial internal carotid artery. J Neurosurg. 1988;68(2):189–97.
27. DiCocco JM, Emmett KP, Fabian TC, Zarzaur BL, Williams JS, Croce MA. Blunt cerebrovascular injury screening with 32-channel multidetector computed tomography: more slices still don't cut it. Ann Surg. 2011;253(3):444–50.
28. Emmett KP, Fabian TC, DiCocco JM, Zarzaur BL, Croce MA. Improving the screening criteria for blunt cerebrovascular injury: the appropriate role for computed tomography angiography. J Trauma. 2011;70(5):1058–65.
29. Paulus EM, Fabian TC, Savage SA, Zarzaur BL, Botta V, Dutton W, et al. Blunt cerebrovascular injury screening with 64-channel multidetector computed tomography: more slices finally cut it. J Trauma Acute Care Surg. 2014;76(2):279–85.
30. Eastman AL, Chason DP, Perez CL, McAnulty AL, Minei JP. Computed tomographic angiography for the diagnosis of blunt cervical vascular injury: is it ready for primetime? J Trauma. 2006;60(5):925–9.
31. Malhotra AK, Camacho M, Ivatury RR, Davis IC, Komorowski DJ, Leung DA, et al. Computed tomographic angiography for the diagnosis of blunt carotid/vertebral artery injury: a note of caution. Ann Surg. 2007;246(4):632–43.
32. Harrigan MR, Weinberg JA, Peaks YS, Taylor SM, Cava LP, Richman J, et al. Management of blunt extracranial traumatic cerebrovascular injury: a multidisciplinary survey of current practice. World J Emerg Surg. 2011;6:11.

11

Epidemiology of spinal injuries in the United Arab Emirates

Michal Grivna[1], Hani O. Eid[2] and Fikri M. Abu-Zidan[2*]

Abstract

Aim: To assess the risk factors, mechanism of injury, and clinical outcome of hospitalized patients with spinal injuries in order to recommend preventive measures.

Methods: Patients with spinal injuries admitted to Al Ain Hospital, United Arab Emirates (UAE) for more than 24 h or who died after arrival to the hospital were studied over 3 years. Demography, location and time of injury, affected body regions, hospital and ICU stay, and outcome were analyzed.

Results: 239 patients were studied, 90 % were males, and 84 % were in the productive years of 25–54. Majority were from the Indian subcontinent (56 %). Road was the most common location for spinal injury (47 %), followed by work (39 %). The most common mechanism of injury was traffic collisions (48 %) followed by fall from height (39 %) and fall from the same level (9 %). UAE nationals were often injured at road and home compared with non-UAE nationals, who were more injured at work ($p < 0.0001$). Patients falling from the same level were older ($p = 0.001$) and predominantly females ($p < 0.0001$) when compared with other mechanisms. Spinal fractures were more common in the lumbar region (57 %). Eleven patients (5 %) sustained paraplegia and five (4 %) patients died.

Interpretation: Traffic injuries and falls were the leading causes for spinal injuries in the UAE. Expatriate males are at high risk for fall from height, UAE national males for traffic injuries and females for falls at the same level at homes. Prevention should focus on traffic and home injuries for UAE nationals and occupational safety for expatriate workers.

Keywords: Spine injury, Fall, Road-traffic crash, Prevention, United Arab Emirates

Introduction

Spinal injury is one of the most devastating injuries having a great impact on patients, their families, and the society [1,2]. It may lead to serious disability when involving the spinal cord with long-term medical complications, including pressure ulcers, autonomic dysreflexia, deep venous thrombosis and pneumonia [3-5]. This significantly impacts rehabilitation and long-term quality of life [4]. People with spinal injury have a high level of distress, depression, anxiety, and suicide attempts because of their lower levels of life satisfaction [6,7]. The costs of spine injuries and their effects on the health care systems are high [8].

United Arab Emirates (UAE), having a predominantly urban population of more than 6 million, is a fast developing country. It is a federation of seven emirates with modern road infrastructure and a high proportion of expatriate workers [9]. Various ethnic groups with sociocultural, religious and educational diversity pose a special challenge for health and safety [10]. In order to propose useful preventive measures, it is necessary to conduct proper epidemiological studies. As there is little information about spine injuries in the Middle East, we aimed to assess the mechanism of injury, severity and outcome of hospitalized spinal injured patients in the UAE in order to give recommendations regarding their prevention.

Patients and methods

Ethics statement

The Local Ethics Committee of Al Ain Health District Area approved the study (UAE RECA/02/44). All patients

* Correspondence: fabuzidan@uaeu.ac.ae
[2]Trauma Group, Department of Surgery, College of Medicine and Health Sciences, UAE University, Al Ain, United Arab Emirates
Full list of author information is available at the end of the article

or their care givers signed a consent form for permitting the use of anonymous data for research or audit.

Setting

Al Ain Hospital is one of the two major hospitals (Al Ain and Tawam Hospitals) in Al Ain City serving a population of about half a million residing in the largest city located in the east of Abu Dhabi Emirate of the UAE [11]. It is a specialized acute care and emergency hospital with 402 beds and more than 35 medical departments and divisions [12]. Around eighty percent of the trauma patients of Al Ain City were treated in Al Ain Hospital during the study period.

Data collection and scoring

All patients who were admitted to Al Ain Hospital for more than 24 h or who have died after admission following their injury were included in Al Ain Hospital Trauma Registry. Data were collected prospectively from March 2003 to March 2006 on a specially designed hard copy form [13]. A full time Trauma Research Fellow collected data on daily basis on the injured patients and followed them up through their hospital stay.

The data of all patients with spinal injury were retrieved from the registry. The demography of the patients, the mechanism and location of their injury, factors reflecting injury severity and outcome including Glasgow Coma Scale (GCS) on arrival, Injury Severity Score (ISS), Intensive Care Unit (ICU) admission, mortality and neurological deficit were studied. The ISS as a global marker of injury severity was calculated manually using the Abbreviated Injury Scale (AIS) 1998 handbook [14].

Statistical analysis

Nationality was categorized into two groups – UAE nationals and non-UAE nationals, because previous studies have shown that injury risks for UAE nationals differ from other nationalities [15,16]. Mechanism of injury was categorized into three groups – traffic-related, fall from height, and fall from the same level. Non parametric statistical methods were used in comparing two or three groups because the numbers of subjects in some of the groups were small. Non-parametric statistical methods are advised in this situation because they compare the ranks, normal distribution is not required, and this has a protective effect for the analysis. [17]. Mann–Whitney U test was used to compare continuous or ordinal data of two groups while Kruskal–Wallis test was used to compare continuous or ordinal data of three groups. Fisher's exact test was used to compare categorical data. Analysis was performed using PASW Statistics 21, SPSS Inc, USA.

Results

There were 239 patients, 215 males (90 %) (male:female ratio was 9:1). The mean (SD) age was 37.5 (12.5) years. Adults in the productive years of 25–54 years were majority (84 %; $n = 201$). Five percent ($n = 12$) were children and youth less than 19 years, and 3 % ($n = 7$) were elderly more than 65 years. Majority were from the Indian subcontinent (55 %; $n = 132$), followed by Arabs (23 %; $n = 54$), UAE nationals (14 %; $n = 34$), and other nationalities 8 % ($n = 19$) (Table 1).

Road was the most common location for spine injury (47 %; $n = 112$), followed by work (39 %; $n = 93$), home (10 %; $n = 23$) and other locations (5 %; $n = 11$). The most common location for injuries for males was road (47 %; $n = 101$) and for females was home (50 %; $n = 12$). UAE nationals were often injured at road and home compared with non-nationals who were injured at work and road ($p < 0.0001$) (Table 2). Traffic-related spine injury was the most common mechanism of injury (48 %; $n = 114$), followed by fall from height (39 %; $n = 94$), fall from same level (9 %; $n = 21$) and other mechanisms, such as falling objects and animal-related injuries (4 %; $n = 10$) (Table 3). Majority of falls fom height occurred at work (85 %; $n = 80$), while majority of falls at the same level occurred at home (68 %; $n = 15$) ($p < 0.0001$) (Table 3). UAE nationals were more injured by traffic and fall from the same level, compared with non-nationals who were more injured by falling from height at work ($p < 0.0001$) (Table 2). Those who had spinal injury at home were significantly older than those who fell from height or were injured by road traffic collisions ($p = 0.001$) (Fig. 1 and Table 3).

The estimated annual incidence of hospitalized spinal injuries in Al Ain City was 17.4/100,000 persons per year. Most of injuries (119/239) occurred during the months of April-August (Fig. 2a). Sunday had the highest incidence of spine injuries (18 %; $n = 43$) and Friday the lowest (9 %; $n = 22$) (Fig. 2b). More than half of the injuries (113/218) occurred during the morning time (8 a.m. -1 p.m.) (Fig. 2c). The mechanism of injury and its location did not affect the time of injury.

Table 1 Hospitalized patients with spine injury by nationality, Al Ain, United Arab Emirates, 2003–2006 ($n = 239$)

	Number	Percent
Pakistan	62	25.9
India	45	18.8
Bangladesh	25	10.5
UAE	34	14.2
Other Arabs	54	22.6
Others	19	7.9
Total	239	100.0

Table 2 Demographic, location, mechanism, severity, and outcome variables of spine injuries by nationality, Al Ain, UAE (n = 239)

Variable		UAE (n = 34)	Non UAE (n = 203)	p-value
Age (years)		30 (7–80)	35.5 (2–70)	0.2
Gender (male)		26 (76.5 %)	187 (92.1 %)	0.01
Location	Home	10 (29 %)	13 (6.4 %)	<0.0001
	Work	1 (3 %)	99 (48.8 %)	
	Road	22 (65 %)	87 (42.8 %)	
	Other	1 (3 %)	4 (2 %)	
Mechanism	Road traffic injury	23 (67.6 %)	90 (44.3 %)	<0.0001
	Fall from height	3 (8.8 %)	90 (44.3 %)	
	Fall from same level	8 (23.5 %)	13 (6.4 %)	
	Other	0	9 (4.5 %)	
Severity	ICU admission	8 (23.5 %)	21 (10.3 %)	0.044
	Hospital stay (days)	6 (1–21)	8 (1–78)	0.005
	GCS	15 (3–15)	15 (3–15)	0.06
	ISS	5 (4–29)	5 (1–38)	0.06
Outcome	Paraplegia	1 (2.9 %)	10 (4.9 %)	1
	Mortality	2 (5.9 %)	3 (1.5 %)	0.14

p = Mann Whitney U test or Fisher's Exact test as appropriate
Data are presented as median (range) or number (%) as appropriate

The most common associated injured anatomical regions were the chest (23 %; n = 56) with highest AIS, followed by upper extremity (22 %; n = 52) and lower extremity (17 %; n = 40) (Table 4). Spinal fractures were more common at the lumbar region (57 %; n = 136).

Twenty nine patients (12 %) had more than one level injured. Eleven patients (5 %) sustained paraplegia, most were associated with lumbar fractures (4/11) (Table 5).

UAE nationals were significantly more admitted to the ICU compared with non-nationals (p = 0.044), and had a shorter hospital stay (p = 0.005). There was a strong trend for statistical difference in GCS (p = 0.06) and ISS (p = 0.06) between UAE and non-UAE nationals. UAE nationals had more severe injuries compared with non UAE nationals. The mean (SD) total hospital stay was 11.4 (11.96) days. Non-nationals were hospitalized longer than UAE nationals (p = 0.005) because they had a higher percentage of paraplegia (Table 2). The median (range) ISS of patients was 5 (1–38). Patients with traffic-related spine injury had higher ISS compared with falls from high or same level (p < 0.0001) (Table 3). Five patients died (2.1 %), all in traffic collisions.

Discussion

Our study has shown that men in the productive age, majority from the Indian subcontinent, are at the highest risk for spinal injuries at work in the UAE. National females were more injured at home by falling at same level, while national males were more injured in traffic collisions. Patients injured in traffic had more severe injuries, were more admitted to the ICU, while patients injured by fall from height had longer hospital stay.

The estimated incidence of spinal injuries in our study (174/million population) was much higher than those reported from other countries [18-20]. The mean age of our patients (37.5 years) was similar to other countries,

Table 3 Demographic, location, mechanism, severity and outcome variables of spine injuries by mechanims, Al Ain, United Arab Emirates, 2003–2006 (n = 239)

Variable		Traffic (n = 114)	Fall from height (n = 94)	Fall at same level (n = 22)	p-value
Age (years)		35 (2–70)	37 (7–64)	50 (25–80)	0.001
Gender (male)		103 (90.4 %)	90 (95.7 %)	14 (63.6 %)	<0.0001
UAE nationality		23 (20.2 %)	3 (3.2 %)	8 (36.4 %)	<0.0001
Location	Home	0	8 (8.5 %)	15 (68.2 %)	<0.0001
	Work	1 (0.9 %)	80 (85.1 %)	5 (22.7 %)	
	Road	111 (97.4 %)	1 (1.1 %)	0	
	Other	2 (1.8 %)	5 (5.3 %)	2 (9.1 %)	
Severity	ICU admission	24 (21.1 %)	6 (6.4 %)	0	0.001
	Hospital stay (days)	8 (1–77)	17.5 (1–57)	5.5 (1–19)	0.11
	GCS	15 (3–15)	15 (4–15)	15 (15–15)	<0.0001
	ISS	8 (1–38)	4 (1–34)	4 (1–9)	<0.0001
Outcome	Paraplegia	6 (5.3 %)	5 (5.3 %)	0	0.8
	Mortality	5 (4.4 %)	0	0	0.13

p = Kruskal–Wallis test or Fisher's Exact test as appropriate
Data are presented as median (range) or number (%) as appropriate
9 patients with other mechanisms were not included in the analysis
Number may not add to 100 % because of missing data

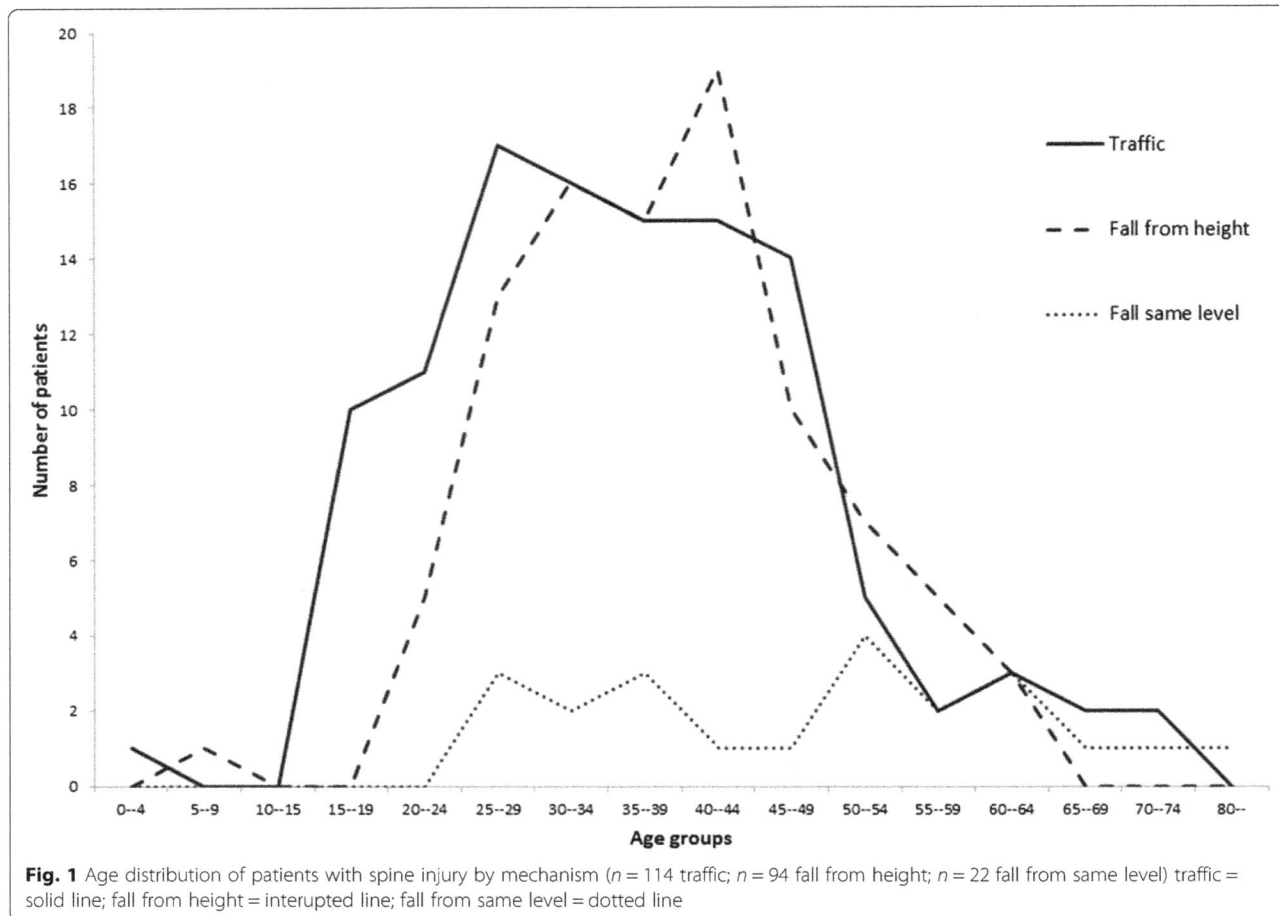

Fig. 1 Age distribution of patients with spine injury by mechanism (*n* = 114 traffic; *n* = 94 fall from height; *n* = 22 fall from same level) traffic = solid line; fall from height = interupted line; fall from same level = dotted line

such as Italy, United States and Pakistan [1,3,5], but lower than Japan and China [21,22] because of the different injury risk in the young UAE population. Patients with traffic spine injuries and fall from height in our study were younger compared with those with fall at the same level.

Similar to others [1,8,23], majority of our injured patients were males. The male:female ratio (9:1) was much higher compared with other countries [1,5,23,24]. The overall male:female ratio in UAE is 2:1 due to the large number of expatriate workers [9].

Traffic-related spine injury was the most common mechanism of injury and occurred in young males in our study, similar to other developed countries [5,8,19,25]. Economic growth and increasing use of motor vehicles with improving road infrastructure in the UAE have been followed by increasing rates of traffic injuries. Restraint use is low and enforcement of traffic safety regulations is not appropriate [10].

Fall from height is the most common cause of spine injury in developing countries [1]. It was the second leading cause in our study. Many expatriate workers from the Indian subcontinent are injured in the

construction industry [26], which was regarded as the most hazardous industry [27]. Immigrant workers often lack safety equipment and safety education in their own language [10].

We identified a daily time peak during the morning hours (8 a.m.–1 p.m.). A study on occupational injuries from Canada reported a daily peak at 11 a.m. possibly due to sleep deprivation [28]. Falls occurred most often on Sundays, first working day in the week in the UAE and less often on Fridays, which is a weekend. The highest monthly incidence of spine injuries in our study was during spring and summer. It is possible that the high outdoor temperatures, which can reach up to 50 °C in the summer, can decrease the vigilance among our population both in the traffic and at work. A study on occupational injuries from Canada [28] reported the highest peak of injuries in August. Spine injuries caused by fall from height occur more at work. A study from Qatar [26] reported that falling from height at construction sites was common with significant effects on the health care system.

Females in our study were more injured at home by falling at the same level. The age of the patients who fell

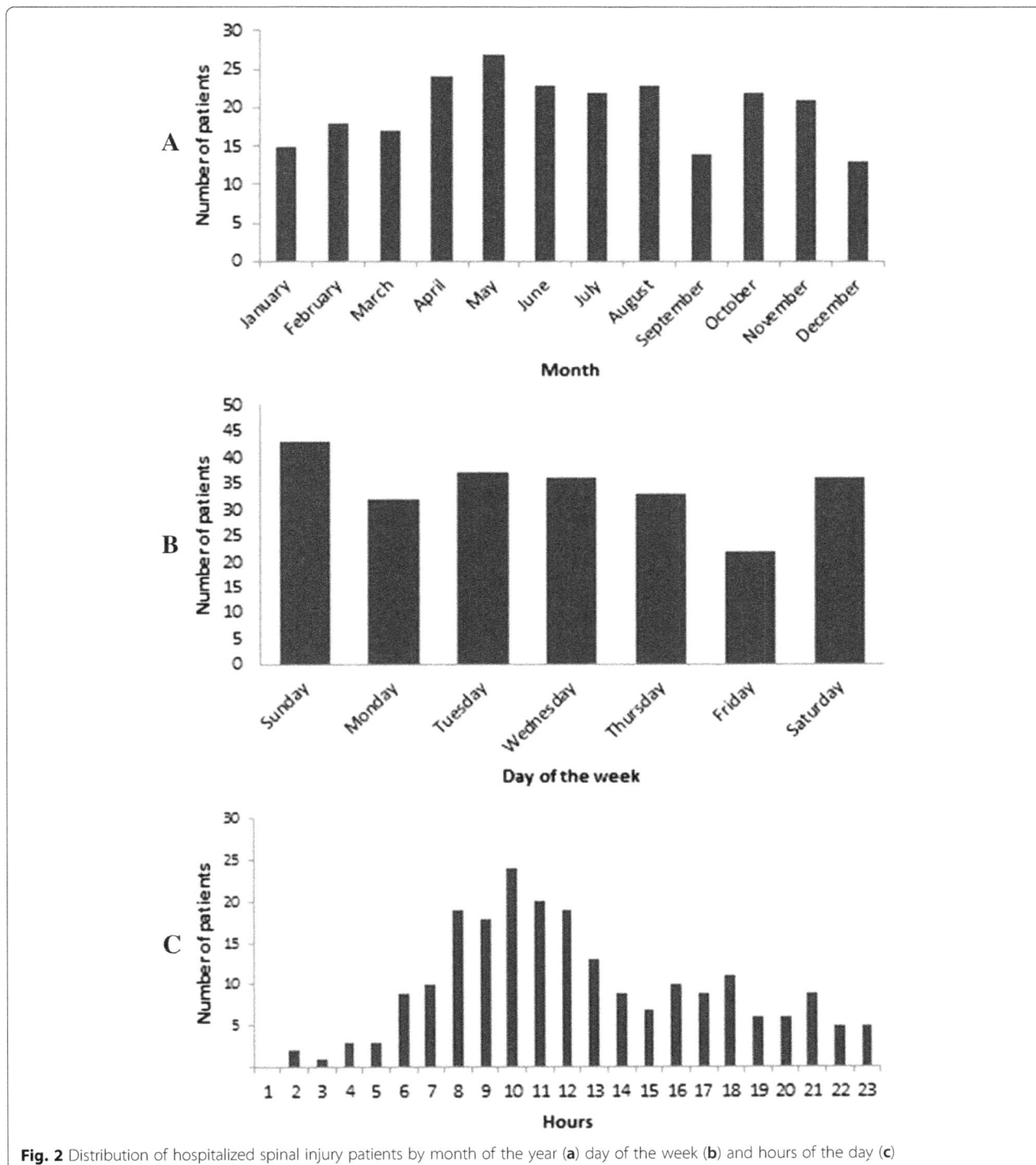

Fig. 2 Distribution of hospitalized spinal injury patients by month of the year (a) day of the week (b) and hours of the day (c)

at the same level was higher compared with other mechanisms. As described elsewhere, falls among elderly can cause serious injuries and death [29]. Hazards in physical environment at home are importact risk factors for falls [30]. We did not record any sport-related spine injury in our study, possibly because high risk sport activities as

diving, skiing or gymnastics are not common in Al Ain City.

Similar to others, the most common region that had spinal fractures in our study was the lumbar region [8]. Cervical spinal fractures are more common in patients injured in traffic, while lumbar spinal fractures are more

Table 4 Associated injured body regions of hospitalized spinal-injured patients, Al Ain, United Arab Emirates, 2003–2006 (n = 239)

Region	Number	%	AIS[a]
Head and Neck	33	13.8	2 (1–4)
Face	20	8.4	1 (1–2)
Chest	56	23.4	3 (1–4)
Abdomen	15	6.3	2 (1–3)
Upper extremity	52	21.7	2 (1–3)
Lower extremity	40	16.7	2 (1–3)
External	4	1.67	1 (1–1)

[a] Data presented as numbers (%) and median (range)

common in falls [8,25]. The transition between the cervical and the thoracic spine has a weak muscular support and is more prone to the acceleration/deceleration impact force during a traffic crash [31]. On the other hand, thoracolumbar junction has a defined muscular structure protecting against distraction forces, but more prone to compression fractures, due to the high pressure on the vertebral body [31]. There is an observed increase in the proportion of complete lumbosacral spine cord injuries because of the progressive increase of falls [23]. It is possible that, with improved traffic safety and increased age of the population, the importance of fall prevention, including prophylaxis of osteoporosis, will increase.

Mortality in our study (2.1 %) was lower than those reported from China (3.4 %) [32], Canada (4 %) [23] or Australia (5.2 %) [24]. All patients who died in our study were injured in traffic collisions. Spinal fractures in road traffic collisions had a higher mortality when compared with falls [25].

The modern traffic design with 2–3 highway lanes in one direction inside Al Ain City with many roundabouts is a high risk for rollover traffic crashes of popular sport utility vehicles leading to the ejection and spine injury of the unrestrained occupants [15]. Seat belt compliance is low in the UAE [15,33]. Proper restraint use may reduce the risk of spine injury and fatality during traffic crashes [34]. The most difficult challenge in the UAE is to

Table 5 Distribution of anatomical regions of spinal fractures

Region	Number	%	Paraplegia	%
Cervical alone	28	11.7	0	
Thoracic alone	46	19.2	2	0.8
Lumbar alone	136	57	4	1.7
Cervical and thoracic	7	3	2	0.8
Cervical and lumbar	3	1.2	0	
Thoracic and lumbar	19	7.9	3	1.3
Total	239	100	11	4.6

change the behavior of the road users [10]. Comprehensive restraint legislation with primary enforcement and culturally appropriate education is a necessity [10].

The high incidence of occupational injuries in the UAE is caused by the large recruitment of workers, especially from Indian subcontinent, and lack of appropriate implementation of safety precautions [10,35]. Occupational setting, such as high construction sites or date palm farms posess a high risk for falls from heights in the UAE. Monitoring of occupational injuries with adequate safety inspections and training is important not only for major employers, but also for smaller entities and farms [10].

Home injury prevention is lacking in the UAE. Due to the hot climate, homes are often built with hard surfaces as marble or tiles. These surfaces do not absorb high impact during falls which increases the risk for injury. Ceilings are high so as to improve cooling. Activities, such as exchanging the electrical bulbs or hanging curtains demand using high ladders and posess a serious fall risk. Popular small carpets at homes without antislippery rubber mat are risk for fall in the elderly in our community. A proper evidence-based architectural design can prevent falls [36].

There are certain limitations in our study. Our study included only patients who were admitted to the hospital for more than 24 h and those who died in the Emergency Department. Patients with more severe spine injuries may have died before arriving to the hospital. Furthermore, our study was based in Al Ain City with less construction sites and lower buildings than Abu Dhabi or Dubai cities. All of this may limit the generalizability of our results for the whole UAE.

It is worthy to note that our data represent the period before 2007 which may not exactly reflect the recent situation. These data were retrieved from Al Ain Hospital Trauma Registry which was the only available trauma registry in our country. It was a specific time limited research project supported by the UAE University. Nevertheless, we think that risk factors for spine injuries in our city did not change since then.

Furthermore, our study is an epidemiological study and not a clinical study. Accordingly we did not stratify our patients by the spinal surgical type and technique [37]. Nevertheless, it is important to highlight that injury prevention is an important integral part of the duties of trauma surgeons. This should include defining injury risk factors, studying the effects of interventional studies on injury prevention, and support health-policy reform through proper research [38-40].

Conclusions

Traffic injuries and falls were the leading causes for spinal injury is the UAE. Expatriate males are at high risk for fall from height, UAE national males from traffic, and females for falls at the same level at homes. Prevention should focus on traffic and home injuries for UAE nationals and occupational safety for expatriate workers.

Competing interest
The authors declare that they have no competing interests.

Authors' contribution
Conceived and designed the experiments: MG HOE FAZ. Retrieved and coded the data: HOE. Analyzed the data: MG HOE FAZ. Wrote the paper: MG FAZ. Critically read the paper: MG HOE FAZ. Approved final version: MG HOE FAZ. All authors read and approved the final manuscript.

Funding
This study was supported by an Interdisciplinary UAE University grant (No. 02-07-8-1/4).

Author details
[1]Institute of Public Health, College of Medicine and Health Sciences, UAE University, Al Ain, United Arab Emirates. [2]Trauma Group, Department of Surgery, College of Medicine and Health Sciences, UAE University, Al Ain, United Arab Emirates.

References
1. Masood Z, Wardug GM, Ashraf J. Spinal injuries: experience of a local neurosurgical centre. Pak J Med Sci. 2008;24:368–71.
2. Chiu WT, Lin HC, Lam C, Chu SF, Chiang YH, Tsai SH. Review paper: epidemiology of traumatic spinal cord injury: comparisons between developed and developing countries. Asia Pac J Public Health. 2010;22:9–18. doi: 10.1177/1010539509355470.
3. Chen D, Apple Jr DF, Hudson LM, Bode R. Medical complications during acute rehabilitation following spinal cord injury–current experience of the Model Systems. Arch Phys Med Rehabil. 1999;80:1397–401.
4. McKinley WO, Gittler MS, Kirshblum SC, Stiens SA, Groah SL. Spinal cord injury medicine. 2. Medical complications after spinal cord injury: Identification and management. Arch Phys Med Rehabil. 2002;83(3 Suppl 1):S58–64. S90–8.
5. Pagliacci MC, Celani MG, Zampolini M, Spizzichino L, Franceschini M, Baratta S, et al. An Italian survey of traumatic spinal cord injury. The Gruppo Italiano Studio Epidemiologico Mielolesioni study. Arch Phys Med Rehabil. 2003;84:1266–75.
6. Post MW, van Leeuwen CM. Psychosocial issues in spinal cord injury: a review. Spinal Cord. 2012;50:382–9.
7. Cao Y, Massaro JF, Krause JS, Chen Y, Devivo MJ. Suicide mortality after spinal cord injury in the United States: injury cohorts analysis. Arch Phys Med Rehabil. 2014;95:230–1.
8. Wang H, Zhang Y, Xiang Q, Wang X, Li C, Xiong H, et al. Epidemiology of traumatic spinal fractures: experience from medical university-affiliated hospitals in Chongqing, China, 2001–2010. J Neurosurg Spine. 2012;17:459–68.
9. National Bureau of Statistics. Population estimates 2006–2010, United Arab Emirates. 2011. [http://www.uaestatistics.gov.ae/ReportDetailsEnglish/tabid/121/Default.aspx?ItemId¼1914&PTID¼104&MenuId¼1].
10. Grivna M, Aw TC, El-Sadeg M, Loney T, Sharif A, Thomsen J, et al. The legal framework and initiatives for promoting safety in the United Arab Emirates. Int J Inj Contr Saf Promot. 2012;19:278–89.
11. United Arab Emirates Census. Population Preliminary results 2005 by age and nationality. Adapted from: Preliminary Results of the General Census for Population, Housing and Establishments, United Arab Emirates 2005. [http://www.zu.ac.ae/library/html/UAEInfo/documents/CensusResults2005.pdf]
12. Al Ain Hospital. [http://www.seha.ae/seha/en/Pages/HospitalDetail.aspx?HospitalId=22]
13. Shaban S, Eid HO, Barka E, Abu-Zidan FM. Towards a national trauma registry for the United Arab Emirates. BMC Res Notes. 2010;3:187.
14. Association of the Advancement of Automotive Medicine. Abbreviated Injury Scale. Barrington, IL: Association for the Advancement of Automotive Medicine; 1998.
15. Grivna M, Eid HO, Abu-Zidan FM. Pediatric and youth traffic-collision injuries in Al Ain, United Arab Emirates: A prospective study. PLoS One. 2013;8:e68636 8.
16. Hefny AF, Eid HO, Abu-Zidan FM: Pedestrian injury in United Arab Emirates. Int J Inj Contr Saf Promot 2014 Apr 10. [Epub ahead of print] doi:10.1080/17457300.2014.884143
17. Munro BH. Selected nonparametric techniques. In: Munro BH, editor. Statistical methods for health care research. 4th ed. New York: Lippincott; 2001. p. 97–121.
18. Otom AS, Doughan AM, Kawar JS, Hattar EZ. Traumatic spinal cord injuries in Jordan–an epidemiological study. Spinal Cord. 1997;35:253–5.
19. Dryden DM, Saunders LD, Rowe BH, May LA, Yiannakoulias N, Svenson LW, et al. The epidemiology of traumatic spinal cord injury in Alberta, Canada. Can J Neurol Sci. 2003;30:113–21.
20. Jackson AB, Dijkers M, Devivo MJ, Poczatek RB. A demographic profile of new traumatic spinal cord injuries: change and stability over 30 years. Arch Phys Med Rehabil. 2004;85:1740–8.
21. Shingu H, Ikata T, Katoh S, Akatsu T. Spinal cord injuries in Japan: a nationwide epidemiological survey in 1990. Paraplegia. 1994;32:3–8.
22. Ning GZ, Yu TQ, Feng SQ, Zhou XH, Ban DX, Liu Y, et al. Epidemiology of traumatic spinal cord injury in Tianjin, China. Spinal Cord. 2011;49:386–90.
23. Kattail D, Furlan JC, Fehlings MG. Epidemiology and clinical outcomes of acute spine trauma and spinal cord injury: experience from a specialized spine trauma center in Canada in comparison with a large national registry. J Trauma. 2009;67:936–43.
24. Tee JW, Chan CH, Fitzgerald MC, Liew SM, Rosenfeld JV. Epidemiological trends of spine trauma: as Australian level 1 trauma centre study. Global Spine J. 2013;3:75–84.
25. Heidari P, Zarei MR, Rasouli MR, Vaccaro AR, Rahimi-Movaghar V. Spinal fractures resulting from traumatic injuries. Chin J Traumatol. 2010;13:3–9.
26. Tuma MA, Acerra JR, El-Menyar A, Al-Thani H, Al-Hassani A, Recicar JF, et al. Epidemiology of workplace-related fall from height and cost of trauma care in Qatar. Int J Crit Illn Inj Sci. 2013;3:3–7.
27. Al-Humaidi HM, Tan FH. Construction safety in Kuwait. Journal of Performance and Constructed Facilities. 2010;24:70–7.
28. Colantonio A, McVittie D, Lewko J, Yin J. Traumatic brain injuries in the construction industry. Brain Inj. 2009;23:873–8.
29. Sterling DA, O'Connor JA, Bonadies J. Geriatric falls: injury severity is high and disproportionate to mechanism. J Trauma. 2001;50:116–9.
30. Marshall SW, Runyan CW, Yang J, Coyne-Beasley T, Waller AE, Johnson RM, et al. Prevalence of selected risk and protective factors for falls in the home. Am J Prev Med. 2005;28:95–101.
31. Leucht P, Fischer K, Muhr G, Mueller EJ. Epidemiology of traumatic spine fractures. Injury. 2009;40:166–72.
32. Feng HY, Ning GZ, Feng SQ, Yu TQ, Zhou HX. Epidemiological profile of 239 traumatic spinal cord injury cases over aperiod of 12 years in Tianjin, China. J Spinal Cord Med. 2011;34:388–94.
33. Barss P, Al-Obthani M, Al-Hammadi A, Al-Shamsi H, El-Sadig M, Grivna M. Prevalence and issues in non-use of safety belts and child restraints in a high-income developing country: lessons for the future. Traffic Inj Prev. 2008;9:256–63.
34. Abbas AK, Hefny AF, Abu-Zidan FM. Seatbelts and road traffic collision injuries. World J Emerg Surg. 2011;6:18.
35. Barss P, Addley K, Grivna M, Stanculescu C, Abu-Zidan F. Occupational injury in the United Arab Emirates: epidemiology and prevention. Occup Med (Lond). 2009;59:493–8.
36. Phoon WO. Epidemiological transition in Asian countries and related health policy issues. Asia Pac J Public Health. 1989;3:139–44.
37. Stahel PF, VanderHeiden T, Flierl MA, Matava B, Gerhardt D, Bolles G, et al. The impact of a standardized "spine damage–control" protocol for unstable thoracic and lumbar spine fractures in severely injured patients: a prospective cohort study. J Trauma Acute Care Surg. 2013;74:590–6.
38. American College of Surgeons. Injury Prevention and Control, https://www.facs.org/quality-programs/trauma/ipc (Accessed on 12th April 2015).
39. Royal Australasian College of Surgeons. Appendix to Policy on Trauma (injury) 2004, Royal Australasian College of Surgeons. 2004, pp: 7.
40. Eid HO, Abu-Zidan FM. Pedestrian injuries–related deaths: a global evaluation. World J Surg. 2015;39:776–81.

12

Prediction of blunt traumatic injuries and hospital admission based on history and physical exam

Alan L. Beal[1]*, Mark N. Ahrendt[3], Eric D. Irwin[3], John W. Lyng[3], Steven V. Turner[2], Christopher A. Beal[2], Matthew T. Byrnes[3] and Greg A. Beilman[2]

Abstract

Background: We evaluated the ability of experienced trauma surgeons to accurately predict specific blunt injuries, as well as patient disposition from the emergency department (ED), based only on the initial clinical evaluation and prior to any imaging studies. It would be hypothesized that experienced trauma surgeons' initial clinical evaluation is accurate for excluding life-threatening blunt injuries and for appropriate admission triage decisions.

Methods: Using only their history and physical exam, and prior to any imaging studies, three (3) experienced trauma surgeons, with a combined Level 1 trauma experience of over 50 years, predicted injuries in patients with an initial GCS (Glasgow Coma Score) of 14–15. Additionally, ED disposition (ICU, floor, discharge to home) was also predicted. These predictions were compared to actual patient dispositions and to blunt injuries documented at discharge.

Results: A total of 101 patients with 92 blunt injuries were studied. 43/92 (46.7 %) injuries would have been missed by only performing an initial history and physical exam ("Missed injury"). A change in treatment, though often minor, was required in 19/43 (44.2 %) of the missed injuries. Only 1/43 (2.3 %) of these "missed injuries" (blunt aortic injury) required surgery. Sensitivity, specificity, and accuracy for injury prediction were 53.2, 95.9, and 92.3 % respectively. Positive and negative predictive values were 53.8 and 95.8 % respectively. Prediction of disposition from the ED was 77. 8 % accurate. In 7/34 (20.6 %) patients, missed injuries led to changes in disposition. "Undertriage" occurred in 9/99 (9.1 %) patients (Predicted for floor but admitted to ICU). Additionally, 8/84 (9.5 %) patients predicted for floor admission were sent home from the ED; and 5/13 (38.5 %) patients predicted for ICU admission were actually sent to the floor after complete evaluations, giving an "overtriage" rate of 13/99 (13.1 %) patients.

Conclusions: In a neurologically-intact group of trauma patients, experienced trauma surgeons would have missed 46. 7 % of the actual injuries, based only on their history and physical exam. Once accurate diagnoses of injuries were completed, usually with the help of CT scans, admission dispositions changed in 20.6 % of patients. Treatment changes occurred in 44.2 % of the missed injuries, though usually minimal. Broad elimination of early imaging studies in alert, blunt trauma patients cannot be advocated.

Keywords: Trauma, Injuries, Triage, Imaging

Abbreviations: BAL, Blood alcohol level; CT, Computed tomography; CXR, Chest X-ray; EAST, Eastern association for the surgery of trauma; ED, Emergency Department; GCS, Glasgow coma score; ICU, Intensive care unit; ISS, Injury severity score; NEXUS, National emergency radiologic utilization study; TRAINS, Traumatic aortic injury score

* Correspondence: Alan.beal@northmemorial.com
[1]North Memorial Medical Center, 3300 Oakdale Ave N, Robbinsdale, MN 55431, USA
Full list of author information is available at the end of the article

Background

Diagnostic accuracy and efficiency are important in the initial trauma evaluation. Goals also include limitation of patients' time spent in the ED, compiling an accurate list of injuries, and making rapid, safe, disposition decisions; i.e.; operating room, ICU, floor or discharge to home. Early and aggressive imaging of the trauma patient, using plain films, ultrasound, and a wide variety of CT scans has become commonplace in the trauma evaluation. The yield of CT scans varies in blunt trauma victims, creating inconsistent recommendations for their use, especially in alert patients [1–3]. We returned to the basics of clinical medicine in this prospective study and evaluated the accuracy of the history and physical exam when carried out by experienced trauma surgeons on a group of awake patients. We also tried to predict the emergency department disposition of these patients, hoping to speed up their admission process.

Methods and study design

The study was reviewed by the North Memorial IRB, and waiver of consent requirements was granted. The study was conducted by three trauma surgeons with similar levels of training and experience. All surgeons completed surgical residencies between 1988 and 1994, and have a combined experience of 56 years at our Level 1 trauma center. A total of 101 non-consecutive blunt trauma patients with a Glasgow Coma Score of 14–15 were evaluated over nine (9) months, prior to completion of any radiologic imaging. Specific injuries were predicted, based only on the history and physical exam. Patients were excluded if any imaging studies, including ultrasonography, had been completed prior to the trauma surgeons' evaluation. Patients underwent collection of medical history and a physical examination, and specific injuries were then predicted in each of eleven (11) categories, using a standardized prediction worksheet. The patient's emergency department disposition was also predicted and recorded prior to imaging studies; i.e., ICU, floor, or discharge to home. "Missed injuries" were defined as those not predicted by the trauma surgeon on the admission prediction worksheet, but eventually diagnosed during the hospitalization. Most patients had multiple imaging studies after predictions had been made. All missed injuries, incorrect diagnoses and incorrect patient dispositions were recorded. Any change in treatment plans were noted for each of the missed injuries.

Sensitivity, specificity, accuracy, as well as positive and negative predictive values was determined for all predicted injuries. The overall accuracy, "overtriage" and "undertriage" rates were determined for the predicted dispositions to the ICU, floor or discharge to home. A comparison of patients' ages and ISS was made between the group with "missed injuries" and those without missed injuries, using a paired t test method. Those patients with a GCS of 14 were compared in the same two groups ("Missed injury vs no missed injury) with those with GCS of 15, using a two-tailed Fisher's exact test.

Results

Table 1 gives a breakdown of the number of patients seen and entered into the study by each surgeon, as well as the number of injuries diagnosed and "missed" by each of them. Table 2 gives basic demographics of the 101 blunt trauma patients.

Table 3 gives details of the three combined surgeons' accuracies in each of the eleven injury categories addressed on the prediction worksheet.

Combined, the surgeons' overall outcome in predicting injuries based on the initial history and physical exam includes a 53.2 sensitivity, 95.9 specificity, 95.8 negative predictive value, and a 53.8 % positive predictive value, for an overall accuracy of 92.3 %.

Results of the predictions for the disposition of the patients are shown in Table 4. A total of 9/84 (10.7 %) patients predicted for a floor admission were instead admitted to the ICU due to their missed injuries ("undertriage"). Also, 8/84 (9.5 %) patients predicted to go to the floor were actually able to go home after their evaluations, while 5/13 (38.5 %) predicted to go to the ICU were able to go to the floor, for an "overtriage" rate of 13/97 (13.4 %). Overall disposition accuracy was 77.8 %.

A total of 43 "missed injuries" occurred in 34 patients. Nine patients each had two missed injuries. The patients with missed injuries had a range of ages from 11–88. The mean age of those patients with missed injuries was older than those with accurate diagnoses (42.8 vs 34.5; $p < 0.03$) There were only two missed injuries in the eight pediatric patients, a clavicle fracture in an 11 year old, and a minimal wrist fracture in a 14 year old.

A total of 6/34 (17.6 %) patients with missed injuries had a GCS of 14, while 4/67 (6.0 %) without missed injuries had GCS of 14. ($p = 0.08$) The mean injury severity score (ISS) of the group with missed injuries was 12.6, as compared to an ISS of 5.7 in those patients without missed injuries. ($p < 0.0001$) Surprisingly, only 4/34 (11.8 %) with missed injuries had elevated blood alcohol levels (BAL) at the time of the initial evaluation.

Table 1 Injuries and missed injuries

Surgeon	# of Pts	Total # of injuries	# of Pts with no injuries	# of missed injuries
Surgeon A	18	17	7	9
Surgeon B	45	46	16	15
Surgeon C	38	29	15	19
Total	101	92	38	43

Table 2 Patient Demographics

Demographics	Data
Sex	Males: $N = 70$ Females: $N = 31$
Age	Mean: 38.1 Range: 3-88
ISS	Mean: 8.0 Range: 0-38
GCS Score	GCS of 15: $N = 91$ GCS of 14: $N = 10$

Table 4 Prediction of Patient Disposition

Predicted disposition	Actual disposition: floor	Actual disposition: ICU	Actual disposition: home
Floor	67	9	8
ICU	5	8	0
Home	0	0	2

Overall, 22/97 (22.7 %) patients had a change in their disposition compared to that predicted. Two patients did not have predictions made at the initial evaluation. Change in admission disposition due to at least one missed injury occurred in 7/34 (20.6 %) patients.. Change in therapy occurred in 19/43 (44.2 %) missed injuries, though most of these treatment changes were modest; e.g., extremity splinting, frequent neurological exam; analgesia. Only one patient required surgery for an injury not predicted by the initial history and physical exam: a blunt thoracic aortic injury.

Table 5 lists the number of missed injuries by categories and whether there were changes in treatment of disposition based on missed injuries.

Only 1/6 of the missed traumatic brain injuries would be considered significant. None of the cervical spine fractures were considered serious, with only one needing a cervical collar. Two of 3 liver injuries were not predicted and both of these patients had short ICU admissions and successful non-operative management. Both of the "missed" pelvic fractures were minor. The surgeons did not predict 8/12 of the thoracolumbar fractures, but none of these fractures required surgery, and only 2 required orthotics. All of the "missed" extremity, clavicular and scapular fractures were modest; none required surgery. Both of the vascular injuries were not suspected on the history and physical. The unilateral vertebral artery injury

was treated with anti-platelet therapy. The blunt thoracic aortic injury required an endovascular stent graft.

Discussion

The history and physical exam can serve an important role in most trauma work-ups. Advanced Trauma and Life Support (ATLS) programs emphasize the use of a history and exam during both the primary and secondary surveys. Treatment of suspected life-threatening injuries can occur based only on the physical exam [4].

For this study, we challenged our most experienced trauma surgeons to prospectively predict injuries, as well as the patients' emergency department (ED) disposition, prior to any imaging studies being completed. Evaluating a group of alert trauma patients (GCS 14–15) and knowing the accuracy of our predictions is a first step in potentially reducing the number of imaging studies, while decreasing patient time spent in the ED. In our study, however, 43/92 (46.7 %) injuries would have been missed if only the history and exam had been used for initial definitive diagnoses ("Missed injury").

The reasons for our high missed injury rate are not clear. By choosing our most experienced surgeons, the impact of the inexperience factor was reduced. Complacence or inattention to detail in the history and physicals may have occurred despite their significant experience. In our institution, the trauma surgeons do not have regular

Table 3 Accuracy of Predicting Injuries with H/P

Injury	TP[1]	FP[2]	TN[3]	FN[4]	Sens[5]	Spec[6]	NPV[7]	PPV[8]	Accur[9]
Brain	3	6	86	6	33.3	93.5	93.5	33.3	88.1
Cervical Fracture	1	4	92	4	20.0	95.8	95.8	20.0	92.1
Rib Fractures	7	9	78	7	50.0	89.7	91.8	43.8	84.2
Pneumothorax	1	1	96	3	25.0	99.0	97.0	50.0	96.0
Solid organ injury	1	4	94	2	33.3	95.9	97.9	20.0	94.1
Pelvic Fracture	4	4	91	2	66.7	97.8	97.8	50.0	94.1
T/L Spine Fracture	3	4	85	8	27.2	95.5	91.4	42.9	87.1
Extremity Fracture	22	6	68	5	81.5	91.9	93.2	78.6	89.1
Clavicle Fracture	5	1	91	4	55.6	98.9	95.8	83.3	95.0
Vascular Injury	0	0	99	2	0	100	98.0	0	98.0
Spinal Cord Injury	2	3	96	0	100	96.7	100	40.0	97.0
Total	49	42	976	43	53.2	95.9	95.8	53.8	92.3

[1]TP True positive, [2]FP False positive, [3]TN True negative, [4]FN False negative, [5]Sens Sensitivity, [6]Spec Specificity, [7]NPV Negative predictive value, [8]PPV Positive predictive value, [9]Accur Accuracy

Table 5 Numbers of "Missed Injuries" by Type

Injury type	N = 43	+Change Rx	+Change disposition
Traumatic Brain Injuries	6	3	3
Cervical Spine Fractures	4	1	0
Ribs/Sternum	7	4	1
Pneumothoraces	3	0	1
Solid Organ Injuries	2	1	0
Pelvic Fractures	2	0	0
Spine Fractures	8	2	0
Extremity Fractures	5	4	0
Clavicle/Scapular Fractures	4	2	0
Vascular	2	2	2

house staff support and remain the frontline decision-makers for our trauma patients. In the modern trauma evaluation, ongoing reliance on imaging studies, such as CT scans, certainly could lead to less focus and concentration on the history and physical exam and erode these clinical skills.

We also identified poor "under/over"-triage rates when relying on the history and physical exam. Since our injury prediction accuracy was unacceptably low, this was likely the major cause for the undertriage rate for patient dispositions.

The injury severity score (ISS) was higher in the 34 patients with missed injuries (12.6 vs 5.7; $p < .0001$). This suggests that the unidentified injuries, or the associated pain, could have been a confounding factor in accurately assessing the extent of injury. The ISS is determined retrospectively by the trauma registrars and thus would not have changed based on our definition of a "missed injury".

The Glasgow Coma Score (GCS) of the two groups (missed injuries vs. no missed injuries) was not significantly different (14.8 vs 14.7). However, 6/34 (17.6 %) patients with missed injuries had a GCS of 14, while only 2/67 (3.0 %) patients without missed injuries had a GCS of 14. ($p = 0.08$). Though not significant, the trend here between differences in mental status could have played a role in the overall accuracy of our history and physical exams.

The mean age of those patients with "missed injuries" was older than those with accurate diagnoses (42.8 vs 34.5: $p < 0.03$). It is not unusual for elderly patients to have abnormal pain thresholds in a variety of clinical scenarios. This could have had an effect on the history and physical exams of our patients.

It did not appear that alcohol played an important role in our diagnoses of injuries. A total of 14/50 (28 %) patients in the group without missed injuries had elevated blood alcohol levels (BAL). Only 4/35 (11.4 %) of patients in the group with "missed injuries" had elevated BAL ($p = 0.10$).

The study was originally designed to have a wider range of clinicians (medical students, surgical interns and critical care fellows) also make predictions in order to gather data from clinicians with a more varied range experiences however their rotations were relatively short and the number of evaluations completed by these clinicians was very small. Given the limited number of surgeons' experiences within this study, it is possible that the accuracy of the predictions cannot be extrapolated to other trauma centers or surgeons. Results from this study indicate that a full evaluation, including imaging, in trauma patients will provide the most beneficial care plan, however further investigations are required to confirm these findings.

A number of studies have addressed the diagnostic accuracy of the history/physical in a variety of traumatic injuries. None have used a small, consistent and experienced group of clinicians, as we did in this study. Many have employed retrospective chart reviews, rather than a prospective approach.

Hoping to reduce the number of CT scans in blunt trauma patients, Tillou, Cryer and colleagues would have missed almost 17 % of injuries with use of their initial clinical evaluation [5]. Even in awake patients with a normal exam and stable hemodynamics, Salim et al. found "clinically significant findings" in 3.5 % of head CT's, 5.1 % of cervical CT's, 7.1 % of abdominal CT's and 19.6 % of chest CT scans. These findings changed patient management in 19 % of the patients [6].

Previous studies of traumatic brain injuries report up to a 20 % rate of abnormal head CT's and a 5 % need for craniotomy, even with a normal clinical exam [7–9]. "The Canadian head CT rule" and the "New Orleans criteria" remain the best predictors of clinically-significant brain injuries in alert patients [10–12].

Clinical criteria to rule out cervical spine injuries have been evaluated. The National Emergency Radiologic Utilization Study (NEXUS) included over 34,000 patients in 21 centers, while the "Canadian C spine rule" prospectively developed clinical criteria to accurately rule out cervical injuries [13, 14]. These studies were the foundation for other more recent recommendations to help reduce the number of imaging studies needed, while simplifying the cervical evaluations in both adults and children [15–19].

The history and exam can be quite accurate for diagnoses in blunt chest injuries in both adults and children, arguing for fewer imaging studies [20–24]. Blunt abdominal trauma diagnoses can be challenging using only the history/physical. Patients with subjective symptoms and positive physical findings, such as bruising and tenderness, will have intra-abdominal injuries in only about 20 % of cases [25, 26]. On the other hand, the incidence of actual injuries with a negative exam is also reported to be up to

20 % [4, 25–32]. Other factors such as distracting injuries, low GCS and alcohol intoxication can affect the accuracy of the physical exam [26, 30, 33]. Physical exam in children has been shown to be more sensitive, but is still challenging without the support of other modalities such as ultrasound [34, 35].

Bedside clinical assessment for pelvic fractures can be sensitive in the alert patient [36]. False negative exams are present in 1-7 % of patients with the appropriate mechanism of injury. Physical exam can sometimes be more sensitive than plain x-rays [37, 38].

An in-depth review of the accuracy of the history/physical in diagnoses of thoracolumbar fractures found conflicting results [39]. Several reports support the premise that the lack of symptoms and tenderness predicts a very low risk for fractures [40, 41]. A prospective, predictive study by Holmes and colleagues supports these findings in alert patients [42]. Diagnostic guidelines for thoracolumbar spine evaluations have been established by the Eastern Association for Surgery of Trauma (EAST) [43]. On the other hand, 20-50 % of these fractures have been reported to have no symptoms or physical findings, even in alert patients [44–46].

Musculoskeletal injuries historically have been the most commonly missed traumatic injuries [47, 48]. The incidence of missed injuries or delayed diagnoses of musculoskeletal trauma has been reported to be from 1.3-39 %, with the higher rates seen in the more severely injured, and especially in those with altered mental status [48–51]. More than 20 % of these missed injuries can be clinically significant [52]. The usefulness of the clinical exam in diagnosis of musculoskeletal trauma has not been widely studied, and available data are mostly from studies of low energy, isolated injuries, often seen in ambulatory patients; e.g., elbow, wrist, hand [53–56].

While a great deal has been written about the evaluation and management of penetrating vascular injuries, blunt vascular trauma has been less well-studied. Blunt arterial injuries comprise only about 20 % of arterial trauma and can present with minimal clinical findings [57]. The mechanism or pattern of injury may be the only factor to make one suspicious for arterial injury. Blunt thoracic aortic injuries rarely have a blood pressure differential between the arms and legs. Even CXR's are normal in 7.3-23 % of those with blunt thoracic aortic injuries [57]. A "traumatic aortic injury score" (TRAINS) has been reported, but relies more on the chest x-ray and the diagnosis of other associated injuries, rather than on the history and exam [58].

Clinical risk factors for a blunt carotid or vertebral artery injury were recently reported in a Western Trauma Association critical decision paper [59]. Unfortunately, up to 20 % of patients with such injuries have none of these risk factors [60]. Emphasizing the importance of timely and accurate diagnoses, the EAST group published practice management guidelines for blunt cerebrovascular injuries, and cite an 80 % morbidity and 40 % mortality rate if neurologic symptoms develop from these injuries [61].

Conclusion

If only a history and physical exam is used for diagnosis in an alert group of trauma patients (GCS 14–15), experienced trauma surgeons at our hospital missed 46.7 % of their injuries. The reasons for these inaccurate clinical predictions are not clear, though the average injury severity score was higher and the age of the patients greater in those with missed injuries. This same approach to predicting a trauma patient's hospital disposition was 77.8 % accurate, with 9.1 % of patients being "undertriaged" to the floor. Due to these results, though many of the "missed" injuries were minor and often did not require a change in treatment, we cannot advocate a broad elimination of early imaging studies, even in alert trauma patients.

Acknowledgments
Not applicable.

Authors' contributions
ALB conceived the project, and participated in the development of the study design, data acquisition, and writing of the manuscript. EDI, MNA, MTB and GAB contributed to study design, and also participated in data acquisition and interpretation. SVT and CAB participated in data analysis and interpretation of the data. ALB, GAB and JWL contributed to the critical review and editing of the manuscript. All authors read and approved of the final manuscript.

Competing interests
The authors declare that they have no competing interests.

Author details
¹North Memorial Medical Center, 3300 Oakdale Ave N, Robbinsdale, MN 55431, USA. ²University of Minnesota, Minnesota, USA. ³North Memorial Medical Center, Minnesota, USA.

References
1. Sampson MA, Colquhoun KB, Hennessy NL. Computed tomography whole body imaging in multi-trauma: 7 years experience;". Clin Radiol. 2006;61:365–9.
2. Millo NZ, Plewes C, Rowe BH, Low G. Appropriateness of CT of the chest, abdomen, and pelvis in motorized blunt force trauma patients without signs of significant injury. AJR Am J Roentgenol. 2011;197:1393–8.
3. Milia D, Brasel K. Current use of CT in the evaluation and management of injured patients. Surg Clinics North Am. 2011;91:233.
4. American College of Surgeons. Advanced Trauma Life Support Student Manual-9th Ed. Chicago: American College of Surgeons; 2012.
5. Tillou A, Cryer HM, et al. Is the use of pan-computed tomography for blunt trauma justified? A prospective evaluation. J Trauma. 2009;67(4):779–87.
6. Salim A, Demetriades D, et al. Whole body imaging in blunt multisystem trauma patients without obvious signs of injury: Results of a prospective study. Arch Surg. 2006;141:468–75.

7. Harnan SE, Goodacre SW, et al. Clinical decision rules for adults with minor head injury: a systematic review. J Trauma. 2011;71:245–51.
8. Stein SC, Ross SE. The value of computed tomographic scans in patients with low-risk head injuries. Neurosurgery. 1990;26:638–40.
9. Shackford SR, et al. The clinical utility of computed tomographic scanning, and neurologic examination in the management of patients with minor head injuries. J Trauma. 1992;33:385–94.
10. Stiell IG, CCC Study Group, et al. The Canadian CT head rule for patients with minor head injury. Lancet. 2001;357:1391–96.
11. Stiell IG, Wells GA, et al. Comparison of the Canadian CT head rule and the New Orleans criteria in patients with minor head injury. JAMA. 2005;294:1511–18.
12. Haydel MJ, DeBlieux PM. Indications for computed tomography in patients with minor head injury. N Engl J Med. 2000;343:100–5.
13. Hoffman JR, NEXUS Group, et al. Validity of a set of clinical criteria to rule out injury to the cervical spine in patients with blunt trauma. N Engl J Med. 2000;343:94–9.
14. Stiell IG, et al. The Canadian C-spine rule for radiography in alert and stable trauma patients. JAMA. 2001;286:1841–48.
15. Stiell IG, Wells DA, et al. The Canadian C-spine rule versus the NEXUS low-risk criteria in patients with trauma. N Engl J Med. 2003;349:2510–8.
16. Stiell IG, Clement CM, et al. Implementation of the Canadian C-spine rule: prospective 12 center cluster randomized trial. BMJ. 2009;339:b4146.
17. Sanchez B, Waxman K, et al. Cervical spine clearance in blunt trauma: Evaluation of a computed tomography-based protocol. J Trauma. 2005;59:179–83.
18. Gonzalez RP, Rodning CB, et al. Clincal examination in complement with computed tomography scan: an effective method for identification of cervical spine injury. J Trauma. 2009;67:1297–304.
19. Viccellio P, Simon H, NEXUS Group, et al. A prospective multicenter study of cervical spine injury in children. Pediatrics. 2001;108:E20.
20. Brink M, Blickman JG, et al. Predictors of abnormal chest CT after blunt trauma: a critical appraisal of the literature. Clin Radiol. 2009;64:272–83.
21. Bokhari F, Barrett J, et al. Prospective evaluation of the sensitivity of physical examination in chest trauma. J Trauma. 2002;53:1135–8.
22. Rodriguez RM, Bjoring A, et al. A pilot study to derive clinical variables for selective chest radiography in blunt trauma patients. Ann Emerg Med. 2006;47:415–8.
23. Paydar P, Sharifian M, et al. The role of routine chest radiography in initial evaluation of stable blunt trauma patients. Am J Emerg Med. 2012;30:1–4.
24. Holmes JF, Kuppermann N, et al. A clinical decision rule for identifying children with thoracic injuries after blunt torso trauma. Ann Emerg Med. 2002;39:492–9.
25. Livingston DH, Malangoni MA, et al. Admission or observation is not necessary after a negative abdominal computed tomographic scan in patients with suspected blunt abdominal trauma: results of a prospective, multi-institutional trial. J Trauma. 1998;44:273–80.
26. Rodriguez A, Shatney CH, et al. Recognition of intra-abdominal injury in blunt trauma victims. A prospective study comparing physical examination with peritoneal lavage. Am Surg. 1982;48:457–9.
27. Nishijima DK, Holmes JF, et al. Does this adult patient have a blunt intra-abdominal injury?'. JAMA. 2012;307:1517–27.
28. Poletti PA, Mermillod B, et al. Blunt abdominal trauma patients: Can organ injury be excluded without performing computed tomography? J Trauma. 2004;57:1072–81.
29. Schauer BA, Holmes JF, et al. Is definitive abdominal evaluation required in blunt trauma victims undergoing urgent extra-abdominal surgery? Acad Emerg Med. 2005;12:707–11.
30. Ferrera PC, Salluzzo RF, et al. Injuries distracting from intra-abdominal injuries after blunt trauma. Am J Emerg Med. 1998;16:145–9.
31. Holmes JF, Kupperman N, et al. Clinical prediction rules for identifying adults at very low risk for intra-abdominal injuries after blunt trauma. Ann Emerg Med. 2009;54:575–84.
32. Richards JR, Derlet RW. Computed tomography and blunt abdominal injury: patient selection based on examination, haematocrit and haematuria. Injury. 1997;28:181–5.
33. Self ML, Dunn E. The benefit of routine thoracic, abdominal, and pelvic computed tomography to evaluate trauma patients with closed head injuries. Am J Surg. 2003;186:609–13.
34. Suthers SE, Tuggle DW, et al. Surgeon-directed ultrasound for trauma is a predictor of intra-abdominal injury in children. Am Surg. 2004;70:164–7.
35. Karom O, LaScala G, et al. Blunt abdominal trauma in children: a score to predict the absence of organ injury. J Pediatr. 2009;154:912–7.
36. Sauerland S, Neugebauer EA, et al. The reliability of clinical examination in detecting pelvic fractures in blunt trauma patients: a meta-analysis. Arch Orthop Trauma Surg. 2004;124:123–8.
37. Salvino CK, Gamelli RL, et al. Routine pelvic x-ray studies in awake blunt trauma patients: a sensible policy? J Trauma. 1992;33:413–6.
38. Gonzalez RP, Bukhalo M, et al. The utility of clinical examination in screening for pelvic fractures in blunt trauma. J Am Coll Surg. 2002;194:121–5.
39. Kirkpatrick AW, McKevitt E. Thoracolumbar spine fractures: is there a problem?". Can J Surg. 2002;45:21–4.
40. Terregino CA, Hughes R, et al. Selective indications for thoracic and lumbar radiography in blunt trauma. Ann Emerg Med. 1995;26:126–9.
41. Hsu JM, Ellis AM, et al. Thoracolumbar fracture in blunt trauma patients: guidelines for diagnosis and imaging. Injury. 2003;34:426–33.
42. Holmes JF, Mower WR, et al. Prospective evaluation of criteria for obtaining thoracolumbar radiographs in trauma patients. J Emerg Med. 2003;24:1–7.
43. Diaz JJ, Cullinane DC, EAST Practice Management Guideline Committee, et al. Practice management guidelines for the screening of thoracolumbar spine fracture. J Trauma. 2007;63:709–18.
44. Cooper C, Rodriguez A, et al. Falls and major injuries are risk factors for thoracolumbar fractures: cognitive impairment and multiple injuries impede the detection of back pain and tenderness. J Trauma. 1995;38:692–6.
45. Meldon SW, Moettus LN. Thoracolumbar spine fractures: clinical presentation and the effect of altered sensorium and major injury. J Trauma. 1995;39:1110–4.
46. Inaba K, Demetriades D, et al. Clinical examination is insufficient to rule out thoracolumbar spine injuries. J Trauma. 2011;70:174–9.
47. Enderson BL, Maull KL. The tertiary trauma survey: a prospective study of missed injury. J Trauma. 1990;30:666–9.
48. Aaland MO, Smith K. Delayed diagnosis in a rural trauma center. Surgery. 1996;120:774–8.
49. Born CT, DeLong WG, et al. Delayed identification of skeletal injury in multisystem trauma: the "missed" fracture. J Trauma. 1989;29:1643–6.
50. Laasonen EM, Kivioja A. Delayed diagnosis of extremity injuries in patients with multiple injuries. J Trauma. 1991;31:257–60.
51. Ward WG, Nunley JA. Occult orthopaedic trauma in the multiply injured patient. J Orthop Trauma. 1991;5:308–12.
52. Pfeifer R, Pape HC. Missed injuries in trauma patients: a literature review. Patient Saf Surg. 2008;23:2.
53. Ballas MT, Mannarino F. Commonly missed orthopedic problems. Am Fam Phys. 1998;15:267–74.
54. Corley FG. Examination and assessment of injuries and problems affecting the elbow, wrist, and hand. Emerg Med Clin North Am. 1984;2:295–312.
55. Darracq MA, Panacek EA, et al. Preservation of active range of motion after acute elbow trauma predicts absence of elbow fracture. Am J Emerg Med. 2007;26:779–82.
56. Lennon RI, Alderson G, et al. Can a normal range of elbow movement predict a normal elbow xray? Emerg Med J. 2007;24:86–8.
57. Baker WE, Wassermann J. Unsuspected vascular trauma: blunt arterial injuries. Emerg Med Clin North Am. 2004;22:1081–98.
58. Mosquera VX, Cuenca JJ, et al. Traumatic aortic injury score (TRAINS): an easy and simple score for early detection of traumatic aortic injuries in major trauma patients with associated blunt chest trauma. Intensive Care Med. 2012;38:1487–96.
59. Biffl WL, Moore FA, et al. Western Trauma Association critical decisions in trauma: Screening for and treatment of blunt cerebrovascular injuries. J Trauma. 2009;67:1150–3.
60. Burlew CC, Biffl WL, et al. Blunt cerebrovascular injuries: redefining screening critieria in the era of noninvasive diagnosis. J Trauma Acute Care Surg. 2012;72:330–5.
61. Bromberg WJ, Vogel TR, et al. Blunt cerebrovascular injury practice management guidelines: the Eastern association for the surgery of trauma. J Trauma. 2010;68:471–7.

13

Metallothionein ameliorates burn sepsis partly via activation of Akt signaling pathway in mice

Keqin Luo[*], Huibao Long, Bincan Xu and Yanling Luo

Abstract

Introduction: Metallothioneins (MTs) are a family of cysteine-rich and low molecular-weight proteins that can regulate metal metabolism and act as antioxidants. Recent studies showed that MTs played a protective role in excessive inflammation and sepsis. However, the role of MTs in burn sepsis remains unclear. This study is designed to investigate the role of MTs in burn sepsis in an experimental mouse model.

Methods: MT-I/II knockout (–/–) mice on a C57BL/6 background and their wild-type (WT) littermates were randomly divided into sham burn, burn, burn sepsis, Zn treated and Zn-MT-2 treated groups. Levels of inflammatory cytokines were measured by enzyme-linked immunosorbent assay (ELISA). Myeloperoxidase (MPO) activity was detected by spectrophotometry. In in vitro study, exogenous MT was added to macrophages that stimulated with serum from burn sepsis mice with or without Akt inhibitor LY294002. The IL-1 β and IL-6 mRNA expression were detected by quantitative real-time polymerase chain reaction. The levels of Akt expression were determined by western blot.

Results: Burn sepsis induced significantly elevated levels of inflammatory cytokines in serum and increased inflammatory infiltration in the liver and lung. These effects were more prominent in MT (–/–) mice than in WT mice. Furthermore, exogenous MT-2 inhibited these elevated inflammatory response in both WT and MT (–/–) mice. MT-2 up-regulated Akt phosphorylation and abrogated the increase of IL-1β and IL-6 mRNA expression from macrophages that stimulated with burn sepsis serum. These effects of MT-2 were abolished in the presence of LY294002.

Conclusion: MT-2 ameliorates burn sepsis by attenuating inflammatory response and diminishing inflammatory organ damage, which is at least partly mediated by activation of Akt signaling pathway.

Keywords: Metallothioneins, Burn, Sepsis, Inflammation, Akt

Introduction

Sepsis remains the leading cause of death in patients who have suffered a severe burn injury, despite advances in antimicrobial therapies have been made [1]. The excessive proinflammatory response after burn is reported to be an important driving factor to the pathogenesis of sepsis [2]. Burn injury initially evokes a pro-inflammatory cascade, if uncontrolled, then subsequent development of systemic inflammatory response syndrome, susceptibility to sepsis, and multiple organ damage would occur, which will largely determine the morbidity and mortality of major burn injuries [3].

Metallothioneins (MTs), characterized by very small molecular weight, high cysteine content, and high affinity to divalent metals, were discovered from horse kidney about five decades ago [4, 5]. In mice, there are four main isoforms of MT: MT-I to MT-IV [6]. MT-I and MT-II are almost expressed in most organs, MT-III is mainly expressed in the brain and reproductive systems,

* Correspondence: keqinluodoc@126.com
Department of Emergency, SunYat-Sen memorial Hospital, Sun Yat-Sen University, 107 yan-jiangxi Road, Guangzhou 510120, China

and MT-IV is mainly seen in stratified squamous epithelial cells [7–9]. In humans, there are 10 functional isoforms of MTs, which can be subdivided into four groups: MT-I, MT-II, MT-III and MT-IV [10].

MTs have been known to exert diverse effects, such as regulating intracellular metal metabolism, protecting cells against oxidative damage, and serving as a reservoir of heavy metals [11]. Recently, MTs are reported to play important roles in many inflammatory conditions or diseases. For example, MTs inhibited the expression of proinflammatory proteins and protected against LPS induced lung injury and multiple organ damage [12]. Moreover, MTs are reported to play beneficial roles in brain inflammation [13], cardiac dysfunction in sepsis [14], and experimental colitis [15]. However, to date, the role of MTs in burn sepsis remains unclear.

In the present study, we hypothesized that MT may play a beneficial role against burn sepsis by inhibiting excessive inflammatory response and attenuating inflammatory organ damage. So we investigated the role of MT in burn sepsis using an experimental mouse model. Specifically, we chose a most commonly used subtype of MTs, Zn-MT-2 for the treatment intervention. Furthermore, we used Zn alone as a control because Zn was reported to display protective effects independent of MT-2 [16]. At last, we discussed whether the effect of MT was mediated by the Akt signaling using an Akt inhibitor 2-(4-Morpholinyl)-8-phenyl-4H-1-benzopyran-4-one hydrochloride (LY294002).

Methods and materials

Animals

MT-I/II double knockout (–/–) mice on a C57BL/6 background and their wild type (WT) littermates (male, 20 ± 1 g, 6–7 weeks old) were purchased from Model Animal Research Center of Nanjing University, Jiangsu, China. Mice were housed conventionally in a constant temperature (25 °C) and humidity (50–60 %), under a 12-h light/dark cycle. Mice were given free access to food and water, and were housed for 7 days before the experiments were started. The research protocol was approved by the Committee of Scientific Research of SunYat-Sen memorial Hospital, Guangzhou, China.

Experimental burn model

WT mice and MT-I/II (–/–) mice were randomly divided into the following groups: sham burn, burn, burn sepsis, Zn treated and Zn-MT-2 treated groups (10 mice in each group). Mice were anesthetized by intraperitoneal injection with 50 mg/kg pentobarbital sodium. The hairs of the dorsal area were removed. To create a full-thickness burn injury, mice were placed in a template immersing 25 % of the total body surface area (TBSA) in 100 °C water for 10 s [17]. Mice were then resuscitated by intraperitoneal injection with 40 mL/kg normal saline and placed in individual cages with free access to food and water. Mice in sham burn group were treated in the same manner except that they were immersed in room temperature water. To create a burn sepsis model, burned mice were subjected to intraperitoneal inoculation of Pseudomonas aeruginosa (2×105 CFU/ml, #27853, American Type Culture Collection, Manassas, VA, USA) at 1 day post burn as previously described [18]. Mice in Zn-MT-2 treated group were intraperitoneal injected with 0.5 mg/kg Zn-MT-2 (#M9542, Sigma-Aldrich, St. Louis, MO) twice a day, starting 1 day post burn immediately after the burn sepsis model was created, till 3 days post burn. Mice in Zn treated group received 35 μg/kg Zn (Because Zn-MT-2 contains 5–8 % Zn) as the same administration manner as Zn-MT-2 treated group. Animals were euthanized at 5 days post burn to assess the proinflammatory cytokines production and neutrophil infiltration in organs.

Myeloperoxidase (MPO) assay

MPO activities in the liver and lung were measured as previously described [19]. Tissue samples were homogenized and centrifuged. 20 ml of the supernatant was incubated with 200 μL of substrate buffer. The optical density changes were read at 460 nm over a 2 min period by a microplate reader. MPO activities were obtained using a standard curve of purified MPO in the kit. Data are presented as units of activity per gram of tissue (U/g).

Enzyme-linked immunosorbent assay (ELISA)

Interleukin (IL)-1β, IL-6, tumor necrosis factors (TNF)-α, and macrophage chemoattractant protein (MCP)-1 levels in serum were detected by commercially available ELISA kits (R&D Systems, Minneapolis, MN). All procedures were performed according to the manufacturer's instruction book.

Cell culture

After 6 days in culture, Raw 264.7 cells (ATCC, Manassas, VA) were stimulated with 10 % serum extracted from burn sepsis mice for 4 h. Cells were either co-cultured with Zn-MT-2 (2 μM, #M9542, Sigma-Aldrich, St. Louis, MO), equivalent concentrations of zinc sulfate, or Zn-MT-2 plus Akt inhibitor LY294002 (5 μM, #L9908, Sigma-Aldrich, St. Louis, MO). The mRNA expression of IL-1β and IL-6 were then detected by quantitative real-time polymerase chain reaction (PCR). Protein levels of Akt and phosphorylated Akt (pAkt) in cell lysates were determined by western blot.

Quantitative real-time PCR

Total RNA was extracted using the RNeasy 96 Kit (QIA-GEN, Hamburg, Germany). The cDNA was synthesized using a Superscript II reverse transcriptase (Invitrogen, Carlsbad, CA) and were amplified using the SYBR green PCR master mix (Applied Biosystems, Foster city, CA). Fluorescence was monitored and analyzed in an ABI 7500 system (Applied Biosystems, Foster city, CA). β-actin was used to normalize the data. All samples were analyzed in duplicate. The cycle threshold (Ct) values were obtained and the fold changes of gene expression were calculated by the $2^{-\Delta\Delta Ct}$ method [20]. The sequences of the primers for IL-1 β were Sense 5'-CTTCAGGCAGGCAGTATC-3' and Antisense 5'-CAG CAGGTTATCATCATCATC-3'. The sequences of the primers for IL-6 were Sense 5'- CGGAGAGGAGACTT CACA -3' and Antisense 5'- CTGTTAGGAGAGCAT TGGAA-3'. The sequences of the primers for intercellular adhesion molecule (ICAM)-1 and vascular cell adhesion molecule (VCAM)-1 were Sense 5'-GGCTGG CATTGTTCTCTA-3', Antisense 5'- TCCTCAGTCAC CTCTACC-3' and Sense 5'-GCGAGTCACCATTGTTC T-3', Antisense 5'- GCCACTGAATTGAATCTCTG-3', respectively. The sequences of the primers for β-actin were Sense 5'-GTCAGAAGGACTCCTATGTG-3' and Antisense 5'- ACGCAGCTCATTGTAGAAG-3'.

Western blot analysis

Protein levels in cell lysates were determined by bicinchoninic acid protein assay kit (Pierce Biotechnology, Rockford, IL). Protein was separated and transferred to a polyvinylidene difluoride membrane. The membranes were blocked and then incubated with anti-Akt (1:1000, # 9272, Cell Signaling Technology, Boston, MA) and anti-Phospho-Akt (Ser473) (1:1000, # 4060, Cell Signaling Technology). The membranes were then incubated with secondary antibody (1:2000; Invitrogen, Carlsbad, CA) for 1 h at room temperature. Immunoreactive bands were detected using an enhanced chemiluminescence reagent (Pierce Biotechnology) and exposed onto Kodak film (Eastman Kodak, Rochester, NY). Glyceraldehyde-3-phosphate dehydrogenase was used as a control. Band densities were quantified using Image J software (National Institutes of Health, Bethesda, MD).

Statistical analysis

Data were expressed as means ± standard deviations (SD). Statistical analysis was performed by using Student's t test or one-way analysis of variance followed by Tukey's test. A p value of less than 0.05 was considered statistically significant. GraphPad prism software V.6.01 for Windows (GraphPad Software, La Jolla, CA) was used for analyses.

Results

Effect of MT on inflammatory cytokines production

Burn sepsis induced profoundly elevated levels of IL-1 β, IL-6, TNF-α, and MCP-1 in serum. The increase of these inflammatory cytokines were more prominent in MT (−/−) mice than in WT mice. Exogenous administration of Zn-MT-2 significantly inhibited these cytokines production after burn sepsis. But administration of Zn alone

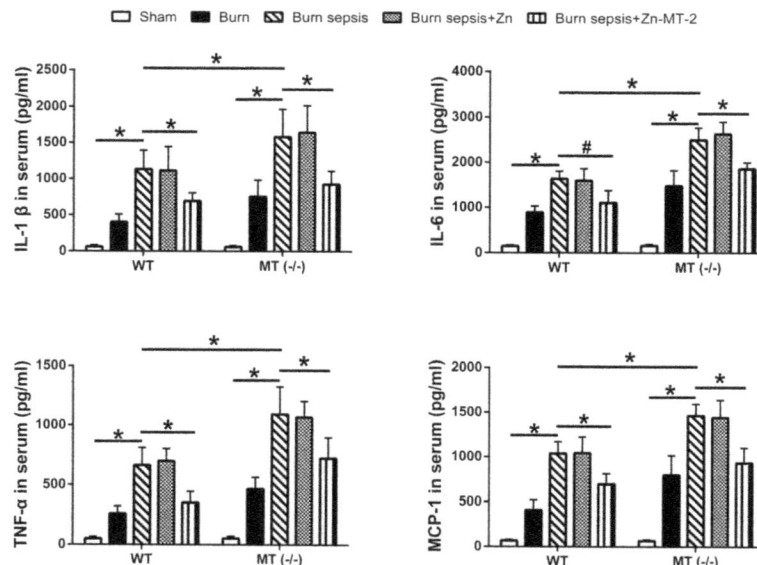

Fig. 1 IL-1β, IL-6, TNF-α, and MCP-1 levels in serum of WT and MT (−/−) mice were detected by ELISA. Data were presented as means ± SD, n = 10 mice/group, *p < 0.01, #p < 0.05

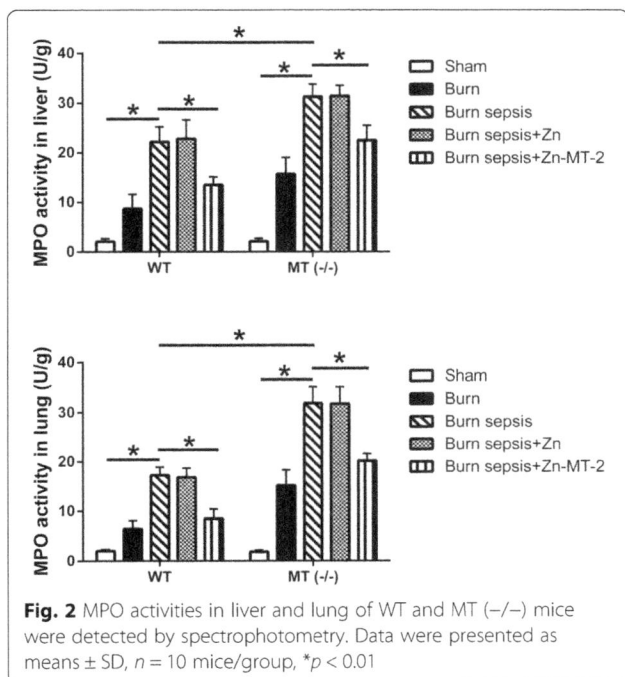

Fig. 2 MPO activities in liver and lung of WT and MT (−/−) mice were detected by spectrophotometry. Data were presented as means ± SD, $n = 10$ mice/group, $*p < 0.01$

had no significant effect on the increase of these inflammatory cytokine levels (Fig. 1).

Effect of MT on neutrophil infiltration in liver and lung

The MPO assay was performed to evaluate the neutrophil infiltration in liver and lung, the two organs that were among the mostly suffered from inflammatory damages after burn sepsis. Burn sepsis induced remarkably increased MPO activities in liver and lung. The increase of MPO activities were more prominent in MT (−/−) mice than in WT mice. Exogenous administration of Zn-MT-2 significantly decreased the MPO activities after burn sepsis. But administration of Zn alone had no significant effect on the increase of MPO activities (Fig. 2).

Effect of MT on adhesive molecule expressions in liver and lung

The mRNA expression of ICAM-1 and VCAM-1 in liver and lung were remarkably elevated after burn sepsis (Fig. 3). These increase of adhesive molecule expressions were more prominent in MT (−/−) mice than in WT mice. Exogenous administration of Zn-MT-2 significantly decreased the adhesive molecule expressions after burn sepsis. But administration of Zn alone had no significant effect on the increase of adhesive molecule expressions.

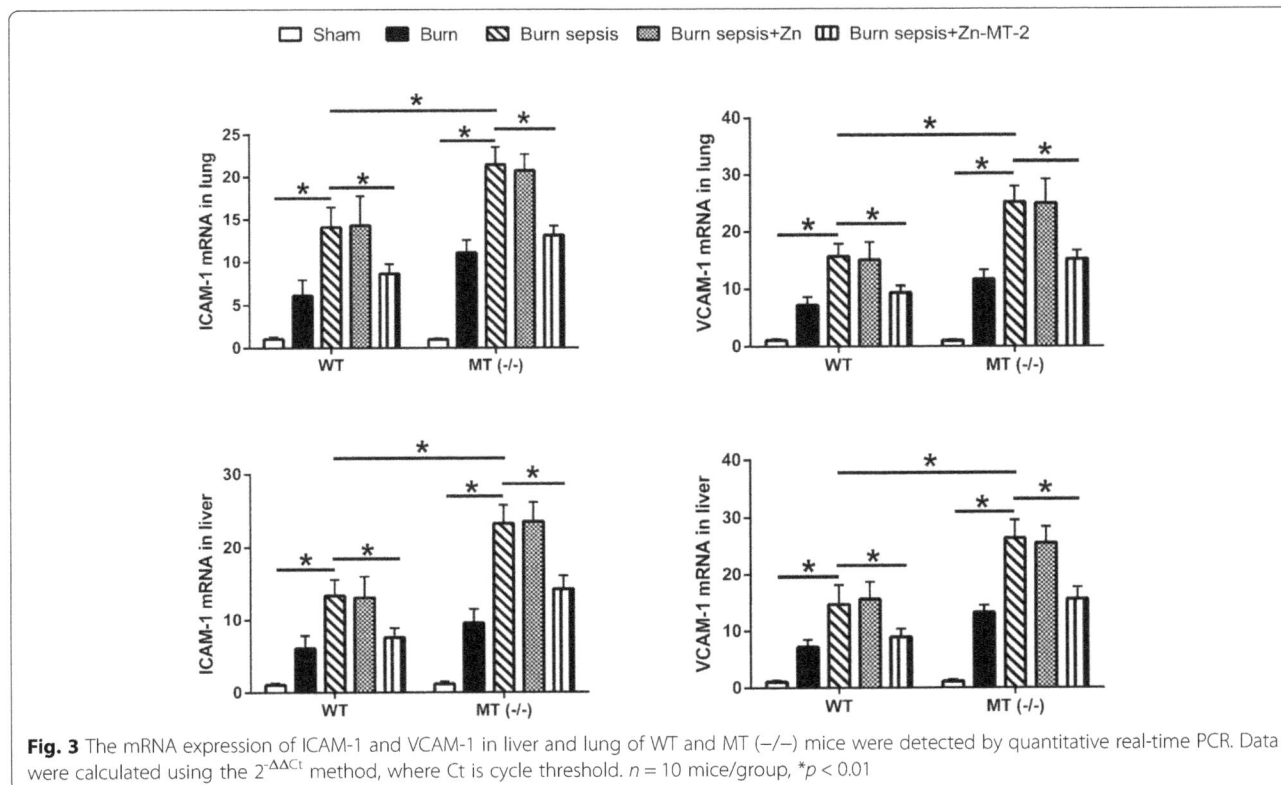

Fig. 3 The mRNA expression of ICAM-1 and VCAM-1 in liver and lung of WT and MT (−/−) mice were detected by quantitative real-time PCR. Data were calculated using the $2^{-\Delta\Delta Ct}$ method, where Ct is cycle threshold. $n = 10$ mice/group, $*p < 0.01$

The effect of MT was at least partly mediated by Akt signaling

The IL-1 β (Fig. 4a) and IL-6 (Fig. 4b) mRNA expression in Raw 264.7 cells were highly elevated after stimulation by burn sepsis serum. Zn-MT-2 upregulated the pAkt to Akt ratio and attenuated the increase of IL-1 β and IL-6 mRNA expression, whereas Zn alone had none of these effects. Moreover, the effects of Zn-MT-2 were abolished in the presence of LY294002.

Discussion

Despite advances have been made in burn prevention, therapy, and rehabilitation, burn sepsis remains a major problem seriously affecting mortality and morbidity. The inflammatory response after burn is necessary for wound healing and host defense. Modest inflammatory response is important for the host to eliminate pathogens and promote wound repair [21]. However, major burns often evoke a systemic inflammatory response syndrome, which lead to reduced resistance to infection, development of

sepsis and damage to multiple organs [22]. Our results in this paper have provided a novel potential therapeutic choice for the prevention of burn sepsis.

MTs have been found playing important roles in many physiologic and pathophysiologic situations ever since their discovery about fifty years ago [11, 23, 24]. Among these various effects of MTs, the role of MTs in inflammation and sepsis is gradually uncovered. MTs can be induced by various inflammatory stimuli and endotoxin challenge [25]. Reciprocally, MTs can regulate inflammatory response and attenuate endotoxemia [26]. MTs have been reported to have a beneficial effect in cardiac dysfunction in sepsis [14], neuroinflammation [27], intestinal inflammation [28], etc. However, the role of MTs in burn sepsis remains unclear.

In the present study, we investigated the role of MTs in burn sepsis using a mouse model. The results showed that MT (−/−) mice demonstrated a more prominent increase of inflammatory cytokine levels and more severe organ damage than WT mice after the sepsis challenge.

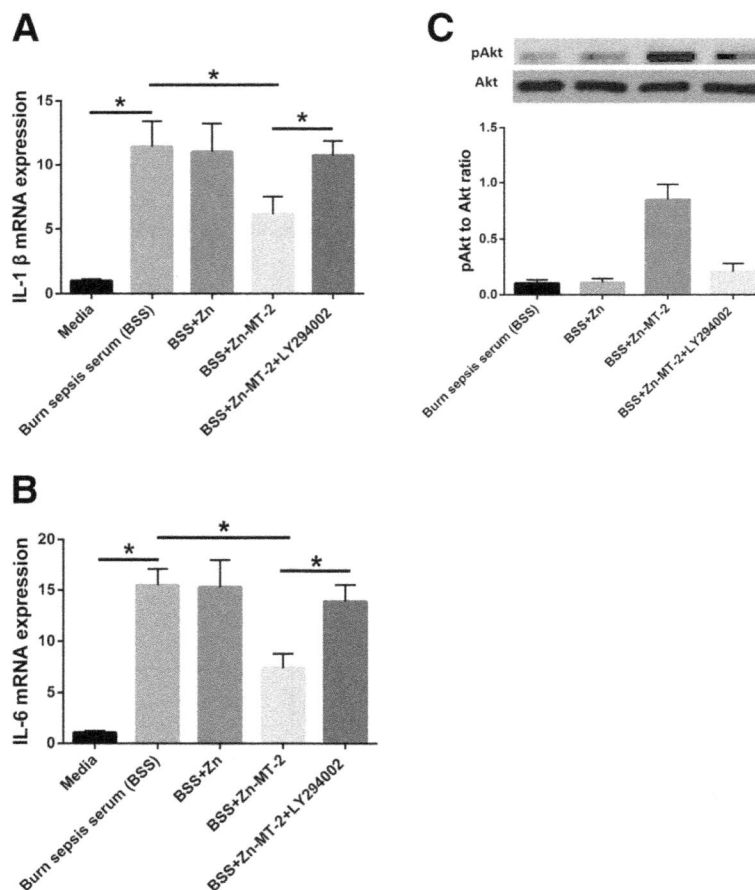

Fig. 4 IL-1β (a) and IL-6 (b) mRNA expression in cell lysates were detected by quantitative real-time PCR. Data were calculated using the $2^{-\Delta\Delta Ct}$ method, where Ct is cycle threshold. c The protein levels of pAkt and Akt were determined by western blot. Data were presented as means ± SD. Results are representative of at least three independent experiments. *$p < 0.01$

Metallothionein ameliorates burn sepsis partly via activation of Akt signaling pathway...

91

These responses were inhibited by Exogenous MT-2 treatment to both MT (−/−) and WT mice, indicating a protective role of MT in burn sepsis.

In mechanistic study, MT-2 upregulated the pAkt to Akt ratio and abrogated the increase of IL-1 β and IL-6 mRNA expression from macrophages that stimulated with burn sepsis serum. The effects of MT-2 were abolished by inhibition of Akt phosphorylation level with LY294002. MT has been reported to prevent cardiac endoplasmic reticulum stress and cell death via activation of Akt signaling pathway. It seemed in this study that, the effect of MT in this mouse burn sepsis model is at least partly through activation of the Akt signaling pathway.

In conclusion, our results in this study provided evidence that MT-2 played a protective role against inflammatory response and organ damage in this mouse burn sepsis model, at least partly through activation of the Akt signaling pathway.

Competing interest

The authors declare that they have no competing interests.

Authors' contributions

LKQ conceived and designed the study. LKQ, LHB, AND XBC performed the experiments. LYL collected and analyzed the data. LKQ and LHB wrote the paper. LHB and LYL reviewed and edited the manuscript. All authors read and approved the manuscript.

References

1. De Blasi RA. Severe sepsis and septic shock. N Engl J Med. 2013;369(21):2062–3. doi:10.1056/NEJMc1312359#SA2.
2. Shigematsu K, Kogiso M, Kobayashi M, Herndon DN, Suzuki F. Effect of CCL2 antisense oligodeoxynucleotides on bacterial translocation and subsequent sepsis in severely burned mice orally infected with Enterococcus faecalis. Eur J Immunol. 2012;42(1):158–64. doi:10.1002/eji.201141572.
3. Grunwald TB, Garner WL. Acute burns. Plast Reconstr Surg. 2008;121(5):311e–9e. doi:10.1097/PRS.0b013e318172ae1f.
4. Lynes MA, Hidalgo J, Manso Y, Devisscher L, Laukens D, Lawrence DA. Metallothionein and stress combine to affect multiple organ systems. Cell Stress Chaperones. 2014;19(5):605–11. doi:10.1007/s12192-014-0501-z.
5. Inoue K, Takano H, Shimada A, Satoh M. Metallothionein as an anti-inflammatory mediator. Mediators Inflamm. 2009;2009:101659. doi:10.1155/2009/101659.
6. Quaife CJ, Findley SD, Erickson JC, Froelick GJ, Kelly EJ, Zambrowicz BP, et al. Induction of a new metallothionein isoform (MT-IV) occurs during differentiation of stratified squamous epithelia. Biochemistry. 1994;33(23):7250–9.
7. Palmiter RD. Molecular biology of metallothionein gene expression. Experientia Suppl. 1987;52:63–80.
8. Masters BA, Quaife CJ, Erickson JC, Kelly EJ, Froelick GJ, Zambrowicz BP, et al. Metallothionein III is expressed in neurons that sequester zinc in synaptic vesicles. J Neuroscience : the official journal of the Society for Neuroscience. 1994;14(10):5844–57.
9. Moffatt P, Seguin C. Expression of the gene encoding metallothionein-3 in organs of the reproductive system. DNA Cell Biol. 1998;17(6):501–10.
10. West AK, Stallings R, Hildebrand CE, Chiu R, Karin M, Richards RI. Human metallothionein genes: structure of the functional locus at 16q13. Genomics. 1990;8(3):513–8.
11. Raudenska M, Gumulec J, Podlaha O, Sztalmachova M, Babula P, Eckschlager T, et al. Metallothionein polymorphisms in pathological processes. Metallomics. 2014;6(1):55–68. doi:10.1039/c3mt00132f.
12. Inoue K, Takano H, Shimada A, Wada E, Yanagisawa R, Sakurai M, et al. Role of metallothionein in coagulatory disturbance and systemic inflammation induced by lipopolysaccharide in mice. FASEB J. 2006;20(3):533–5. doi:10.1096/fj.05-3864fje.
13. Manso Y, Adlard PA, Carrasco J, Vasak M, Hidalgo J. Metallothionein and brain inflammation. J Biol Inorg Chem. 2011;16(7):1103–13. doi:10.1007/s00775-011-0802-y.
14. Ceylan-Isik AF, Zhao P, Zhang B, Xiao X, Su G, Ren J. Cardiac overexpression of metallothionein rescues cardiac contractile dysfunction and endoplasmic reticulum stress but not autophagy in sepsis. J Mol Cell Cardiol. 2010;48(2):367–78. doi:10.1016/j.yjmcc.2009.11.003.
15. Tsuji T, Naito Y, Takagi T, Kugai M, Yoriki H, Horie R, et al. Role of metallothionein in murine experimental colitis. Int J Mol Med. 2013;31(5):1037–46. doi:10.3892/ijmm.2013.1294.
16. Itoh N, Kimura T, Nakanishi H, Muto N, Kobayashi M, Kitagawa I, et al. Metallothionein-independent hepatoprotection by zinc and sakuraso-saponin. Toxicol Lett. 1997;93(2–3):135–40.
17. Shen CA, Fagan S, Fischman AJ, Carter EE, Chai JK, Lu XM, et al. Effects of glucagon-like peptide 1 on glycemia control and its metabolic consequence after severe thermal injury–studies in an animal model. Surgery. 2011;149(5):635–44. doi:10.1016/j.surg.2010.11.017.
18. Liu QY, Yao YM, Yu Y, Dong N, Sheng ZY. Astragalus polysaccharides attenuate postburn sepsis via inhibiting negative immunoregulation of CD4 + CD25(high) T cells. PLoS One. 2011;6(6):e19811. doi:10.1371/journal.pone.0019811.
19. Xiao M, Li L, Li C, Zhang P, Hu Q, Ma L, et al. Role of autophagy and apoptosis in wound tissue of deep second-degree burn in rats. Acad Emerg Med. 2014;21(4):383–91. doi:10.1111/acem.12352.
20. Schmittgen TD, Livak KJ. Analyzing real-time PCR data by the comparative C(T) method. Nat Protoc. 2008;3(6):1101–8.
21. Klein MB, Silver G, Gamelli RL, Gibran NS, Herndon DN, Hunt JL, et al. Inflammation and the host response to injury: an overview of the multicenter study of the genomic and proteomic response to burn injury. J Burn Care Res. 2006;27(4):448–51. doi:10.1097/01.BCR.0000227477.33877.E6.
22. Lord JM, Midwinter MJ, Chen YF, Belli A, Brohi K, Kovacs EJ, et al. The systemic immune response to trauma: an overview of pathophysiology and treatment. Lancet. 2014;384(9952):1455–65. doi:10.1016/S0140-6736(14)60687-5.
23. Raymond AD, Gekonge B, Giri MS, Hancock A, Papasavvas E, Chehimi J, et al. Increased metallothionein gene expression, zinc, and zinc-dependent resistance to apoptosis in circulating monocytes during HIV viremia. J Leukoc Biol. 2010;88(3):589–96. doi:10.1189/jlb.0110051.
24. Coyle P, Philcox JC, Carey LC, Rofe AM. Metallothionein: the multipurpose protein. Cell Mol Life Sci. 2002;59(4):627–47.
25. Sakaguchi S, Iizuka Y, Furusawa S, Ishikawa M, Satoh S, Takayanagi M. Role of Zn(2+) in oxidative stress caused by endotoxin challenge. Eur J Pharmacol. 2002;451(3):309–16.
26. Kimura T, Itoh N, Takehara M, Oguro I, Ishizaki J, Nakanishi T, et al. MRE-binding transcription factor-1 is activated during endotoxemia: a central role for metallothionein. Toxicol Lett. 2002;129(1–2):77–84.
27. Manso Y, Carrasco J, Comes G, Adlard PA, Bush AI, Hidalgo J. Characterization of the role of the antioxidant proteins metallothioneins 1 and 2 in an animal model of Alzheimer's disease. Cell Mol Life Sci. 2012;69(21):3665–81. doi:10.1007/s00018-012-1045-y.
28. Devisscher L, Hindryckx P, Olievier K, Peeters H, De Vos M, Laukens D. Inverse correlation between metallothioneins and hypoxia-inducible factor 1 alpha in colonocytes and experimental colitis. Biochem Biophys Res Commun. 2011;416(3–4):307–12. doi:10.1016/j.bbrc.2011.11.031.

14

Microbial colonization of open abdomen in critically ill surgical patients

Suvi Kaarina Rasilainen[1*], Mentula Panu Juhani[2] and Leppäniemi Ari Kalevi[2]

Abstract

Introduction: This study was designed to describe the time-course and microbiology of colonization of open abdomen in critically ill surgical patients and to study its association with morbidity, mortality and specific complications of open abdomen. A retrospective cohort analysis was done.

Methods: One hundred eleven consecutive patients undergoing vacuum-assisted closure with mesh as temporary abdominal closure method for open abdomen were analyzed. Microbiological samples from the open abdomen were collected. Statistical analyses were performed using Fisher's exact test for categorical variables. Mann-Whitney U test was used when comparing number of temporary abdominal closure changes between colonized and sterile patients. Kaplan-Meier analysis was done to calculate cumulative estimates for colonization. Cox regression analyses were performed to analyze risk factors for colonization.

Results: Microbiological samples were obtained from 97 patients. Of these 76 (78 %) were positive. Sixty-one (80 %) patients were colonized with multiple micro-organisms and 27 (36 %) were cultured positive for candida species. The duration of open abdomen treatment adversely affected the colonization rate. Thirty-three (34 %) patients were colonized at the time of laparostomy. After one week of open abdomen treatment 69, and after two weeks 76 patients were colonized with cumulative colonization estimates of 74 % and 89 %, respectively. Primary fascial closure rate was 80 % (61/76) and 86 % (18/21) for the colonized and sterile patients, respectively. The rate of wound complications did not significantly differ between these groups.

Conclusions: Microbial colonization of open abdomen is associated with the duration of open abdomen treatment. Wound complications are common after open abdomen, but colonization does not seem to have significant effect on these. The high colonization rate described herein should be taken into account when primarily sterile conditions like acute pancreatitis and aortic aneurysmal rupture are treated with open abdomen.

Keywords: Open abdomen, Laparostomy, Temporary abdominal closure, Microbial colonization

Introduction

The management of several acute surgical conditions with open abdomen (OA) has become more accepted and widely used [1]. More recently, this strategy has been applied to the treatment of critical surgical illnesses such as secondary peritonitis and severe acute pancreatitis with the aim of preserving intra-abdominal circulation and viability of the abdominal organs [2–5]. OA or laparostomy often serves as a life-saving intervention to treat or prevent abdominal compartment syndrome (ACS) or intra-abdominal hypertension (IAH) [6–8]. Nevertheless,

OA is associated with increased risk of complications, such as enteroathmospheric fistulae (EAF) [9–11], intra-abdominal sepsis or abscesses, wound complications and incisional hernias [12, 13]. In critically ill surgical patients, infective complications associated with OA are more frequent than with trauma patients [14]. The most effective strategy to reduce the risk of complications is to achieve primary fascial closure as soon as possible [15].

Temporary abdominal closure (TAC) methods have become more sophisticated and several recent studies have confirmed the benefits of negative pressure wound therapy systems to achieve primary fascial closure [16–18]. Combining the vacuum effect with mechanical traction using a temporary mesh (vacuum-assisted closure with

---
* Correspondence: rasilainensuvi@gmail.com
[1]Department of Abdominal Surgery, Jorvi Hospital, Turuntie, 150 Espoo, Finland
Full list of author information is available at the end of the article

mesh, VACM) has been shown to achieve primary fascial closure rates of about 90 % [19–21].

The rate and timing of microbial colonization of the open abdomen is not known. It has previously been suggested that negative-pressure wound therapy would have an antimicrobial effect when treating severe peritonitis with OA [22, 23]. In addition, a recent review suggested that this therapy has a favorable anti-inflammatory role in OA after ACS [24].

This study was designed to describe the time-course and microbiology of colonization of the open abdomen in critically ill surgical patients treated with VACM as the TAC method. Furthermore, the implications of colonization of the OA on morbidity, mortality and the specific complications of OA were studied.

Material and methods

This is a retrospective analysis of hospital records of 111 consecutive patients treated at a single institution for OA using the VACM as the TAC method. The study period was about 5 years, from July 2008 until June 2013. The study was conducted in accordance with the principles of the Declaration of Helsinki. The institutional review board of hospital approved the protocol.

Definitions and procedures

Prophylactic OA was used for the indications described in our previous study [21], i.e. in anticipation of high risk for the development of IAH or ACS with fascial closure at the initial laparotomy or planned relaparotomy.

Intra-abdominal pressure (IAP) was measured by the Foley bladder-catheter manometer technique (Holtech Medical, Charlottenlund, Denmark). ACS was defined as IAP over 20 mmHg with simultaneous new organ dysfunction [25].

The VACM method has been described previously [19, 21]. Briefly, a commercially available vacuum-assisted wound closure system was used (V.A.C.® Abdominal Dressing System; KCI, San Antonio, Texas, USA). First, the viscera were covered with a perforated polyethylene sheet followed by the suturing of an oval-shaped polypropylene mesh to the fascial edges. The mesh was then covered with a polyurethane sponge. Finally, an occlusive film was applied on top, perforated locally in the middle, and linked to a suction device to create continuous negative pressure. TAC changes were performed every two to three days. Except for three patients, all dressing changes were performed in the operating theatre. At the first TAC change, the mesh was divided in the midline and tightened with continuous suture after inserting a new inner polyethylene sheet. The fascia was closed when tension-free closure was considered possible. The closure was performed with either interrupted 1-Vicryl (Ethicon, Johnson&Johnson,

Somerville, New Jersey, USA) sutures or continuous 1-PDS (Ethicon, Johnson&Johnson).

The antimicrobial treatment of patients with OA is implemented in accordance with their diagnosis. According to our clinical protocols and unless contraindications, patients with ruptured abdominal aortic aneurysm (RAAA/AAA) or severe acute pancreatitis (SAP) are primarily treated with prophylactic i.v. cefuroxime. Patients with peritonitis get an empiric combination of i.v. cefuroxime and metronidatsole.

Wound complications

All postoperative wound complications were analysed. These included superficial infections treated with leaving the skin open at the fascial closure or by reopening the skin for superficial lavage. Deeper infections with intra-abdominal abscesses were separately analysed. Fascial ruptures, either partial or of full wound length, after successful primary fascial closure were studied.

Microbiological analysis

Samples for bacterial and fungal cultures from the surface of the viscera and deeper intra-abdominal areas were collected from 97 of the 111 patients during the TAC changes. Most patients had several samples taken at consecutive TAC changes. A semiquantitative analysis was performed for all samples. The colonization was considered multi-microbial if the cultures turned positive for more than one pathogen at any time-point during the OA treatment.

Statistical analysis

Statistical analyses were performed using Fisher's exact test for categorical variables. Mann-Whitney U test was used when comparing number of TAC changes between colonized and sterile patients. Kaplan-Meier analysis was done to calculate cumulative estimates for colonization. Cox regression analyses were performed to analyze risk factors for colonization.

Results

Patient characteristics

A total of 120 critically ill surgical patients were treated with OA between July 2008 and June 2013. Nine of these were managed mainly with a plastic silo (Bogota Bag) or commercial VAC without mesh as the TAC method, and were excluded. The remaining 111 patients treated with VACM as the TAC method were included in the analysis. The indications for OA included ACS, IAH, inability to close the abdomen mostly due to intra-abdominal swelling and/or bowel dilatation, and prophylactic OA as described above. Detailed patient characteristics are summarized in Table 1.

Table 1 Patient characteristics

Age years (mean, range)	60,1 (22-88)
Sex ratio (male)	77 (69.4 %)
Diagnosis	
Severe acute pancreatitis	19 (17.1 %)
Peritonitis	38 (34.2 %)
AAA/RAAA/aortic dissection$^{\varphi}$	28 (25.2 %)
Other*	26 (23.4 %)
Indication for laparostomy	
ACS$^{\$}$	38 (34.2 %)
Inability to close the abdomen	36 (32.4 %)
Prophylactic	31 (27.9 %)
IAH$^{£}$	6 (5.4 %)

$^{\varphi}$AAA = abdominal aortic aneurysm, RAAA = ruptured abdominal aortic aneurysm
*Other dg included: bowel ischemia (3), ileus (4), incarserated hernia (2), fascial dehiscence (3), postoperative hemorrage or abdominal trauma (7), other infection (5: sepsis, botulinism, salmonella, aortic prosthesis infection), pancreatitis after organ transplantation (1), metastatic hemoperitoneum (1)
$^{\$}$ACS = abdominal compartment syndrome
$^{£}$IAH = intra-abdominal hypertension

Colonization of the open abdomen

Ninety-seven of the 111 patients had samples taken for bacterial and fungal cultures from the OA. Seventy-six (78 %) patients had positive bacterial culture at least in one sample. Sixty one (80 %) were colonized with multiple micro-organisms and 27 (36 %) were cultured positive for candida species. The median time to colonization from laparostomy was two days. The duration of the OA adversely affected the colonization rate. Thirty-three (34 %) patients were colonized at the time of laparostomy. After one week and two weeks with OA, 69 and 76 patients were colonized with cumulative colonization estimates of 74 % and 89 %, respectively (Fig. 1). Both patients with SAP or RAAA/AAA were significantly less primarily colonized ($p = 0.001$ and $p = 0.002$, respectively) compared to the overall study population. Instead, patients with peritonitis had a significantly greater amount of primary colonization ($p = 0.001$). Figure 2 shows Kaplan-Meier curve of appearance of new microbes after beginning of open abdomen treatment.

Cox regression analysis was performed to study potential risk factors of colonization of the open abdomen. Table 2 shows that other diagnosis than RAAA/AAA had significantly higher risk for colonization during OA treatment. Also, patients with positive intra-abdominal culture taken during the first laparotomy had significantly lower risk for additional colonization during the TAC treatment (Table 3).

Gram-positive cocci (56/76, 74 %) and Gram-negative bacilli (36/76, 47 %) species were most frequently found in the colonized open abdomens. In detailed analysis of patients with peritonitis ($N = 37$), we detected the spectrum

of colonizing microbes to change in 16 cases. The new microbes found at later TAC changes mostly represented candida species, enterococci (mostly faecium) and staphylococcus epidermidis. The spectrum of pathogens represented by the colonized patients is presented in Table 4.

Primary fascial closure

Eighty-three out of 97 patients (86 %) with bacterial samples taken survived to abdominal closure. Sixty-five (78 %) of these patients were colonized with micro-organisms. Fourteen patients died with open abdomen. Among them the colonization rate was similar 11/14 (79 %), $p = 1.00$.

Seventy-nine of the 83 surviving patients (95 %) achieved primary fascial closure. Among patients with colonization and surviving to abdominal closure ($n = 65$) the fascia was successfully closed in 61 (92 %) patients, whereas fascia was successfully closed in all 18 patients with sterile abdomen ($p = 0.572$). All four patients with unsuccessful primary fascial closure were colonized with multiple micro-organisms. A median of 4 (IQR 2-5.5, range 1-19) TAC changes were needed to achieve successful primary closure among the colonized patients, while 3 (IQR 2-4, range 1-6) changes were sufficient in the group of sterile patients. ($p = 0.120$).

Morbidity
Fascial dehiscence and wound complications

Fascial dehiscence after successful primary fascial closure was observed in 7 % (4/61) of the colonized patients. 1 out of 18 patients (6 %) with sterile open abdomen had fascial rupture ($p = 1.000$). Three of these were partial (the sterile patient and two colonized patients) and two (both colonized) had a full-length fascial rupture.

Fifteen of the 61 patients (25 %) with successful primary fascial closure of a colonized open abdomen developed a wound complication, and the wound complication rate in patients colonized with multiple micro-organisms was similar, 29 % (14/48). In contrast, in the group of patients with sterile open abdomen, 3 out of 18 (17 %) patients were diagnosed with a wound complication after closure ($p = 0.750$). Three out of 61 patients (5 %) with colonization developed a deep intra-abdominal abscess after successful primary fascial closure.

Enteroatmospheric fistula (EAF)

Thirteen patients developed an EAF. In 11 patients the colonization was detected at a median of 8 days (range 2-16) before the development of an EAF, whereas in two patients colonization of the OA occurred after the detection of EAF. Thus, the rate of EAF was 15 % (11/74) among the colonized and 9 % (2/23) among the sterile patients ($p = 0.727$).

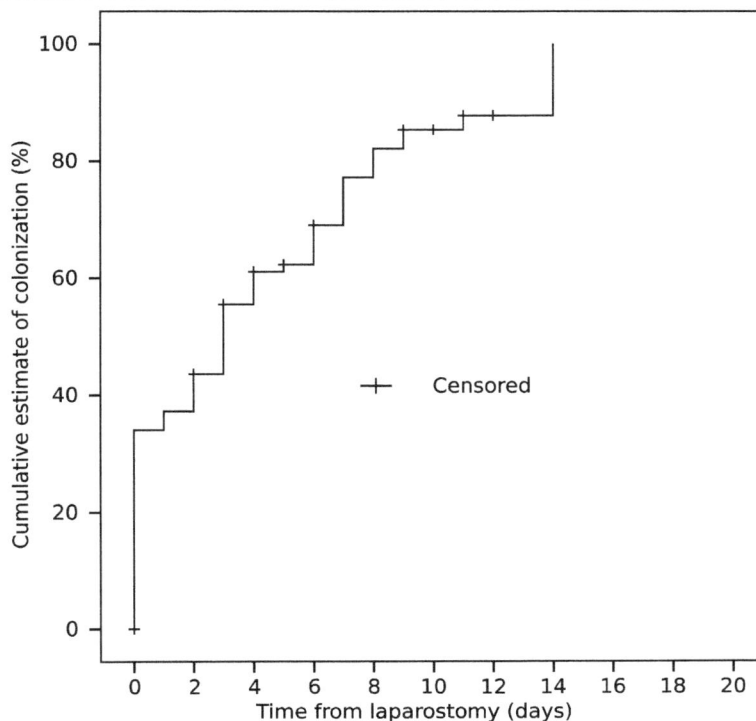

Fig. 1 A Kaplan-Meyer plot for colonization of the open abdomen. The time point of the last and negative microbial sample is marked with a plus sign (=censored)

A median of five TAC changes were performed to the patients, who developed an EAF. In contrast, patients without EAF underwent three (median) TAC changes during the OA treatment, ($p = 0.073$). The duration of primary ICU stay (8 vs 12 days, median) and the re-admission rate (15 % vs. 14 %) were similar for patients with or without an EAF, respectively.

Specifically, 7 of the 28 patients with acute aortic pathology treated with open abdomen developed an infective complication (3/7 EAF, 2/7 prosthesis infection and 2/7 both). All were detected in colonized open abdomens. All five patients with an EAF died during the same hospitalization period. The two patients with a chronic prosthesis infection survived.

Mortality
Thirty-one of 97 patients (32 %) with available microbiological samples died during their hospital stay period. Fourteen patients (45 %) died before abdominal closure. The in-hospital mortality rate of patients with colonized or sterile OA was 27 % (21/76) and 48 % (10/21), respectively ($p = 0.112$). Three out of 10 (30 %) of the sterile patients and 11/21 (52.4 %) of the colonized patients died with OA, $p = 0.280$. The higher mortality among the sterile patients is explained by the uneven distribution of diagnoses between the groups. Only 7/36 patients (19 %) with peritonitis died during the same hospitalization period

compared with 11/20 patients (55 %) with acute aortic pathology ($p = 0.015$). There were no patients with secondary peritonitis in the sterile group. Instead RAAA patients represented 50 % of deaths in the sterile group.

Discussion
The decision to treat a patient with open abdomen is often of forced or life-saving nature [7]. The duration of the OA plays a key role in the development of the known complications of this therapy. In general, the shorter the period of OA, the fewer are the complications [16]. The goal is to achieve rapid primary closure of the fascia [26]. As reported previously, the vacuum assisted closure with mesh (VACM) is a safe and efficient method to temporally cover the abdominal contents and to achieve primary fascial closure during the same hospitalization period [19–21]. The VACM method was used in the present study and the overall rate of primary fascial closure (81 %) reached the same level as in earlier studies.

Time spent with OA also predisposes the patient to microbial colonization. Although covered with occlusive negative pressure dressings, the laparostomy wound creates a potential route for pathogens to enter the abdominal cavity. In a recent study Pliakos et al. [27] showed in 39 patients with severe abdominal sepsis treated with open abdomen and VAC that 54 % of the patients

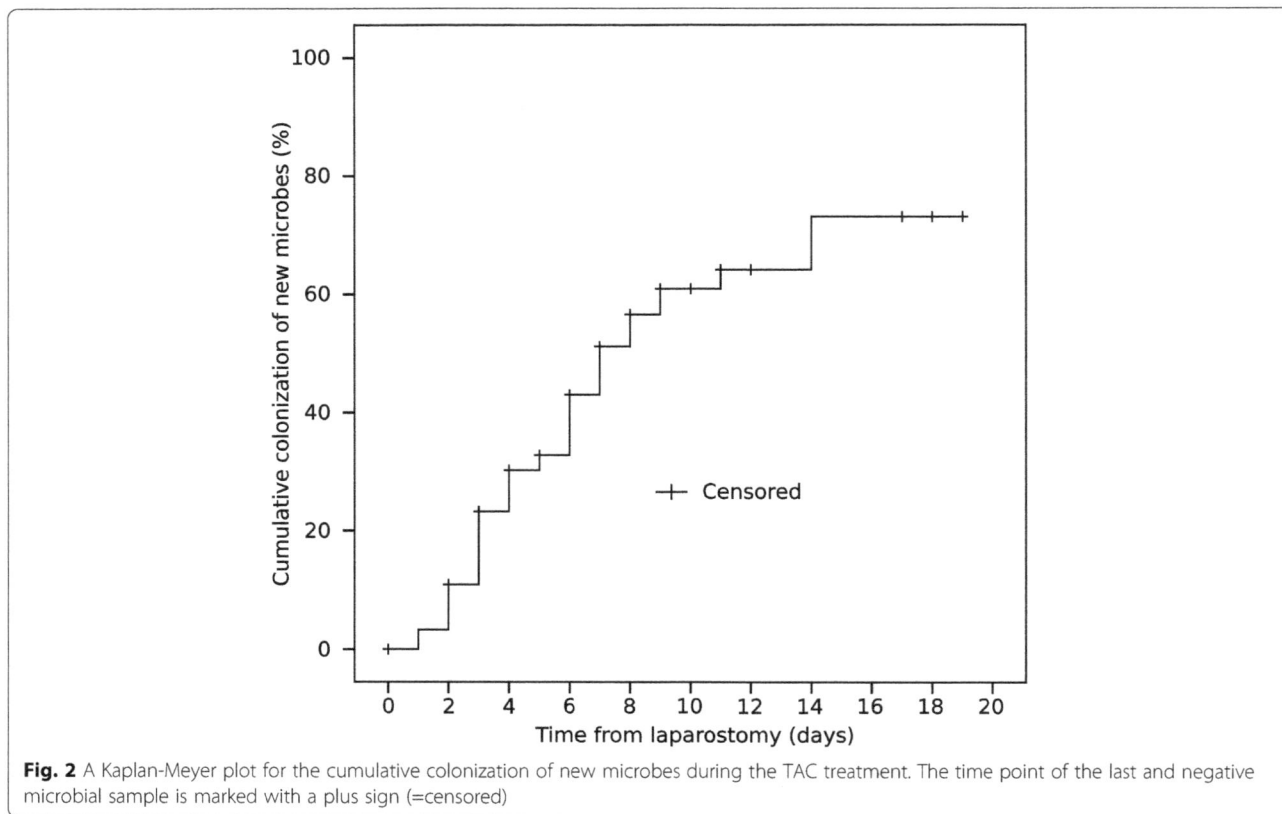

Fig. 2 A Kaplan-Meyer plot for the cumulative colonization of new microbes during the TAC treatment. The time point of the last and negative microbial sample is marked with a plus sign (=censored)

developed a hospital-acquired peritoneal infection during the VAC-treatment. We observed a similar trend with 34 % of patients being colonized at the primary laparostomy and 89 % after two weeks of OA treatment, although a significant number of our patients had initially a non-contaminated surgical field. Patients, with RAAA/AAA had significantly lower risk for colonization than patients with other diagnosis. This may indicate that intestinal pathology and acute pancreatitis could predispose to translocation of intestinal bacteria into open abdomen. Patients, with primary colonization had significantly lower risk for acquiring new microbes into open abdomen. This may be related to administration of broad-spectrum antibiotics in these patients.

In our study the TAC changes were predominantly performed under sterile operation room conditions. In combination with the disease-altered physiology, fluid resuscitation and invasive monitoring, the patient is at increased risk to be colonized with micro-organisms via several routes. The positive correlation between the duration of the OA and its microbial colonization reported in this study was also shown by Pliakos et al as a significant association of increased incidence of hospital-acquired peritoneal infection with the length of OA treatment, intensive care unit stay and overall hospitalization. In addition, our

Table 2 Risk factors for colonization of open abdomen*

	Hazard ratio	95 % CI	p-value
Diagnosis			
Aortic pathology	reference		
SAP[£]	2.4	1.01–5.82	0.048
Peritonitis	5.8	2.10–16.23	0.001
Other diagnosis	3.3	1.30–8.44	0.012

*Patients without primary colonization (n = 64) were included. Preoperative abdominal compartment syndrome and diagnosis were included in backward stepwise Cox regression analysis
[£]SAP = severe acute pancreatitis

Table 3 Risk factors for colonization of open abdomen with new pathogens*

	Hazard ratio	95 % CI	p-value
Diagnosis			0.005
Aortic pathology	reference		
SAP[£]	2.15	0.92–5.04	0.077
Peritonitis	5.69	2.18–14.84	<0.001
Other diagnosis	2.79	1.14–6.84	0.025
Primary colonization	0.068	0.023–0.20	<0.001

*All patients with at least one follow-up culture during open abdomen were included (n = 91). Preoperative abdominal compartment syndrome, primary colonization and diagnosis were included in backward stepwise Cox regression analysis
[£]SAP = severe acute pancreatitis

Table 4 Bacterial and fungal cultures

	Number	Percentage of colonized patients (76)
Gram-negative bacilli	43	57
E. coli	21	28
Pseudomonas aeruginosa	10	13
Klebsiella pneumoniae	7	9
Klebsiella oxytoca	4	5
Morganella morganii	3	4
Stenotrophomonas maltophilia	5	7
Enterobacter cloacae	6	8
Proteus vulgaris	1	1
Serratia marcescens	2	3
Serratia liquefaciens	1	1
Burkholderia cepacia	1	1
Gram-positive cocci	54	71
Enterococcus faecalis	24	32
Enterococcus faecium	33	43
Staphylococcus epidermidis	15	20
Staphylococcus haemolyticus	5	7
Coag.neg. staphylococcus	22	29
Streptococcus viridans	2	3
Enterococci (unspecific)	2	3
Gram-positive bacilli	8	11
Bacillus cereus	5	7
Clostridium species (unspecific)	1	1
Clostridium perfringens	2	3
Lactobacillus	1	1
Fungi	27	36
Candida albicans	24	32
Candida glabrata	6	8
Candida dubliensis	2	3
Candida crusei	1	1
Geotrichum candidum		
Anaerobes	19	25
Bacteroides fragilis	13	17
Gram-positive bacilli	3	4
Gram-negative bacilli	2	3
Difteroid	4	5

study shows that colonization is associated with the number of TAC changes.

As pointed out by Pliakos et al., and also showing a trend in this study, microbial colonization reduces the chances of delayed primary fascial closure. We also observed that colonization is associated with an elevated rate of fascial dehiscence and increased number of wound complications after successful primary fascial closure.

These adverse effects were most frequent in patients colonized with multiple micro-organisms. However, these differences did not reach statistical significance.

The spectrum of colonizing microbes is extensive, and albeit important, it is sometimes challenging to identify the potentially clinically harmful pathogens. In a review by Solomkin and Mazuski [28] the authors point out that the consequences of treatment failure of a severely septic abdomen and of hospital-acquired intra-abdominal infections might be more significant compared to milder infections and thus recommend empiric use of broad spectrum antibiotics. More resistant flora predominate in hospital-acquired intra-abdominal infections. These include Enterococci, E. coli, Proteus species, Klebsiella, Ps. aeruginosa, Enterobacter species and Candida species [29, 30], all of which were detected as colonizing pathogens also in the present study. Pliakos et al showed predominance of intestinal bacteria in the OAs of patients treated for peritonitis [27] many of these also belonging to the previously mentioned families of resistant microbes. In particular, postoperative isolation of Enterococci, observed as the most commonly cultured pathogens from the OAs in the present study, has been associated with treatment failure and death [31, 32]. Furthermore, patients with hospital-acquired intra-abdominal infections and especially with postoperative infections have been reported to be at increased risk for Candida peritonitis [33]. In this study Candida species were observed in 33 % of the colonized patients confirming the vulnerability of the critically ill surgical patients to fungal infections.

Pathologic processes leading to OA mostly represent severe, catabolic conditions [34, 35] that reduce the patients' resources to combat not only against infective but also against mechanical challenges. These include decreased tolerance for repeated operative management, which was recently evidenced in a study on 517 trauma patients treated for OA. They reported that an increasing number of abdominal re-explorations independently predict the occurrence of fistula and other infective complications [36]. We observed a similar phenomenon in our material of critically ill surgical patients of whom 13 developed an EAF, all of which had undergone more operations than patients without fistula. Although EAFs developed more often into colonized than into a sterile OAs, the difference was not statistically significant.

In view of the morbidity associated with OA, it is important to emphasize that reducing the need for OA by using all conservative means to reduce intra-abdominal hypertension as outlined in the consensus statement of the World Society of the Abdominal Compartment Syndrome [37] including percutaneous drainage of ascites should be exhausted before surgical decompression and OA. In addition, minimizing operation time, monitoring physiological parameters and avoiding excess fluid resuscitation at index operation help to reduce tissue edema and the need for OA.

In contrast to complicated intra-abdominal infections, severe acute pancreatitis and acute aortic pathology represent primarily sterile conditions often managed with OA in order to avoid or treat ACS. Nonetheless, infective complications of OA have been described in these patients. Sörelius et al recently published a subgroup study based on their former work of 30 patients treated with OA after repair of elective or ruptured AAA [38]. Two patients developed an EAF, two were diagnosed with a prosthesis infection and one with an aorto-enteric fistula. Patients with aortic pathology, especially acute aneurysmal rupture, often require extensive fluid resuscitation both pre- and postoperatively. This issue was also studied by Bradley et al. in 517 trauma patients [36]. They concluded that large-volume fluid resuscitation independently predicts the development of infective complications including EAF. In our material, all infective complications (EAFs and prosthesis infections) developed into colonized open abdomens. All five patients with an EAF died during the same hospitalization period and the two patients with a chronic prosthesis infection survived. These mortality figures are in line with those published by Sörelius et al [38] and highlight the severity of the infectious complications in this patient group. In the present study, no EAFs were detected among patients with SAP, but two pancreatic fistula developed later on and both for patients with colonized OA. Thus, collection of microbial samples from the OA and strict follow-up of infection parameters could be useful in predicting the development of both acute devastating and chronic complications. Similar follow-up measures were discussed and recommended by Solomkin and Mazuski [28] in the treatment of intra-abdominal sepsis.

Conclusions

In conclusion, colonization of OA is associated with the duration of the OA treatment. It may adversely affect the primary fascial closure rate and is associated with the development of infective complications in critically ill surgical patients. Negative-pressure TAC therapy does not seem to protect patients from bacterial growth in the OA cavity. A high risk of colonization should be taken into account when treating primarily sterile conditions like acute pancreatitis and aortic aneurysm repair with OA.

Abbreviations

ACS: Abdominal compartment syndrome; EAF: Entroathmospheric fistula; IAH: Intra-abdominal hypertension; IAP: Intra-abdominal pressure; OA: Open abdomen; RAAA/AAA: Ruptured abdominal aortic aneurysm/abdominal aortic aneurysm; SAP: Severe acute pancreatitis; TAC: Temporary abdominal closure; VACM: Vacuum-assisted closure with mesh.

Competing interests
The authors declare that they have no competing interests.

Authors' contributions
SR participated in designing the study, collected the data, participated in analyzing and interpreting the data, drafted the manuscript. PM participated in designing the study, analyzed and interpreted the data, participated in critical revision of the manuscript. AL participated in designing the study, critically revised the manuscript, gave final approval of the version to be published. All authors read and approved the final manuscript.

Acknowledgements
This study was financially supported only by a Helsinki University Hospital research grant for emergency abdominal-surgery.

Author details
[1]Department of Abdominal Surgery, Jorvi Hospital, Turuntie, 150 Espoo, Finland. [2]Department of Abdominal Surgery, Helsinki University Central Hospital, Helsinki, Finland.

References
1. Ivatury RR. Update on open abdomen management: achievements and challenges. World J Surg. 2009;33:1150–3.
2. Duff JH, Moffat J. Abdominal sepsis managed by leaving abdomen open. Surgery. 1981;90:774–8.
3. Bosscha K. Open management of abdomen and planned reoperations in severe bacterial peritonitis. Eur J Surg. 2000;166:44–9.
4. Steinberg D. On leaving the peritoneal cavity open in acute generalized suppurative peritonitis. Am J Surg. 1979;137:216–20.
5. Jansen JO, Loudon MA. Damage control surgery in a non-trauma setting. Br J Surg. 2007;94:789–90.
6. Ivatury RR, Diebel L, Porter JM, Simon RJ. Intra-abdominal hypertension and the abdominal compartment syndrome: review. Surg Clin North Am. 1997;77:783–800.
7. Leppäniemi A. Laparostomy: why and when? Crit Care. 2010;14:216.
8. Schein M, Saadia R, Decker GG. The open management of the septic abdomen. Surg Gynecol Obstet. 1986;163:587–92.
9. Evenson RA, Fischer JE. Treatment of enteric fistula in open abdomen. Chirurg. 2006;77:594–601.
10. Ramsay PT, Meija VA. Management of enteroatmospheric fistulae in the open abdomen. Am Surg. 2010;76:637–9.
11. Marinis A, Gkiokas G, Argyra E, Fragulidis G, Polymeneas G, Voros D. "Enteroatmospheric fistulae" – gastrointestinal openings in the open abdomen: a review and recent proposal of a surgical technique. Scand J Surg. 2013;102:61–8.
12. Miller RS, Morris Jr JA, Diaz Jr JJ, Herring MB, May AK. Complications after 344 damage control open celiotomies. J Trauma. 2005;59:1371–4.
13. Leppäniemi A, Tukiainen E. Planned hernia repair and late abdominal wall reconstruction. World J Surg. 2012;36:511–5.
14. Tsuei BJ, Skinner JC, Bernard AC, Kearney PA, Boulanger BR. The open peritoneal cavity: etiology correlates with the likelihood of fascial closure. Am Surg. 2004;70:652–6.
15. Vogel TR, Diaz JJ, Miller RS, May AK, Guillamondequi OD, Guy JS, et al. The open abdomen in trauma; do infectious complications affect primary abdominal closure? Surg Infect (Larchmt). 2006;7:433–41.
16. Garner GB, Ware DN, Cocanour CS, Duke JH, McKinley BA, Kozar RA, et al. Vacuum-assisted wound closure provides early fascial reapproximation in trauma patients with open abdomen. Am J Surg. 2001;182:630–8.
17. Stonerock CE, Bynoe RP, Yost MJ, Nottingham JM. Use of a vacuum-assisted closure device to facilitate abdominal closure. Am Surg. 2003;69:1030–4.
18. Barker DE, Kaufman HJ, Smith LA, Ciraulo DL, Richart CL, Burns RP. Vacuum pack technique of temporary abdominal closure: a 7-year experience with 112 patients. J Trauma. 2000;48:201–6.
19. Petersson U, Acosta S, Björck M. Vacuum-assisted wound closure and mesh-mediated fascial traction—a novel technique for late closure of the open abdomen. World J Surg. 2007;31:2133–7.
20. Acosta S, Bjarnason T, Petersson U, Pålsson B, Wanhainen A, Svensson M, et al. Multicentre prospective study of fascial closure rate after open

abdomen with vacuum and mesh-mediated fascial traction. Br J Surg. 2011;98:735–43.

21. Rasilainen SK, Mentula PJ, Leppäniemi AK. Vacuum and mesh-mediated fascial traction for primary closure of the open abdomen in critically ill surgical patients. Br J Surg. 2012;99:1725–32.

22. Amin AI, Shaikh IA. Topical negative pressure in managing severe peritonitis: a positive contribution? World J Gastroenterol. 2009;15:3394–7.

23. Horwood J, Akbar F, Maw A. Initial experience of laparostomy with immediate vacuum therapy in patients with severe peritonitis. Ann R Coll Surg Engl. 2009;91:681–7.

24. Shah SK, Jimenez F, Letourneau PA, Walker PA, Moore-Olufemi SD, Stewart RH, et al. Strategies for modulating the inflammatory response after decompression from abdominal compartment syndrome. Scand J Trauma Resusc Emerg Med. 2012;3:20–5.

25. Malbrain ML, Cheatham ML, Kirkpatrick A, Sugrue M, Parr M, De Waele J, et al. Results from the international conference of experts on intra-abdominal hypertension and abdominal compartment syndrome. I Definitions Intensive Care Med. 2006;32:1722–32.

26. Goussous N, Kim BD, Jenkins DH, Zielinski MD. Factors affecting primary fascial closure of the open abdomen in the nontrauma patient. Surgery. 2012;152:777–83.

27. Pliakos I, Michalopoulos N, Papavramidis TS, Arampatzi S, Diza-Mataftsi E, Papavramidis S. The effect of vacuum-assisted closure in bacterial clearance of the infected abdomen. Surg Infect (Larchmt). 2014;15:18–23.

28. Solomkin JS, Mazuski J. Intra-abdominal sepsis: newer interventional and antimicrobial therapies. Infect Dis Clin North Am. 2009;23:593–608.

29. Montravers P, Gauzit R, Muller C, Marmuse JP, Fichelle A, Desmonts JM. Emergence of antibiotic-resistant bacteria in cases of peritonitis after intra-abdominal surgery affects the efficacy of empiric antimicrobial therapy. Clin Infect Dis. 1996;23:486–94.

30. Montravers P, Dupont H, Gauzit R, et al. Candida as a risk factor for mortality in peritonitis. Crit Care Med. 2006;34:646–52.

31. Burnett RJ, Haverstock DC, Dellinger EP, Reinhart HH, Bohnen JM, Rptstein OD, et al. Definition of the role of enterococcus in intraabdominal infection: analysis of a prospective randomized trial. Surgery. 1995;118:716–21.

32. Sitges-Serra A, López MJ, Girvent M, Almirall S, Sancho JJ. Postoperative enterococcal infection after treatment of complicated intra-abdominal sepsis. Br J Surg. 2002;89:361–7.

33. Eggimann P, Francioli P, Bille J, Schneider R, Wu MM, Chapuis G, et al. Fluconazole prophylaxis prevents intra-abdominal candidiasis in high-risk surgical patients. Crit Care Med. 1999;27:1066–72.

34. Rotondo MF, Schwab CW, McGonical MD, Phillips 3rd GR, Fruchterman TM, Kauder DR, et al. 'Damage control': an approach for improved survival in exsanguinating penetrating abdominal injury. J Trauma. 1993;35:375–82.

35. Diaz Jr JJ, Cullinare DC, Dutton WD, Jerome R, Bagdonas R, Bilaniuk JW, et al. The management of open abdomen in trauma and emergency general surgery: part 1—damage control: review. J Trauma. 2010;68:1425–38.

36. Bradley MJ, Dubose JJ, Scalea TM, Holcomb JB, Shrestha B, Okoye O, et al. Independent predictors of enteric fistula and abdominal sepsis after damage control laparotomy: results from the prospective AAST Open Abdomen registry. JAMA Surg. 2013;148:947–54.

37. Kirkpatrick AW, Roberts DJ, De Waele J, Jaeschke R, Malbrain ML, De Keulenaer B, et al. Pediatric Guidelines Sub-Committee for the World Society of the Abdominal Compartment Syndrome. Intra-abdominal hypertension and the abdominal compartment syndrome: updated consensus definitions and clinical practice guidelines from the World Society of the Abdominal Compartment Syndrome. Intensive Care Med. 2013;39:1190–206.

38. Sörelius K, Wanhainen A, Acosta S, Svensson M, Djavani-Gidlund K, Björck M. Open abdomen treatment after aortic aneurysm repair with vacuum-assisted wound closure and mesh-mediated fascial traction. Eur J Vasc Endovasc Surg. 2013;45:588–94.

15

Learning curve after rapid introduction of laparoscopic appendectomy: are there any risks in surgical resident participation?

Eszter Mán, Tibor Németh, Tibor Géczi, Zsolt Simonka and György Lázár*

Abstract

Background: With the spread of the minimally invasive technique, laparoscopic appendectomy (LA) is performed with increasing frequency with excellent results. The method provides surgical residents with an excellent opportunity to learn basic laparoscopic skills and prepares them for more complex interventions.

Methods: We evaluated the results of 600 laparoscopic appendectomies performed by 5 surgical residents (Group A) and 5 consultant surgeons (Group B) between 2006 and 2009. Comparing the two groups based on patient demographics, duration of surgery, operation time depending on the severity of inflammation, intraoperative blood loss, conversion rate, hospital stay in days, and postoperative complications. We also assessed the extent to which the minimum of 20 surgeries to be performed in the learning curve period as recommended by the EAES corresponds to our experience. SPPS 20 was used for the statistical analysis.

Results: Six hundred laparoscopic appendectomies were performed in the study period (Group A: $n = 319$; Group B: $n = 281$). A significant difference was found between the two groups in duration of surgery during the learning curve period and when comparing the duration of LA surgeries in the learning curve period with the duration of later surgeries in both groups. The operation time in case of more severe inflammation also showed a significant difference when comparing with simple appendicitis operation time.

Conclusions: The rapid introduction of laparoscopy involves few risks, the surgery is also performed with sufficient safety by surgical residents, and it provides them with an excellent opportunity to learn the basic laparoscopy skills.

Keywords: Laparoscopic surgery, Residency, Learning curve, Operative time, Complications

Background

In recent years, the minimally invasive technique has been used in emergency surgery in ever increasing numbers [1]. The most common urgent surgical condition to be treated with a laparoscopic method nowadays is acute appendicitis [2]. Laparoscopic appendectomy is proved to have numerous advantages over open surgery (more rapid recovery, less postoperative pain, a decrease in the need for medications and in complications from wound infections, and better cosmetic results). In addition, the procedure is reliable and safe for the treatment of this condition [3].

In many Western countries, appendectomies outside the day-shift hours are performed by surgical residents under the supervision of a consultant [4]. This is therefore the first type of laparoscopic surgery residents learn; they thus learn the basics of the minimally invasive surgical technique and may develop the basic skills they can use in later, more complex surgeries [5].

Several studies have assessed the results of laparoscopic appendectomies performed by resident surgeons (duration of surgery, hospital stay, and conversion rate) [6, 7]. It can therefore be concluded that laparoscopic appendectomy is a safe method both in the case of residents and in that of consultants. Other studies have reported that the complication rate is higher for surgeries carried out by residents [8]. Several studies have also focused on the learning curve, that is, how many

* Correspondence: gylazar@gmail.com
Department of Surgery, University of Szeged, Szőkefalvi-Nagy Béla u. 6, H-6720 Szeged, Hungary

surgeries are required for a surgical resident to be able to perform laparoscopic surgeries independently. These studies estimate that 20 to 30 surgeries should be performed during the learning curve [9, 10]. According to the European Association of Endoscopic Surgery (EAES) recommendation, this number is 20 [11].

At our clinic, laparoscopic appendectomy was introduced in 2006, and, over a mere six months, a complete change in approach regarding the treatment of acute appendicitis occurred, with the minimally invasive method becoming the primary approach in treating this condition. In our study, we compared resident surgeries with those performed by consultants in terms of efficacy and safety by analyzing the results of the initial, learning curve period. We also assessed the extent to which the 20 surgeries recommended by the EAES in the learning curve period correspond to our own results and experience.

Methods

Laparoscopic appendectomy was introduced at our clinic in 2006 over a mere six months. In our retrospective study, we evaluated the results of surgeries performed by 5 residents (Group A – young resident colleagues with 2 to 3 years of surgical experience at the beginning of the study) and 5 consultants (Group B – consultant group, colleagues with 8 to 9 years of surgical experience) in the learning curve period (20 surgeries as recommended by the EAES) and in the period after that (up to Dec. 31, 2009) during routine use. Therefore, subgroups within groups A and B were created: A1 – residents, B1 – consultants in the learning curve period, A2 – residents, and B2 – consultants in the period of routine use.

The steps for the laparoscopic appendectomy were the following:

Step 1 – a pneumoperitoneum was created using a Veress needle via the umbilical access. In the case of a former abdominal operation, the umbilical trocar was introduced with the open technique (n = 27). We positioned the optical trocar in the umbilicus and two additional trocars under direct vision in the midline suprapubic area (5 mm) and left iliac fossa (10 mm).
Step 2 – exploration of the abdominal cavity, isolation of the appendix. Irrigation, suction and sampling for microbiological investigation, if necessary.
Step 3 – skeletisation of the mesoappendix with monopolar diathermy, clipping the appendicular artery with metal clips (two proximal clips, one distal clip).
Step 4 – clipping the base of the appendix using Hem-o-lok clips (two proximal clips, one distal clip). In 8 cases, when the XL Hem-o-lok clip could not encircle the base of the appendix, we used an Endostapler (n = 6) or Endoloops (n = 2) (Group A: 2 Endostapler, 1 loop; Group B: 4 Endostapler, 1 loop). The distribution of

these appendix closure methods did not differ between the groups.
Step 5 – extraction of the appendix using an Endobag through a lateral 10 mm trocar.

During emergency surgical care, the head surgeon on duty (with minimum surgical experience of 10 years) was responsible for the care at the clinic, and it was that person who decided on indication for surgery and, randomly, on the surgeon who would perform the operation. In all cases, the assistant surgeon scrubbed in, actually participated in the surgical intervention, supervised the procedure, and, naturally, gave advice to the operating surgeon, if needed, but did not "take over" the procedure.

Each resident had completed a two-week "Basic laparoscopic skills course" (training box, live animals) and had already assisted in other laparoscopic procedures (cholecystectomy, laparoscopic hernia repair, laparoscopic hiatal hernia repair, etc.). Each consultant was a more experienced laparoscopic surgeon who regularly performed other surgical procedures independently (cholecystectomy, hernia repair, etc.). Before the introduction of laparoscopic appendectomy, each surgeon was provided with theoretical training to learn the details of the technique. In both groups, the assistant was an older consultant on duty, who had the most experience in both conventional and laparoscopic procedures.

Results were evaluated for a total of 600 patients (Group A, $n = 319$ – A1: $n = 100$, A2: $n = 219$; Group B, $n = 281$ – B1: $n = 100$, B2: $n = 181$). Patient selection and data collection were performed retrospectively through an analysis of our computer database (Medsolution System) and the documentation for the patients. All patients over the age of 18 who underwent laparoscopic appendectomy in the study period were included, and none of the patients were excluded from our study.

The groups were compared based on general patient demographics (age, gender, comorbidities, and ASA score), duration of surgery, operation time depending on the severity of inflammation, intraoperative blood loss, conversion rate, hospital stay in days, negative appendectomy rate, and number of complications (early, late).

Statistical analysis

SPSS 20 was used for the statistical analysis—the durations of surgery were compared with a two-sample t-test, the complications were compared with Fisher's exact test, and the effect of inflammation on the duration of surgery was determined by analysis of variance. A significance level of $p < 0.05$ was used.

Results

Data was evaluated for 600 patients in total between 2006 and 2009. The mean age of the patients was 38.4 years

(A1: 39.6, A2: 39.3, $p = 0.321$; B1: 39.1, B2: 35.9, $p = 0.273$). Gender distribution: A1 – female: $n = 53$, male: $n = 47$; A2 – female: $n = 119$, male: $n = 100$; B1 – female: $n = 65$, male: $n = 35$; B2 – female: $n = 98$, male: $n = 83$. Regarding comorbidities (ASA score III to IV, severe cardiac disease, COPD, DM, underlying tumor disease, and chronic renal failure): A1: $n = 10$, A2: $n = 16$, $p = 0.393$; B1: $n = 12$, B2: $n = 16$, $p = 0.281$. We may thus consider these patient groups homogeneous (Table 1).

We evaluated intraoperative blood loss in the two main groups: it was 55 mL in Group A and 45 mL in Group B, and there was no significant difference ($p = 0.664$). In Group A, conversion was required in 18 cases (5.6 %) (adhesions due to prior surgeries [$n = 6$], perforated, gangrenous appendix, the stump of which could not be treated safely with laparoscopy [$n = 12$]), while this number was 21 (7.4 %) in Group B (adhesions [$n = 13$], the stump could not be treated safely due to severe inflammation [$n = 6$], extreme obesity [$n = 1$], mesenteric injury during insufflation [$n = 1$]; $p = 0.321$). We also assessed whether the conversion rate was higher in the learning curve period: conversion was required in 14 out of 200 surgeries (7 %) in LC period subgroups A1 (residents) and B1 (consultants), while this number was 25 out of 400 (6.25 %) in routine use subgroups A2 (residents) and B2 (consultants), without a significant difference between the early and late period ($p = 0.522$). Also, there was no significant difference in hospital stay between the groups (3.21 vs. 3.84 days, $p = 0.391$, non-perforated group: Group A: 2.34 days, Group B: 2.13 days. Perforated group: Group A 4.78 days, Group B: 4.98 days). The two groups did not differ in negative appendectomy rate (NAR, 8.5 % vs. 7.8 %, $p = 0.835$) either (Table 2).

As to duration of surgery, we evaluated whether there was a difference during the learning curve period

Table 1 Demographics by subgroup

	A1 ($n = 100$)	A2 ($n = 219$)	p
Gender (n)			
Female	53	119	0.283
Male	47	100	0.326
Age (years)	39.6	39.3	0.895
Comorbidities(n)	10	16	0.384
	B1 ($n = 100$)	B2 ($n = 181$)	p
Gender (n)			
Female	65	98	0.438
Male	35	83	0.245
Age (years)	39.1	35.9	0.263
Comorbidities(n)	12	16	0.654

A1: residents during the learning curve, A2: residents after the learning curve, B1: consultants during the learning curve, B2: consultants after the learning curve

Table 2 Comparison of clinical datas in Groups A and B

	A ($n = 200$)	B ($n = 400$)	p
Blood loss (ml)	55	45	0.664
Conversion rate (n, %)	18 (5.6 %)	21 (7,4 %)	0.321
Hospital stay (days)			
Non perforated appendicitis	2.34	2.13	0.812
Perforated appendicitis	4.78	4.98	0.734
Negative appendectomy rate (NAR, %)	8.5 %	7,8 %	0.835

A: residents, B: consultants

between residents (A1) and consultants (B1), if there was a difference between the two groups after the learning curve (A2 vs. B2), and how duration of surgery changed over time in the case of residents and in that of consultants (A1 vs. A2, B1 vs. B2). We also investigated the effect of the severity of inflammation on operation time in each subgroup.

The mean duration of surgery was 74.6 min in Group A1 (residents LC period), 57.3 min in Group A2 (residents routine use period), 64.13 min in Group B1 (consultants LC period) and 53.38 min in Group B2 (consultants routine use period) (Fig. 1).

When comparing the mean duration of surgery between residents and consultants in the learning curve period, a significant difference was found between the groups (A1 – residents: 74.6 min vs. B1 – consultants: 64.13 min, $p < 0.05$). The same was observed when comparing the groups after the learning curve period (A2 – residents: 57.3 min vs. B2 – consultants: 53.38 min, $p < 0.05$).

In the two main groups, we compared the change in duration of surgery, the learning "dynamic": in Group A, the duration of surgery decreased from 74.6 min to 57.3 min ($p < 0.05$), while a drop from 64.13 min to 53.38 min was observed in Group B ($p < 0.05$) (Fig. 2).

When investigating the effect of the severity of inflammation on operation time, we founda significant difference between the subgroups. In Group A (residents), operation time was 61.4 min for early appendicitis with less severe inflammation (catarrhal, phlegmonous) vs. 74.8 min for severe inflammation (gangrenous, perforated) ($p < 0.05$) (Fig. 3).

This value was 53.4 min vs. 68.5 min for Group B (consultants) ($p < 0.05$) (Fig. 4).

In the learning curve period, operation time was 58.49 min for early appendicitis and 70.12 min with severe inflammation; in the routine use period, it was 56.13 min vs. 63.34 min. We found that the severity of the inflammation affected the duration of the operation significantly when comparing Groups A and B in the LC period vs. routine use period.

The groups were also compared in terms of complications during and after the learning curve period. Early

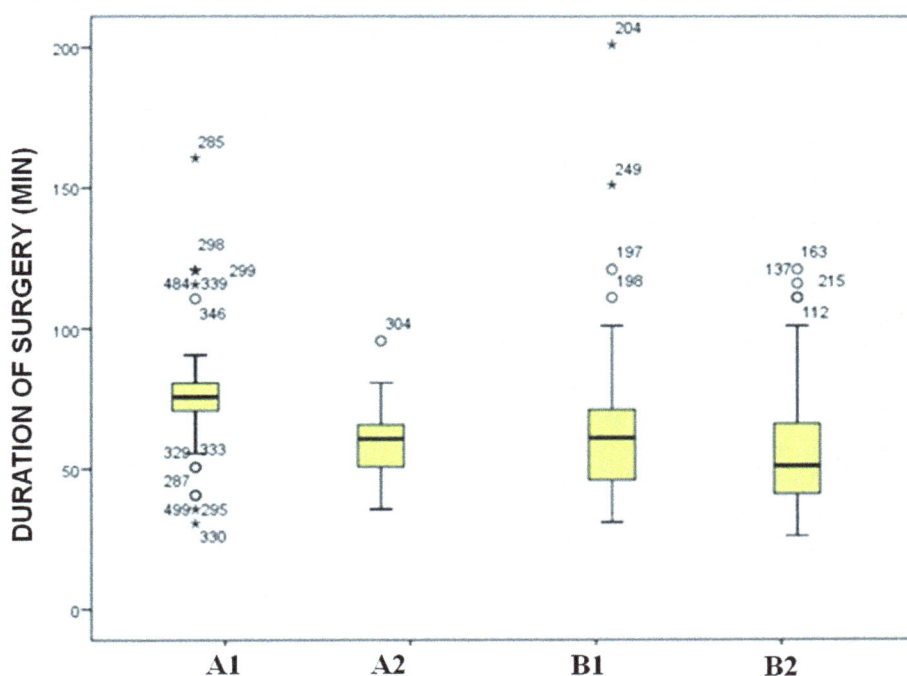

Fig. 1 Duration of surgery by subgroup. A1: residents during the learning curve; A2: residents after the learning curve; B1: consultants during the learning curve; B2: consultants after the learning curve

(within 30 days) major (bleeding, ileus, abscess, and thermal injury that require reoperation) and minor complications (wound infection), and late (after 30 days) complications (postoperative hernia) were assessed. There was no mortality. The types and occurrence of complications are shown in Table 3.

In comparing the frequency of complications between subgroups A1 (residents) and B1 (consultants) (5 vs. 9; 5 % vs. 9 %), it can be concluded that the occurrence of complications in the learning curve period was independent of surgical experience ($p = 0.238$)

In comparing subgroups A2 (residents) and B2 (consultants) after the learning curve period (10 vs. 17; 4.5 % vs. 9.3 %), the number of complications was lower in the case of the younger group, but the difference was not statistically significant. The analysis of the same question using Fisher's exact test did not reveal a correlation between surgical experience and number of complications.

We used an Endostapler (n = 6) or Endoloops (n = 2) (Group A: 2 Endostapler, 1 loop; Group B: 4 Endostapler, 1 loop). The distribution of these appendix closure methods did not differ between the groups. The mean operation time in the groups was the following: Endostapler – Group A: 48.4 min; Group B: 44.2 min; Endoloops – Group A: 84.6 min; Group B: 67.3 min. We found a significant difference in the duration of surgery *when comparing the Endostapler and Endoloop groups (p < 0.01). As the number of these cases were low, they did not affect the mean operation time in Group A or B significantly: Group A operation time using only Hem-o-lok clips: 65.67 min vs. using Endoloops/Endostapler as well: 65.95 min; Group B operation time using only Hem-o-lok clips: 58.325 min vs. using Endoloops/Endostapler as well: 58.755 min (Data not shown).*

Discussion

The minimally invasive technique is used worldwide for numerous surgery types with excellent results. The open and laparoscopic techniques have been compared in numerous studies, and many advantages have been confirmed for the latter (less postoperative pain, faster recovery, lower rate of surgical infections, better cosmetic result, and less need for medication) [12–14]. It is now also generally accepted that many of the cases with severe inflammation, and even perforation, can be treated safely with laparoscopy [15, 16].

The minimally invasive technique was also introduced rapidly at our clinic, over a period of six months in 2006, and it completely superseded the open method. Considering the fact that appendicitis is an urgent surgical condition, it is treated in many cases by young resident surgeons outside the day-shift hours under the supervision of a consultant. Numerous studies

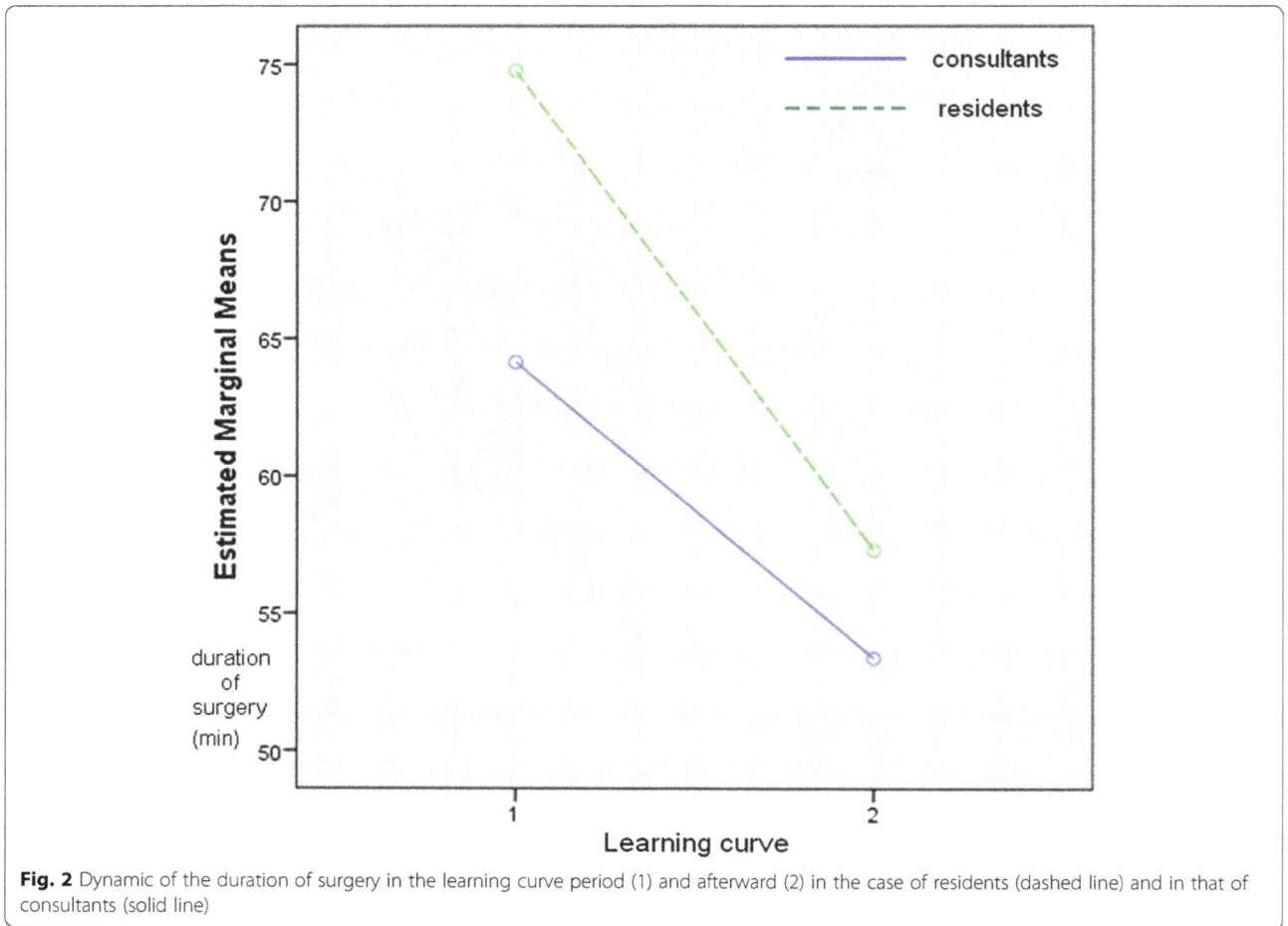

Fig. 2 Dynamic of the duration of surgery in the learning curve period (1) and afterward (2) in the case of residents (dashed line) and in that of consultants (solid line)

have analyzed the results of laparoscopic appendectomies performed by resident surgeons. The factors evaluated were duration of surgery, hospital stay in days, complications, and conversion rate.

In our study, we also evaluated these data, comparing the results achieved by residents with the results of the surgeries performed by consultants. In addition, the results of laparoscopic appendectomies performed by the two groups were compared in the learning curve period and thereafter.

Several studies have focused on the learning curve, that is, how many laparoscopic interventions under supervision are required for a resident to be able to perform surgeries independently. The learning curve period for laparoscopic appendectomy is short; a working group has found that 2.5 procedures on average are sufficient for independent practice [17]. Other studies recommend 30 surgeries [9]. Based on the 1994 EAES recommendation, in the case of laparoscopic appendectomy, 20 surgeries are to be performed under supervision in the learning curve period for independent practice, and this is supported by several studies [5, 10, 11]. Based on our

own experience, this number of surgeries is mandatory for a resident to be able to perform appendectomy independently. After the learning curve period (20 surgeries), there was a significant difference in mean duration of surgery both in the consultant group and the resident group (64.13 vs. 53.38 min and 74.6 vs. 57.3 min, respectively, $p < 0.05$). According to our results, the severity of the inflammation affected operation time significantly.

The mean hospital stay in days is a good measure of laparoscopic experience, as this period is longer in the case of a prolonged, complicated surgery. A similar objective parameter is conversion rate. In our study, there was no significant difference between the learning curve period and the period after that either in hospital stay or in conversion rate, nor was there any difference when comparing young surgeons with consultants. Conversion rate, therefore, was independent of laparoscopic experience. It was determined by the severity of the inflammation. Similarly to reports from other studies, conversion was required when the stump could not be treated safely because of the severity of the inflammation [5, 18].

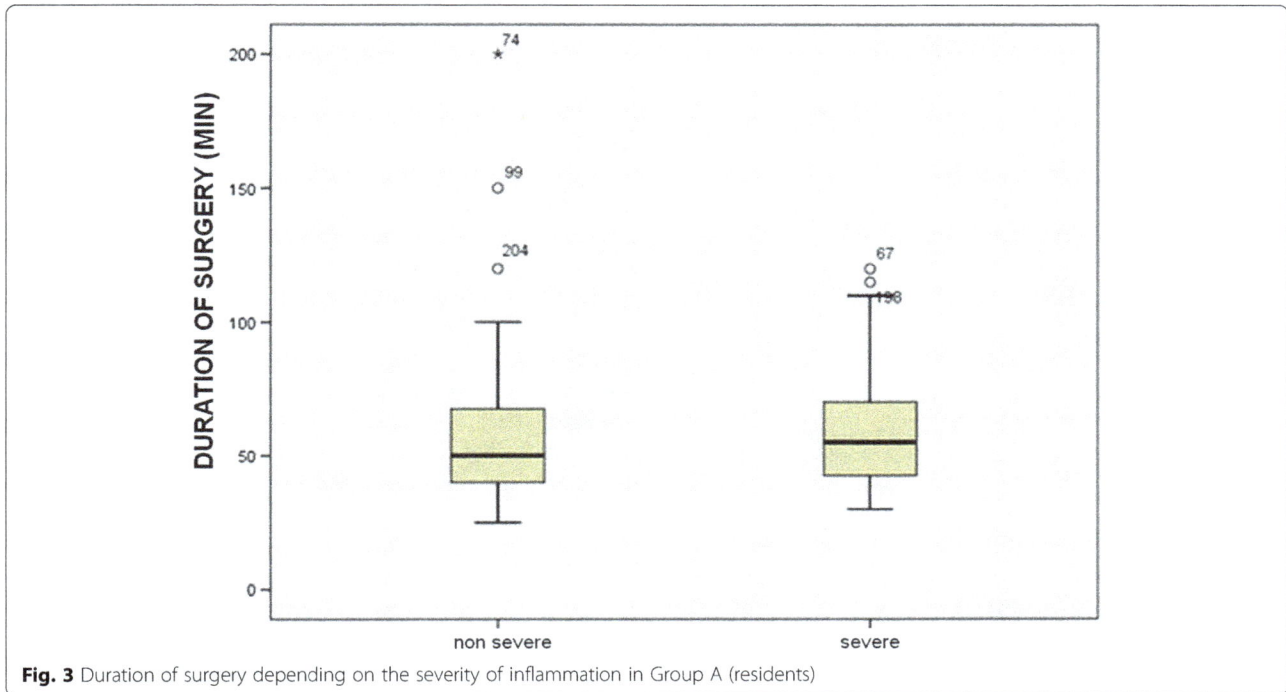

Fig. 3 Duration of surgery depending on the severity of inflammation in Group A (residents)

Since, according to our results, there was no difference in the frequency of complications between subgroups A1 (residents) and B1 (consultants) (5 vs. 9; 5 % vs. 9 %), the occurrence of complications in the learning curve period was independent of surgical experience ($p = 0.238$).

When comparing subgroups A2 (residents) and B2 (consultants) after the learning curve period (10 vs. 17; 4.5 % vs. 9.3 %), the number of complications was lower in the case of the younger group; however, this drop was not statistically significant. In a recent multicenter US

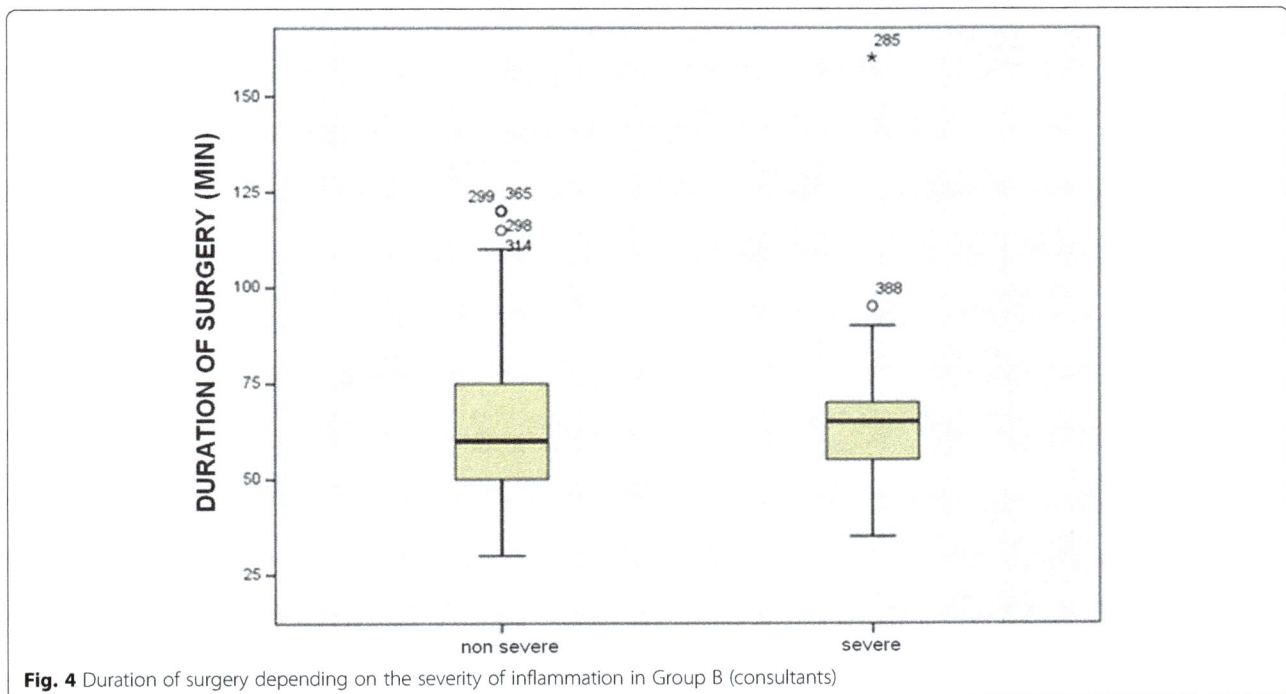

Fig. 4 Duration of surgery depending on the severity of inflammation in Group B (consultants)

Table 3 Complications by subgroups

	A1 (n = 100)	A2 (n = 219)	B1 (n = 100)	B2 (n = 181)
Early				
Major				
Ileus	0	1	0	2
Abscess	1	1	2	1
Bleeding	1	1	2	2
Minor				
(Wound infection)	3	5	3	9
Late	–	2	2	2
Total (n,%)	5 (5 %)	10 (4.6 %)	9 (9 %)	17 (9.3 %)

A1: residents during the learning curve, A2: residents after the learning curve,
B1: consultants during the learning curve, B2: consultants after the learning curve

study, the data for 54,467 appendectomies performed between 2005 and 2009 was analyzed. It was found that the duration of surgery is significantly longer and the number of major postoperative complications significantly higher in the case of surgeries performed by residents [8]. Our sample size was much smaller, but we only observed a difference between the groups in duration of surgery. In the learning curve period, it was 74.6 min in subgroup A1 (residents) and 64.13 min in subgroup B1 (consultants) ($p < 0.05$), while it was 57.3 min in subgroup A2 (residents) and 53.38 min in B2 (consultants) after the learning curve period ($p < 0.05$). In the two main groups, we compared the change in duration of surgery, the "dynamics" of learning: in Group A, duration of surgery decreased from 74.6 min to 57.3 min ($p < 0.05$), while in Group B, a drop from 64.13 min to 53.38 min was found ($p < 0.05$). It is interesting that the decrease in duration of surgery after the learning curve period was greater among residents. As they performed an increasing number of surgeries, they used the laparoscopic instruments with ever greater confidence, and both the surgeon performing the surgery and the surgical staff felt more confident in the laparoscopic situation [19, 20]. The more rapid improvement observed in the case of residents may be caused by the fact that, for many of them, laparoscopy was the primary surgical technique for appendectomy, as they had begun working in a period when the number of open appendectomies performed was small.

Except for a few cases, we used Hem-o-lok clips for the closure of the appendix stump. Based on our experience, the time required to use Hem-o-lok clips is shorter than that involved in using Endoloops. It is also much easier for young surgeons with less experience, so we consider it a safer procedure. Endostaplers are easy to use, but their cost-effectiveness is low; on the other hand, Endoloops or

endoscopic sutures represent a reliable, safe and cheap technique for closing the appendix base in the hands of an experienced laparoscopic surgeon. However, especially for residents in the learning curve period, it is a very challenging method, which can lengthen the operation time considerably. That is why we use Hem-o-lok clips as a gold standard for closing the stump of the appendix.

Use of a standardised technique described in a step-by-step manner can easily be learned by residents and may contribute to an improvement in outcomes [21]. This low-cost technique can also enable young residents to learn advanced laparoscopic skills in laparoscopic appendectomy, even in cases of complicated appendicitis.

Based on our experience, the algorithm for the safe introduction of laparoscopic appendectomy is the following:

1. *Basic skills training: a two-week "Basic laparoscopic skills" course (with a training box and live animals) at the beginning of residency.*
2. *First assistance: assisting in laparoscopic procedures (appendectomy, cholecystectomy, laparoscopic hernia repair and laparoscopic hiatal hernia repair) to acquire the basic skills and learn the standardised technique.*
3. *Practising the standardised appendectomy technique during the learning curve period (first 20 cases) under the supervision of a consultant surgeon proficient in both laparoscopic and open techniques.*
4. *Starting appendectomies independently.*

This is another reason why learning this basic technique is so important—it is encountered by residents in large numbers, and it may be of great assistance during their training to prepare them for subsequent, more complex laparoscopic surgeries. In many countries, residents must participate in laparoscopic training first, with the basic surgery types practiced on simulators. According to some studies, this training decreases subsequent intraoperative complications [22, 23]. Others suggest that real procedures performed in the OR are required for the actual development of skills and for the resident to become a professional surgeon [24].

According to a US survey, a large proportion of residents feel that they did not perform a sufficient number of laparoscopic procedures during their residency and therefore do not feel secure when they have to perform surgery independently [25, 26]. As a result, in 2007–2008, the Accreditation Council of Graduate Medical Education increased the mandatory number of laparoscopic surgeries to be performed during residency training: from 25 to 60 for simpler, so-called basic procedures, and from 9 to 25 for more complex, advanced procedures [26].

With the spread of laparoscopy, increased attention must be paid to the training of residents, and there is a need to implement standardized training models, as it is clear that, in our case, laparoscopic appendectomy is a technique that can also be used safely by residents in the learning curve period—naturally under the supervision of a consultant. Learning this technique provides the residents with a valuable opportunity to perform more difficult, more complex laparoscopic surgeries with adequate safety in the future.

Conclusions

Based on our experience laparoscopic appendectomy is a technique that can also be used safely by residents in the learning curve period as well. The rapid introduction of laparoscopy involves few risks, the surgery is also performed with sufficient safety by surgical residents. Comparing the resident and the consultant group based on patient demographics, intraoperative blood loss, conversion rate, hospital stay in days, and postoperative complications we did not find significant difference.

Abbreviations

EAES: European Association of Endoscopic Surgery; LC: learning curve; NAS: negative appendectomy rank.

Competing interests

The authors declare that they have no competing interests.

Authors' contributions

EM carried out the design of the study, made the patients' data collection, made the statistical analysis and drafted the manuscript. TN, TG helped in the patients' data collection, ZS helped to draft the manuscript. GL conceived of the study, and participated in its design and coordination and helped to draft the manuscript. All authors read and approved the final manuscript.

References

1. Kirshtein B, Roy-Shapira A, Lantsberg L, Mandel S, Avinoach E, Mizrahi S. The use of laparoscoy in abdominal emergencies. Surg Endosc. 2003;17:1118–24. doi:10.1007/s00464-002-9114-1.
2. Peiser JG, Greenberg D. Laparoscopic versus open appendectomy: results of a retrospective comparison in an Israeli hospital. Isr Med Assoc J. 2002;4:91–4.
3. Long KH, Bannon MP, Zietlow SP, Helgeson ER, Harmsen WS, Smith CD, Ilstrup DM, Baerga-Varela Y, Sarr MG, Laparoscopic Appendectomy Interest Group. A prospective randomized comparison of laparoscopic appendectomy with open appendectomy: clinical and economic analyses. Surgery. 2001;129:390–400. doi:10.1067/msy.2001.114216.
4. Hedrick T, Turrentine F, Sanfey H, Schirmer B, Friel C. Implications of laparoscopy on surgery residency training. Am J Surg. 2009;197:73–5. doi:10.1016/j.amjsurg.2008.08.013.
5. Pandey S, Slawik S, Cross K, Soulsby R, Pullyblank AM, Dixon AR. Laparoscopic appendectomy: a training model for laparoscopic right hemicolectomy? Colorectal Dis. 2007;9:536–9.
6. Sweeny KJ, Dillon M, Johnston SM, Keane FB, Conlon KC. Training in laparoscopic appendectomy. World J Surg. 2006;30:358–63. doi:10.1007/s00268-005-0311-7.
7. Yaghoubian A, de Virgilio C, Lee SL. Appendicitis outcomes are better at resident teaching institutions: a multi-institutional analysis. Am J Surg. 2010;200:810–3. doi:10.1016/j.amjsurg.2010.07.028.
8. Scarborough JE, Bennett KM, Pappas TN. Defining the impact of resident participation outcomes after appendectomy. Ann Surg. 2012;255:577–82. doi:10.1097/SLA.0b013e3182468ed9.
9. Kim SY, Hong SG, Roh HR, Park SB, Kim YH, Chae GB. Learning curve for a a laparoscopic appendectomy by a surgical trainee. J Korean Soc Coloproctol. 2010;26:324–8. doi:10.3393/jksc.2010.26.5.324.
10. Jaffer U, Cameron AE. Laparoscopic appendectomy: a junior trainee's learning curve. JSLS. 2008;12:288–91.
11. Neugebauer E, Troidl H, Kum CK, Eypasch E, Miserez M, Paul A. The E.A.E.S. Consensus Developement Conferences on laparoscopic cholecystectomy, appendectomy and hernia repair. Consensus statements – September 1994. The Educational Committee of the European Association for Endoscopic Surgery. Surg Endosc. 1995;9:550–63.
12. Paterson HM, Quadan M, de Luca SM, Nixon SJ, Paterson-Brown S. Changing trends in surgery for acute appendicitis. Br J Surg. 2008;95:363–8. doi:10.1002/bjs.5961.
13. Caravaggio C, Hauters P, Malvaux P, Landenne J, Janssen P. Is laparoscopic appendectomy an effective procedure? Acta Chir Belg. 2007;107:368–72.
14. Craus W, Di Giacomo A, Tommasino U, Frezza A, Festa G, Cricri AM, Mosella G. [Laparoscopic appendectomy and laparotomy appendectomy: comparison of methods. Article in Italian]. Chir Ital. 2001;53:327–37.
15. Yau KK, Siu WT, Tang CN, Yang G, Li MK. Laparoscopic versus open appendectomy for complicated appendicitis. J Am Coll Surg. 2007;205:60–5. doi:10.1016/j.jamcollsurg.2007.03.017.
16. Pokala N, Sadhasivam S, Kiran RP, Parithivel V. Complicated appendicitis –is the laparoscopic approach appropriate? A comparative study with the open approach: outcome in a community hospital setting. Am Surg. 2007;73:737–41.
17. Noble H, Gallagher P, Campbell WB. Who is doing laparoscopic appendectomies and who taught them? Ann R Coll Surg Engl. 2003;85:331–3. doi:10.1308/003588403769162459.
18. Perry Z, Netz U, Mizrahi S, Lanstberg L, Kirshtein B. Laparoscopic appendectomy as an initial step in independent laparoscopic surgery by surgical residents. J Laparoendosc Adv Surg Tech. 2010;20:447–50. doi:10.1089/lap.2009.0430.
19. Shabtai M, Rosin D, Zmora O, Munz Y, Scarlat A, Shabtai EL, Zakai BB, Natour M, Ben-Haim M, Ayalon A. The impact of a resident's seniority on operative time and length of hospital stay for laparoscopic appendectomy. Surg Endosc. 2004;18:1328–30. doi:10.1007/s00464-003-9216-4.
20. Dagash H, Chowdhury M, Pierro A. When can I be proficient in laparoscopic surgery? A systematic review of the evidence. J Pediatr Surg. 2003;38:720–4. doi:10.1016/j.jpsu.2003.50192.
21. Di Saverio S, Mandrioli M, Sibilio A, Smerieri N, Lombardi R, Catena F, Ansaloni L, Tugnoli G, Masetti M, Jovine E. A cost-effective technique for laparoscopic appendectomy: outcomes and costs of a case-control prospective single-operator study of 112 unselected consecutive cases of complicated acute appendicitis. J Am Coll Surg. 2014;218(3):e51–65. doi:10.1016/j.jamcollsurg.2013.12.003.
22. Sanfey H, Ketchum J, Bartlett J, Markwell S, Meier AH, Williams R, Dunnington G. Verification of proficiency in basic skills for postgraduate year 1 residents. Surgery. 2010;148:759–67. doi:10.1016/j.surg.2010.07.018.
23. Sanfey H, Dunnungton G. Verification of proficiency: a prerequisite for clinical experience. Surg Clin North Am. 2010;90:559–67. doi:10.1016/j.suc.2010.02.008.
24. McFadden CL, Cobb WS, Lokey JS, Cull DL, Smith DE, Taylor SM. The impact of a formal minimally invasive service on the resident's ability to achieve new ACGME guidelines for laparoscopy. J Surg Educ. 2007;64:420–3. doi:10.1016/j.jsurg.2007.06.013.
25. Park A, Kavic SM, Lee TH, Heniford BT. Minimally invasive surgery: the evolution of fellowship. Surgery. 2007;140:506–13. doi:10.1016/j.surg.2007.07.009.
26. Unawane A, Kamyab A, Patel M, Flynn JC, Mittal VK. Changing paradigms in minimally invasive surgery training. Am J Surg. 2013;205:284–8. doi:10.1016/j.amjsurg.2012.10.018.

16

Prediction of mortality in patients with colorectal perforation based on routinely available parameters

Takehito Yamamoto[1*], Ryosuke Kita[2], Hideyuki Masui[2], Hiromitsu Kinoshita[2], Yusuke Sakamoto[2], Kazuyuki Okada[2], Junji Komori[2], Akira Miki[2], Kenji Uryuhara[2], Hiroyuki Kobayashi[2], Hiroki Hashida[2], Satoshi Kaihara[2] and Ryo Hosotani[2]

Abstract

Introduction: Even after surgery and intensive postoperative management, the mortality rate associated with colorectal perforation is high. Identification of mortality markers using routinely available preoperative parameters is important.

Methods: We enrolled consecutive patients with colorectal perforation who underwent operations from January 2010 to January 2015. We divided them into a mortality and survivor group and compared clinical characteristics between the two groups. Additionally, we compared the mortality rate between different etiologies: malignant versus benign and diverticular versus nondiverticular. We used the χ^2 and Mann–Whitney U tests and a logistic regression model to identify factors associated with mortality.

Results: We enrolled 108 patients, and 52 (48 %) were male. The mean age at surgery was 71 ± 13 years. The postoperative mortality rate was 12 % (13 patients). Multivariate logistic regression analysis showed that a high patient age (odds ratio [OR], 1.09; 95 % confidence interval [CI], 1.020–1.181) and low preoperative systolic blood pressure (OR, 0.98; 95 % CI, 0.953–0.999) were independent risk factors for mortality in patients with colorectal perforation. In the subgroup analysis, there was no significant difference between the malignant and benign group (11.8 % vs. 23.9 %, respectively; $p = 0.970$), while the diverticular group had a significantly lower mortality rate than the nondiverticular group (2.6 % vs. 17.1 %, respectively; $p = 0.027$).

Conclusions: Older patients and patients with low preoperative blood pressure had a high risk of mortality associated with colorectal perforation. For such patients, operations and postoperative management should be performed carefully.

Keywords: Colorectal perforation, Mortality marker, Prognostic factor

Introduction

Colorectal perforation causes widespread dissemination of bacteria throughout the intra-abdominal space and easily leads to panperitonitis and septic shock. Septic shock is responsible for disseminated intravascular coagulation and organ failure. Therefore, the mortality rate associated with colorectal perforation is considered to be high. The Complicated Intra-Abdominal infections Worldwide Observational (CIAOW) study, a large multicenter observational study that included 1898 patients undergoing surgery or interventional drainage for complicated intra-abdominal infections performed by Sartelli et al. [1], indicated that colonic nondiverticular perforation was a source of infection that was significantly correlated with patient mortality. Many other studies also analyzed the mortality of colorectal perforation, and the reported mortality rate ranged from 6 to 33 % [2–10]. Immediate surgical management of colorectal perforation is necessary, and preoperative knowledge of the severity of colorectal perforation and risk factors for mortality is

* Correspondence: tkht26@me.com
[1]Department of Surgery, Kitano Hospital, The Tazuke Kofukai Medical Research Institute, 2-4-20 Ogimachi, Kita-ku, Osaka 530-8480, Japan
Full list of author information is available at the end of the article

Prediction of mortality in patients with colorectal perforation based on routinely available...

109

also important. Patients with severe peritonitis should undergo preoperative preparations for high-quality postoperative intensive care. Additionally, adequate information about the likelihood of mortality should be provided to the patient and his or her family before the operation.

A number of studies have reported several risk factors for mortality associated with colorectal perforation, such as age, sex, the serum protein level, and the serum creatinine level [2, 5, 7, 8]. However, most such studies involved small samples or were performed many years ago. For example, Alvarez et al. [2] enrolled 114 patients from 1986 to 2005, and Kriwanek et al. [7] enrolled 112 patients from 1979 to 1992. These study periods were too long and included many old cases. On the other hand, a recent study by Shimazaki et al. [8] was performed from 1998 to 2011, but they enrolled just 42 patients. We consider that postoperative intensive care techniques are progressing year by year, and a study enrolling many patients within a short period is necessary in this field. Our institution has a large emergency care unit and serves as the core emergency medicine facility in the region; thus, many patients with colorectal perforation present at our institution every year. Therefore, we analyzed mortality markers in consecutive patients with colorectal perforation who underwent operations in our institution.

Patients and methods
Data collection
We analyzed consecutive patients with colorectal perforation who underwent emergent surgery from January

2010 to January 2015 at a single center. All patients underwent surgery within 24 h of diagnosis. The primary outcome was mortality after surgery. The patients were divided into a mortality group and a survivor group, and we analyzed the factors associated with mortality. Mortality was defined as death of colorectal perforation within 2 months after surgery. The patients' clinical characteristics were reviewed, including age, sex, body mass index, comorbidities, preoperative laboratory data, etiology, and site of perforation.

Additionally, we divided the patients into two groups according to etiology (malignant versus benign and diverticular versus nondiverticular) and compared the mortality rates between these groups. Furthermore, as a subgroup analysis, we analyzed risk factors associated with mortality in the nondiverticular group alone.

The preoperative white blood cell counts were dichotomized into $\geq 4000/\mu L$, <4000 to $\leq 12,000/\mu L$, and $>12,000/\mu L$, and the preoperative body temperature was dichotomized into $\leq 36\ °C$, $36\ °C$ to $\leq 38\ °C$, and $>38\ °C$, which reflect the criteria for systemic inflammatory response syndrome criteria [11]. Other variables were evaluated as continuous variables.

Diagnosis
Colorectal perforation was diagnosed by two or more surgeons and radiologists according to the following criteria: a) the presence of symptoms indicating panperitonitis, such as severe abdominal pain and nausea; b) the presence of signs of peritoneal irritation such as muscular defense and rebound tenderness, indicating

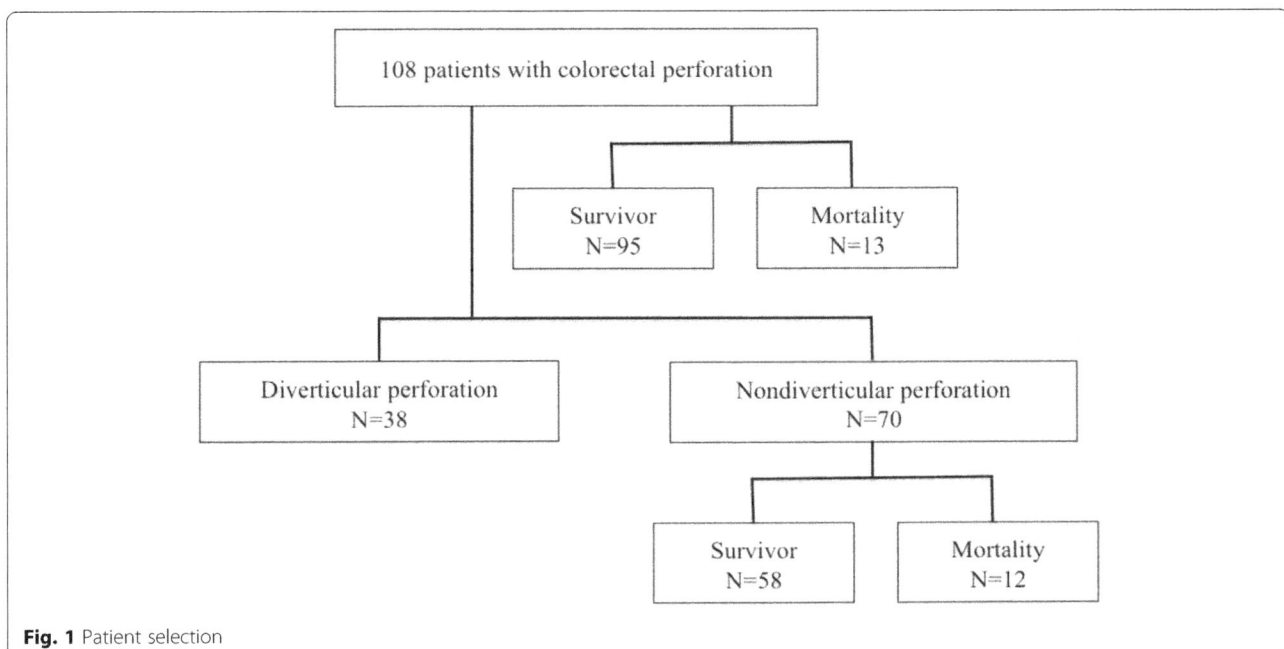

Fig. 1 Patient selection

panperitonitis; and c) the presence of free air on pre-operative computed tomography. Abdominal radiography findings were not useful in diagnosing colorectal perforation and were not included in the diagnostic criteria. All perforations were diagnosed preoperatively and confirmed intraoperatively.

Statistical analyses

Continuous variables are presented as mean ± standard deviation or median (range), and categorical variables are expressed as number and percentage. We used the χ^2 and Mann–Whitney U tests and a logistic regression model to assess the associations between outcomes and clinical characteristics. The factors with a significant relationship in the univariate analyses were subsequently used in the multivariate regression models. The effect of a factor was presented as the odds ratio (OR) and its 95 % confidence interval (CI). All statistical analyses were conducted by one physician (T.Y.) using JMP 10 (SAS Institute Inc., Cary, NC, USA). A p value of <0.05 was considered statistically significant.

The protocol for this study was approved by our hospital's institutional review board. Informed consent was waived because of the historical cohort nature of the study.

Results

Patient selection is shown in Fig. 1. We enrolled 108 patients, whose clinical characteristics are presented in Table 1. Their mean age at surgery was 71 ± 13 years, and 52 (48 %) were male. The etiology of the perforation was a diverticulum ($n = 38$), cancer ($n = 17$), fecal impaction ($n = 17$), iatrogenic ($n = 12$), inflammatory disease ($n = 5$), trauma ($n = 2$), rectal prolapse ($n = 1$), and idiopathic ($n = 16$). All perforative fecal impactions were caused by colorectal obstruction and obstructive colitis by retention of feces and chronic constipation, which were confirmed intraoperatively. Iatrogenic perforations included perforations due to colonoscopy and radiographic contrast enemas, and inflammatory diseases included cytomegalovirus-induced colitis, ulcerative colitis, Behçet's disease, and colitis caused by radiation therapy for rectal cancer.

The postoperative mortality rate was 12 % (13 patients). The clinical characteristics between the survivor group and mortality group are compared in Table 2. The patients were significantly older in the mortality group than in the survivor group (79 ± 8 vs. 70 ± 13 years, respectively; $p = 0.009$). The mean preoperative systolic blood pressure was significantly lower in the mortality group than in the survivor group (96 vs. 130 mmHg, respectively; $p = 0.004$). The mean preoperative serum creatinine level was significantly higher in the morality group than in the survivor group (2.0 ± 1.4 vs. 1.1 ± 1.2 mg/dl,

Table 1 Clinical characteristics of patients

Variables	
Age (years)	71 ± 13
Male	52 (48.1)
Body mass index (kg/m²)	21.5 ± 4.6
Chemotherapy	8 (7.4)
Steroid use	25 (23.1)
Diabetes mellitus	7 (6.5)
Body temperature >38.0 °C or <36.0 °C	34 (31.4)
Systolic blood pressure (mmHg)	127 (50–188)
Heart rate (/min)	98 (54–144)
White blood cells >12,000 or <4000 (/μL)	50 (46.2)
C-reactive protein (mg/dl)	11.7 ± 10.7
Albumin (mg/dl)	2.8 ± 0.8
Creatinine (mg/dl)	1.2 ± 1.2
Perforation etiology	
Diverticulum	38 (35.2)
Cancer	17 (15.7)
Fecal impaction	17 (15.7)
Iatrogenic	12 (11.1)
Inflammatory disease	5 (4.6)
Trauma	2 (1.9)
Rectal prolapse	1 (0.9)
Idiopathic	16 (14.8)
Perforation site	
Cecum	8 (7.4)
Ascending colon	4 (3.7)
Transverse colon	7 (6.5)
Descending colon	6 (5.6)
Sigmoid colon	70 (64.8)
Rectum	13 (12.0)
Stoma creation	84 (77.8)
Length of operation (min)	179 ± 57
Blood loss (g)	219 (0–3112)
Hospital stay (d)	19 (4–185)

Data are presented as mean ± standard deviation, median (range), or n (%)

respectively; $p = 0.004$). Logistic regression analysis using the potential risk factors for mortality determined by univariate analysis (patient age, preoperative systolic blood pressure, and preoperative serum creatinine level) showed that patient age (OR, 1.09; 95 % CI, 1.020–1.181) and preoperative systolic blood pressure (OR, 0.98; 95 % CI, 0.953–0.999) were independent risk factors for mortality in patients with colorectal perforation (Table 3). Figures 2 and 3 compare these two factors between the survivor group and mortality group.

Table 2 Comparison of clinical characteristics between the survivor and mortality groups

Variables	Survivor	Mortality	p value
	n = 95	n = 13	
Age (years)	70 ± 13	79 ± 8	0.009*
Male	48	4	0.181
Body mass index (kg/m^2)	21.8 ± 4.7	19.5 ± 3.3	0.080
Chemotherapy	6	2	0.242
Steroid use	20	5	0.163
Diabetes mellitus	5	2	0.169
Body temperature >38.0 °C or <36.0 °C	30	4	
Systolic blood pressure (mmHg)	130 (60–188)	96 (50–173)	0.004*
Heart rate (/min)	96 (54–144)	110 (75–133)	0.074
White blood cells >12,000 or <4000 (/µL)	45	5	0.546
C-reactive protein (mg/dl)	12.4 ± 11.0	6.8 ± 6.8	0.171
Albumin (mg/dl)	2.9 ± 0.8	2.5 ± 0.7	0.058
Creatinine (mg/dl)	1.1 ± 1.2	2.0 ± 1.4	0.004*
Perforation etiology			0.275
Diverticulum	37	1	
Cancer	15	2	
Fecal impaction	13	4	
Iatrogenic	11	1	
Inflammatory disease	4	1	
Trauma	2	0	
Rectal prolapse	1	0	
Idiopathic	12	4	
Perforation site			0.055
Cecum	7	1	
Ascending colon	3	1	
Transverse colon	7	0	
Descending colon	3	3	
Sigmoid colon	62	8	
Rectum	13	0	
Stoma creation	72	12	0.179
Length of operation (min)	177 ± 55	187 ± 73	0.581
Blood loss (g)	200 (0–3112)	347 (0–1000)	0.248

Data are presented as mean ± standard deviation, median (range), or n
*p < 0.05

Table 3 Multivariate logistic regression analysis of risk factors for mortality of colorectal perforation

Variables	Odds ratio	95 % Confidence interval	p value
Age	1.09	1.020–1.181	0.008*
Systolic blood pressure	0.98	0.953–0.999	0.039*
Creatinine	1.43	0.918–2.206	0.107

*p < 0.05

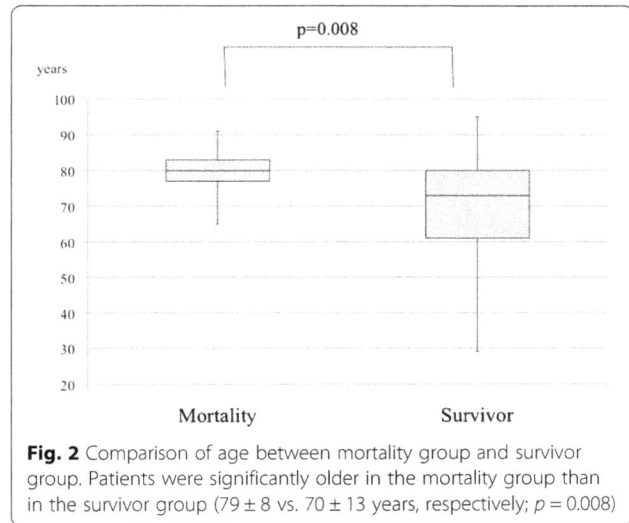

Fig. 2 Comparison of age between mortality group and survivor group. Patients were significantly older in the mortality group than in the survivor group (79 ± 8 vs. 70 ± 13 years, respectively; p = 0.008)

The comparison of the mortality rate between the malignant and benign groups is shown in Fig. 4. There was no significant difference in the mortality rate between the two groups (11.8 % vs. 23.9 %, respectively; p = 0.970). The comparison of the mortality rate between the diverticular and nondiverticular groups is shown in Fig. 5. The mortality rate in the diverticular group was significantly lower than that in the nondiverticular group (2.6 % vs. 17.1 %, respectively; p = 0.027).

The results of subgroup analysis in the nondiverticular group (n = 70) are shown in Tables 4 and 5. In the univariate analysis, older age, lower systolic blood pressure, higher heart rate, and higher serum creatinine level were significantly associated with mortality, and the multivariate analysis showed that age alone was a significant mortality marker (OR, 1.09; 95 % CI, 1.013–1.182).

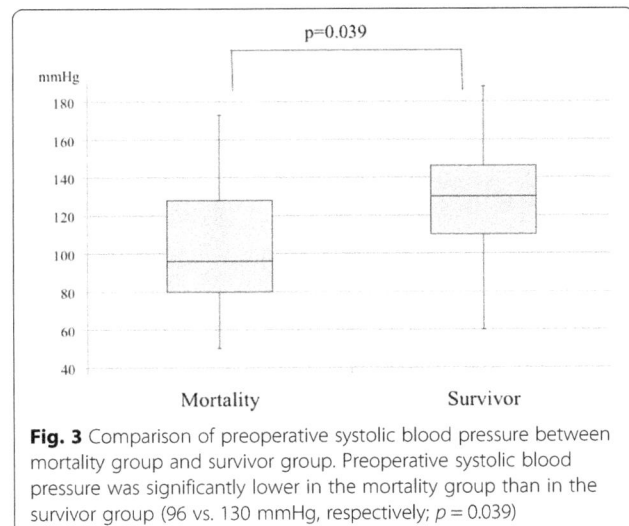

Fig. 3 Comparison of preoperative systolic blood pressure between mortality group and survivor group. Preoperative systolic blood pressure was significantly lower in the mortality group than in the survivor group (96 vs. 130 mmHg, respectively; p = 0.039)

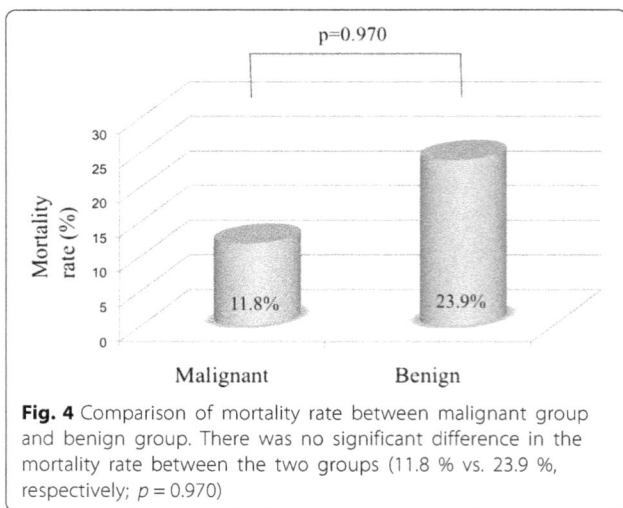

Fig. 4 Comparison of mortality rate between malignant group and benign group. There was no significant difference in the mortality rate between the two groups (11.8 % vs. 23.9 %, respectively; $p = 0.970$)

Discussion

Despite progress in postoperative management, the prognosis of colorectal perforation remains quite poor. Fecal panperitonitis easily causes septic shock, disseminated intravascular coagulation, and multiple organ failure. Prediction of mortality using routinely and easily available preoperative parameters is important to provide adequate information about the likelihood of postoperative death to patients and their families and prepare for intensive postoperative management in case of the need for rescue.

Our study indicates that higher age and a lower preoperative systolic blood pressure are independent risk factors for mortality in patients with colorectal perforation. Like our study, Kriwanek et al. [7] and Alvarez et al. [2] also indicated that higher age was significantly associated with mortality in patients with colorectal perforation. Our study also indicates that colorectal

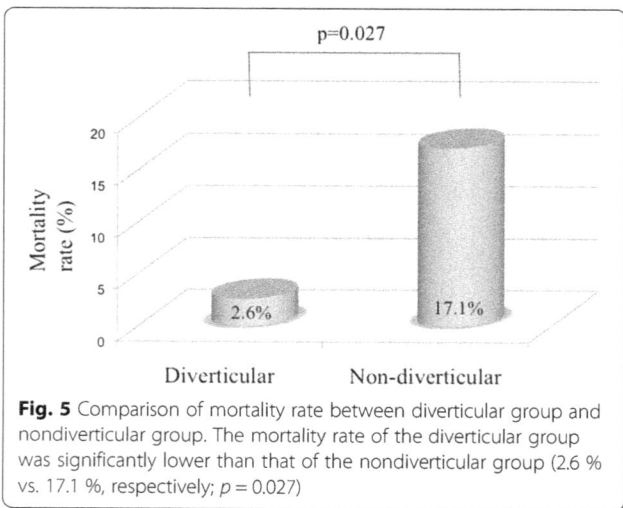

Fig. 5 Comparison of mortality rate between diverticular group and nondiverticular group. The mortality rate of the diverticular group was significantly lower than that of the nondiverticular group (2.6 % vs. 17.1 %, respectively; $p = 0.027$)

Table 4 Comparison of clinical characteristics between the survivor and mortality groups in the nondiverticular group

Variables	Survivor	Mortality	p value
	$n = 58$	$n = 12$	
Age (years)	72 ± 12	81 ± 7	0.008[*]
Male	25	4	0.532
Body mass index (kg/m²)	20.4 ± 4.0	19.4 ± 3.4	0.428
Chemotherapy	4	2	0.271
Steroid use	10	4	0.228
Diabetes mellitus	4	2	0.271
Body temperature >38.0 °C or <36.0 °C	14	3	0.950
Systolic blood pressure (mmHg)	131 (60–188)	95 (50–173)	0.004[*]
Heart rate (/min)	93 (54–144)	110 (75–133)	0.031[*]
White blood cells >12,000 or <4000 (/μL)	29	4	0.288
C-reactive protein (mg/dl)	10.8 ± 11.7	6.3 ± 6.9	0.624
Albumin (mg/dl)	2.8 ± 0.8	2.5 ± 0.7	0.142
Creatinine (mg/dl)	1.1 ± 1.1	1.7 ± 0.9	0.010[*]
Perforation site			0.113
Cecum	4	1	
Ascending colon	2	1	
Transverse colon	6	0	
Descending colon	3	3	
Sigmoid colon	31	7	
Rectum	12	0	
Stoma creation	47	11	0.374
Length of operation (min)	177 ± 58	185 ± 76	0.749
Blood loss (g)	222 (0–1372)	326 (0–1000)	0.492

Data are presented as mean ± standard deviation, median (range), or n
[*] $p < 0.05$

perforation caused by a nondiverticular etiology is associated with higher mortality than diverticular perforation. Sartelli et al. [1] also indicated in their multicenter trial that nondiverticular perforation was significantly associated with mortality among abdominal infectious diseases. Although these data do not delineate the pathophysiology of this relationship, one could theorize that in patients with diverticular perforation, the size of

Table 5 Multivariate logistic regression analysis of risk factors for mortality of colorectal perforation in the nondiverticular group

Variables	Odds ratio	95 % Confidence interval	p value
Age	1.09	1.013–1.182	0.018[*]
Systolic blood pressure	0.98	0.949–1.001	0.064
Heart rate	1.01	0.977–1.055	0.453
Creatinine	1.18	0.633–2.076	0.559

[*] $p < 0.05$

the perforation is generally smaller than that of perforations of other causes, and this can interrupt the spreading of feces to the peritoneal space, leading to a better prognosis. In this retrospective study, we were not able to obtain adequately detailed information about the size and shape of the perforations and were thus unable to confirm this hypothesis. Further investigations are necessary in this respect.

However, the usefulness of a number of risk score systems has been reported in this field. Sugimoto et al. [10] and Horiuchi et al. [5] reported that a higher Acute Physiology and Chronic Health Evaluation II (APACHE II) score was significantly associated with mortality in patients with colorectal perforation. The APACHE II scoring system was developed by Knaus et al. [12] in 1985 and comprises 12 parameters, including blood pressure, body temperature, respiratory rate, and several laboratory data. The severity of each parameter is classified into nine stages from −4 to +4. We considered that the calculation of this score was too complicated for colorectal perforation in the emergency setting. Bielecki et al. [3] and Kriwanek et al. [7] indicated the usefulness of the Mannheim peritonitis index (MPI) for prediction of mortality in patients with colorectal perforation. The MPI was developed by Linder et al. [13] in 1987 and has since been used to predict mortality associated with peritonitis. One parameter of this scoring system, namely the preoperative duration of peritonitis, is sometimes difficult to determine, especially in patients with impaired consciousness. Whether peritonitis is diffuse or focal may also be difficult to ascertain. We considered the fact that both scoring systems were developed approximately 30 years ago and that recent progress has been made in intensive postoperative management regimens, including the use of several medications such as antibiotics. For this reason, we did not use these scoring systems. We consider that the optimal parameters should be able to be easily determined; therefore, in our analysis, we selected parameters that can be determined easily and routinely in the emergent setting. Ishizuka et al. [14] indicated that the Physiologic and Operative Severity Score for the enUmeration of Mortality (POSSUM) was a sensitive system for predicting mortality associated with colorectal perforation. This scoring system was presented in the early 1990s by Copeland et al. [15, 16], and it is reportedly a useful predictor of postoperative mortality. It includes all parameters that were considered to be associated with mortality in the present study: age, preoperative blood pressure, and preoperative serum creatinine level. However, we were unable to retrospectively analyze one parameter of this scoring system, namely respiratory history; we were therefore unable to determine its usefulness.

The serum procalcitonin level is reportedly a useful marker for the diagnosis and severity of peritonitis according to several studies [17–20]. Pupelis et al. [19] analyzed 222 patients and found that higher procalcitonin levels were associated with an increased risk for septic shock. Additionally, Shimazaki et al. [8] indicated that the serum lactate level could be a predictive marker for mortality in patients with colorectal perforation. They indicated in their retrospective analysis that the postoperative serum lactate level was an independent risk factor for mortality in these patients. These parameters are not routinely determined in our institution. The usefulness of these factors should be analyzed in further investigations.

There were several limitations in this study. First, the operative and postoperative management was performed by different doctors and was thus inconsistent in quality. Additionally, this study was conducted at a single center, and the number of patients was small. A large-scale multicenter study should be performed to confirm our findings.

Conclusions

Patient age and preoperative blood pressure are useful for prediction of postoperative mortality in patients with colorectal perforation. For older patients and patients with lower blood pressure, adequate information about this higher mortality rate should be provided to the patients and their family members, and postoperative management should be carefully performed.

Competing interests
The authors declare that they have no competing interests.

Authors' contributions
TY designed the study, acquired the data, analyzed and interpreted the data, and drafted and revised the manuscript. H Kobayashi helped to acquire the data and revise the manuscript. RK, HM, H Kinoshita, YS, KO, JK, AM, KU, HH, SK, and RH helped to revise the manuscript. All authors read and approved the final manuscript.

Author details
[1]Department of Surgery, Kitano Hospital, The Tazuke Kofukai Medical Research Institute, 2-4-20 Ogimachi, Kita-ku, Osaka 530-8480, Japan. [2]Kobe City Medical Center General Hospital, 2-1-1 Minatojima-Minamimachi, Chuoku, Kobe 650-0047, Japan.

References
1. Sartelli M, Catena F, Ansaloni L, Coccolini F, Corbella D, Moore EE, et al. Complicated intra-abdominal infections worldwide: the definitive data of the CIAOW Study. World J Emerg Surg. 2014;9:37.
2. Alvarez JA, Baldonedo RF, Bear IG, Otero J, Pire G, Alvarez P, et al. Outcome and prognostic factors of morbidity and mortality in perforated sigmoid diverticulitis. Int Surg. 2009;94:240–8.
3. Bielecki K, Kaminski P, Klukowski M. Large bowel perforation: morbidity and mortality. Tech Coloproctol. 2002;6:177–82.
4. Biondo S, Ramos E, Deiros M, Rague JM, De Oca J, Moreno P, et al. Prognostic factors for mortality in left colonic peritonitis: a new scoring system. J Am Coll Surg. 2000;191:635–42.

5. Horiuchi A, Watanabe Y, Doi T, Sato K, Yukumi S, Yoshida M, et al. Evaluation of prognostic factors and scoring system in colonic perforation. World J Gastroenterol. 2007;13:3228–31.

6. Komatsu S, Shimomatsuya T, Nakajima M, Amaya H, Kobuchi T, Shiraishi S, et al. Prognostic factors and scoring system for survival in colonic perforation. Hepatogastroenterology. 2005;52:761–4.

7. Kriwanek S, Armbruster C, Beckerhinn P, Dittrich K. Prognostic factors for survival in colonic perforation. Int J Colorectal Dis. 1994;9:158–62.

8. Shimazaki J, Motohashi G, Nishida K, Ubukata H, Tabuchi T. Postoperative arterial blood lactate level as a mortality marker in patients with colorectal perforation. Int J Colorectal Dis. 2014;29:51–5.

9. Shinkawa H, Yasuhara H, Naka S, Yanagie H, Nojiri T, Furuya Y, et al. Factors affecting the early mortality of patients with nontraumatic colorectal perforation. Surg Today. 2003;33:13–7.

10. Sugimoto K, Sato K, Maekawa H, Sakurada M, Orita H, Ito T, et al. Analysis of the efficacy of direct hemoperfusion with polymyxin B-immobilized fiber (PMX-DHP) according to the prognostic factors in patients with colorectal perforation. Surg Today. 2013;43:1031–8.

11. Bone RC, Balk RA, Cerra FB, Dellinger RP, Fein AM, Knaus WA, et al. Definitions for sepsis and organ failure and guidelines for the use of innovative therapies in sepsis. The ACCP/SCCM Consensus Conference Committee. American College of Chest Physicians/Society of Critical Care Medicine. Chest. 1992;101:1644–55.

12. Knaus WA, Draper EA, Wagner DP, Zimmerman JE. APACHE II: a severity of disease classification system. Crit Care Med. 1985;13:818–29.

13. Linder MM, Wacha H, Feldmann U, Wesch G, Streifensand RA, Gundlach E. The Mannheim peritonitis index. An instrument for the intraoperative prognosis of peritonitis. Chirurg. 1987;58:84–92.

14. Ishizuka M, Nagata H, Takagi K, Horie T, Kubota K. POSSUM is an optimal system for predicting mortality due to colorectal perforation. Hepatogastroenterology. 2008;55:430–3.

15. Copeland GP, Jones D, Walters M. POSSUM: a scoring system for surgical audit. Br J Surg. 1991;78:355–60.

16. Copeland GP, Sagar P, Brennan J, Roberts G, Ward J, Cornford P, et al. Risk-adjusted analysis of surgeon performance: a 1-year study. Br J Surg. 1995;82:408–11.

17. Yang SK, Xiao L, Zhang H, Xu XX, Song PA, Liu FY, et al. Significance of serum procalcitonin as biomarker for detection of bacterial peritonitis: a systematic review and meta-analysis. BMC Infect Dis. 2014;14:452.

18. Ivancevic N, Radenkovic D, Bumbasirevic V, Karamarkovic A, Jeremic V, Kalezic N, et al. Procalcitonin in preoperative diagnosis of abdominal sepsis. Langenbecks Arch Surg. 2008;393:397–403.

19. Pupelis G, Drozdova N, Mukans M, Malbrain ML. Serum procalcitonin is a sensitive marker for septic shock and mortality in secondary peritonitis. Anaesthesiol Intensive Ther. 2014;46:262–73.

20. Reith HB, Mittelkotter U, Wagner R, Thiede A. Procalcitonin (PCT) in patients with abdominal sepsis. Intensive Care Med. 2000;26 Suppl 2:S165–9.

17

Validity of predictive factors of acute complicated appendicitis

Yuki Imaoka[1,2*], Toshiyuki Itamoto[1], Yuji Takakura[1], Takahisa Suzuki[1], Satoshi Ikeda[1] and Takashi Urushihara[1]

Abstract

Background: Our previous retrospective study revealed the three preoperative predictors of complicated appendicitis (perforated or gangrenous appendicitis), which are body temperature ≥37.4 °C, C-reactive protein ≥4.7 mg/dl, and fluid collection surrounding the appendix on computed tomography. We reported here an additional prospective study to verify our ability to predict complicated appendicitis using the three preoperative predictors and thus facilitate better informed decisions regarding emergency surgery during night or holiday shifts.

Methods: We prospectively evaluated 116 adult patients who underwent surgery for acute appendicitis from January 2013 to October 2014. Ninety patients with one or more predictive factors of complicated appendicitis underwent immediate surgery regardless of the time of patient's presentation. Twenty-six patients had no predictive factors and thus were suspected to have uncomplicated appendicitis. Of the 26 patients, 14 who presented to our hospital during office hours underwent immediate surgery. The other 12 patients who presented to our hospital at night or on a holiday underwent short, in-hospital delayed surgery during office hours.

Results: All patients with no predictive factors had uncomplicated appendicitis, whereas 37 %, 81 %, and 100 % of patients with one, two, or all three factors, respectively, were diagnosed with complicated appendicitis. The emergency operation rate decreased from 83 % before to 58 % after adopting this scoring system, but no significant differences in postoperative complication rates and hospitalization periods were observed.

Conclusions: The above-mentioned preoperative factors predictive of complicated appendicitis preoperatively are useful for emergency surgical decisions and reduce the burdens on surgeons and medical staff.

Keywords: Acute appendicitis, Predictive factor, Emergency surgery

Background

Acute appendicitis is the most well-known acute abdominal disease. However, not all diagnosed cases of acute appendicitis require emergency surgery. Non-operative management is recommended for uncomplicated appendicitis [1], but preoperative distinction between uncomplicated and complicated disease is challenging. In addition, cases of complicated appendicitis, which include perforated appendicitis and gangrenous appendicitis, may progress to acute peritonitis, a condition that necessitates emergency surgery regardless of the time of development. This emergent nature presents additional complications, as our hospital is staffed by young surgical residents (3–5 years after graduation) at night and over holidays, who examine patients and make decisions regarding the indications for emergency surgeries (e.g., appendectomy). In contrast, the short-term risk of perforation in cases of uncomplicated appendicitis, such as catarrhal and cellulitis appendicitis is low, and these cases can be treated conservatively with antibiotics until sufficient on-duty medical staffs are available to perform surgery. In addition, some of these cases can continue receiving conservative treatment with antibiotics [2–4].

To address the challenge presented by the emergent nature of some appendicitis cases, we performed a retrospective study in which we considered three factors, a body temperature ≥37.4 °C, C-reactive protein (CRP) level ≥4.7 mg/dl, and fluid collection surrounding the appendix on computed tomography (CT), as potential preoperative

---

* Correspondence: ub044982kkr@yahoo.co.jp
[1]Department of Gastroenterological Surgery, Hiroshima Prefectural Hospital, 5-54, Ujinakanda, Minami-ku, Hiroshima 734-00041, Japan
[2]Department of Gastroenterological and Transplant Surgery, Applied Life Sciences, Institute of Biomedical & Health Sciences, Hiroshima University, 1-2-3, Kasumi, Minami-ku, Hiroshima 734-8551, Japan

factors predictive of complicated appendicitis [5]. Herein, we report an additional prospective study to verify our ability to predict complicated appendicitis using these factors and thus facilitate better informed decisions regarding emergency surgery during night or holiday shifts.

Methods

Our strategies of the diagnostic strategies of and for acute appendicitis are shown in Fig. 1. Clinical suspicion of acute appendicitis is made based on the routine use of Alvarado [6] and appendicitis inflammatory response (AIR) scores [7]. In the absence of contraindication to CT use such as pregnancy, CT scans are performed for patients with an Alvarado score ≥ of 5 or more and/or AIR score ≥ of 2 or more, if patients had no contraindication of use of CT scan such as pregnancy. A diagnosis of acute appendicitis is given if the patient has when positive CT findings on all of the following CT findings: a short appendix diameter greater than >6 mm, a thickened wall of the appendix, and absence of gas in the appendicular lumen. Decisions to surgery was performed when the patient was positive for at least one of the following findings: the existence of peritoneal irritation, a short appendix diameter ≥10 mm, stone in the appendix root, and ascites around the appendix or Douglas fossa. Patients without these factors received non-operative treatment.

We prospectively evaluated 116 patients who underwent surgery for acute appendicitis from January 2013 to October 2014 in this study. Patients who were treated successfully with antibiotics were excluded. Out of the 116 patients, 90 patients who had one or more factors predictive of complicated appendicitis underwent the immediate surgery regardless of the time of the patients' visited to our hospital. Twenty-six patients had no predictive factors and thus, whose appendicitis were suspected to have be uncomplicated appendicitis. Out of

the 26 patients, 14 patients who presented to our hospital during office hours underwent the immediate surgery. The other 12 patients who presented to our hospital at night or on a holiday underwent delayed surgery during office hours (Fig. 2).

Histopathologically, catarrhal appendicitis was defined as the apparent enlargement of lymphoid follicles in the appendix mucosa, and cellulitis appendicitis was defined as neutrophil infiltration into all layers. Gangrenous appendicitis was defined as neutrophil infiltration and muscle layer necrosis, and perforated appendicitis was defined as necrosis and perforation in all layers. Complicated appendicitis was defined as a pathologically proven gangrenous or perforated appendix. Our strategies for patients with acute appendicitis indicated for surgery included immediate operation for patients with suspicion of complicated appendicitis and short, in-hospital delay for patients with suspicion of uncomplicated appendicitis.

JMP statistical software (JMP® 11; SAS Institute Inc., Cary, NC, USA) was used for the statistical analysis. A p-value ≤0.05 was considered statistically significant. Pearson's chi-square test was used to determine the significance of differences between dichotomous groups. Fisher's exact test was used when a table included a cell with an expected frequency of <5.

Results

The prospective study included 65 male (56 %) and 51 female patients (44 %). The general patient characteristics are shown in Table 1. The mean patient age was 44.5 years, with a range of 14–90 years. Overall, 52 (45 %) of the 116 patients had uncomplicated appendicitis: 2 had pathologically proven catarrhal appendicitis and 50 had pathologically proven cellulitis appendicitis. The remaining 64 patients (55 %) had complicated

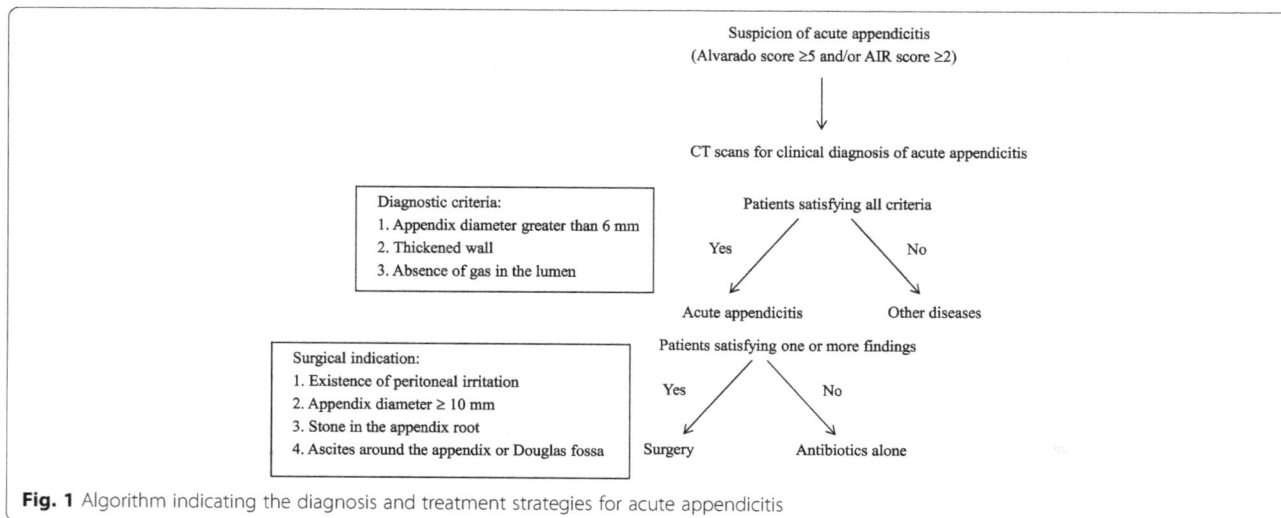

Fig. 1 Algorithm indicating the diagnosis and treatment strategies for acute appendicitis

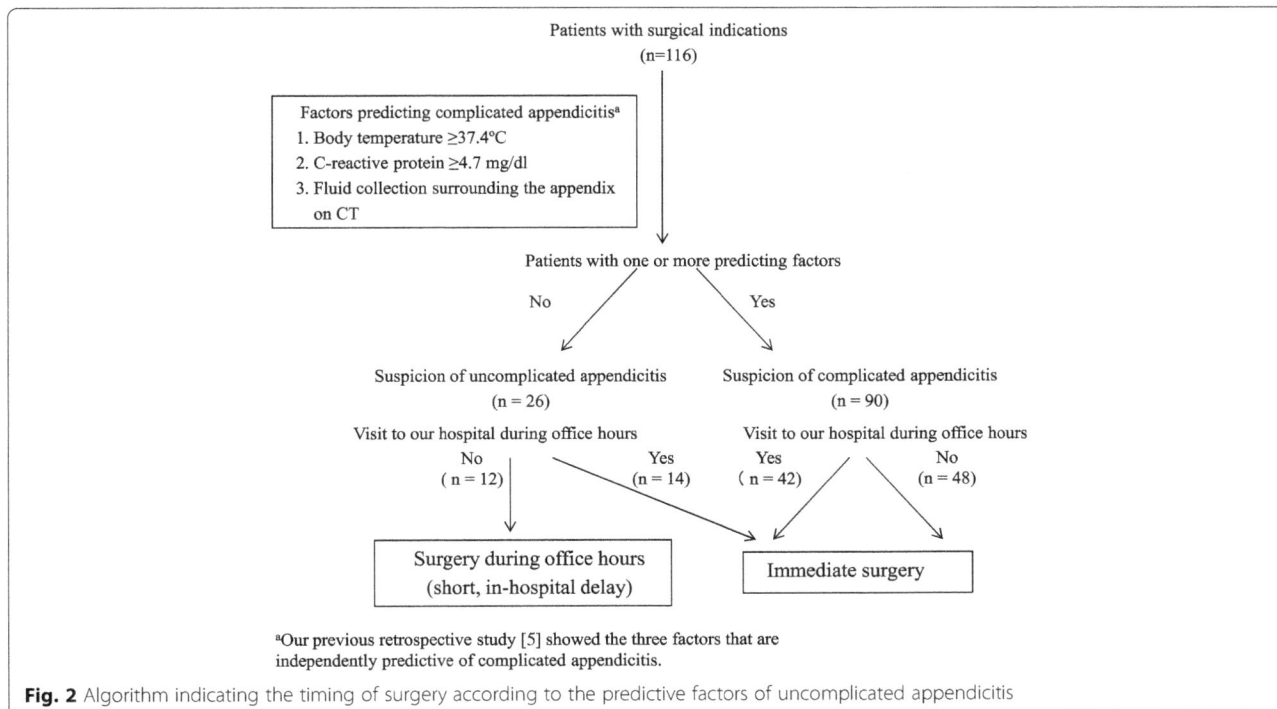

Fig. 2 Algorithm indicating the timing of surgery according to the predictive factors of uncomplicated appendicitis

appendicitis. All patients without any of the three predictive factors (body temperature ≥ 37.4 °C, CRP level ≥ 4.7 mg/dl, and fluid surrounding the appendix on CT) had uncomplicated appendicitis. In contrast, 37 %, 81 %, and 100 % of the patients with one, two, or all three factors, respectively, were proved pathologically to have complicated appendicitis (Table 2).

During the prospective study conducted after adopting this scoring system, 35 (58 %) of the 60 patients admitted to the hospital at night or over a holiday underwent immediate surgery. This represented a decrease of 25 percentage points from the immediate surgery rate of 83 % during the retrospective study period of January 2009 to December 2012 (172 cases). However, there were no significant differences in the postoperative complication rate and hospitalization period between the prospective and retrospective studies (Tables 3 and 4).

Discussion

The Alvarado and AIR scores are standardized diagnostic approaches in evaluating patients with suspected acute appendicitis, using only clinical signs and symptoms and laboratory values. Di Saverio et al. suggested that the combination of scores might significantly reduce the risk of overpredicting acute appendicitis and reach a diagnostic performance as highly reliable as a CT scan, thus avoiding the routine use of CT [8]. Moreover, they emphasized that both scores were the only independent predictive factors of non-operative management failure with antibiotics for uncomplicated appendicitis [8].

The treatment of patients with complicated intra-abdominal infection involves both timely source control and antimicrobial therapy [9]. Clinical trials have demonstrated the successful treatment of acute appendicitis

Table 1 Patient characteristics

Mean age (ranges), years	44.5 (14–90)
Male/female	65/51
During office hour/at night or on a holiday[a]	56/60
Body temperature (°C)	37.4 (35.8–40)
WBC (/μl)	12000 (2700–25700)
CRP (mg/dl)	5.15 (0.2–36.0)
Fluid collection surrounding appendix +/-	66/50
Uncomplicated/complicated	52/64
Operation	
Laparotomy	71
Laparoscopy	42
Ileocecal resection	3

[a]The time when the patients presented to our hospital

Table 2 Relationship between the number of predictive factor and the severity of appendicitis

Number of predictive factor	0	1	2	3
Uncomplicated (n = 52)	26 (100 %)	19 (63 %)	7 (19 %)	0 (0 %)
Complicated (n = 64)	0 (0 %)	11 (37 %)	29 (81 %)	24 (100 %)
Total (n = 116)	26	30	36	24

Table 3 Pathological findings and postoperative outcomes

	January 2009 to December 2012 (172 cases, retrospective study) [5]	January 2013 to October 2014 (116 cases, prospective study)	p-Value
Severity of appendicitis (uncomplicated/ complicated)	120/52	52/64	<0.01
Hospital stay	5 (3–31)	4 (3–22)	N.S.
Postoperative complications	26 (15 %)	21 (18 %)	N.S.

Pathological findings of the resected appendix and postoperative outcomes compared with those of previously published retrospective data
N.S., not significant

with antibiotics [4, 10–12]. Notably, not all cases of appendicitis can be treated surgically, especially cases involving catarrhal appendicitis [13], and unnecessary surgeries should be avoided in light of the risk complications such as ileus (1.2 % of cases) and abdominal hernia (0.68 % of cases) [14]. However, cases of complicated appendicitis, such as perforated appendicitis and gangrenous appendicitis, can potentially progress to acute peritonitis, which necessitates emergency surgery. Cases of complicated appendicitis with localized abscesses, however, present a lower risk of progression to acute peritonitis, allowing surgery to be delayed until normal office hours, and recent studies of this protocol, or interval appendectomy, have confirmed the safety of this approach [3, 15].

The surgical indication criteria for acute appendicitis in our department are shown in Fig. 1. Some of the patients with uncomplicated appendicitis and all of the patients with complicated appendicitis had surgical indication according to our criteria. Although cases of complicated appendicitis should be treated immediately, it remains a question whether cases of uncomplicated appendicitis indicated for surgical treatment should be treated immediately even at night or on a holiday.

Table 4 Immediate operation rates at night or on holiday

	January 2009 to December 2012 (172 cases, retrospective study) [5]	January 2013 to October 2014 (116 cases, prospective study)	p-Value
During office hour/at night or on a holiday[a]	113/59	56/60	< 0.01
Immediate operation rates at night or on holiday	49 (83 %)	35 (58 %)	< 0.01

Results of intentional prevention from immediate surgery at night or on a holiday compared with those of retrospective study when without the intention
[a]The time when the patients presented to our hospital

Although several previous reports have discussed factors associated with the diagnosis of acute appendicitis, the ability of preoperative factors in predicting the presence of complicated appendicitis is not easy to verify [6, 16–18]. However, Atema et al. [19] reported that the scoring system accurately predicted the complicated appendicitis using a maximum possible score of 22 points based on clinical and CT features and a model was created that included age, body temperature, duration of symptoms, white blood cell count, C-reactive protein level, and presence of extraluminal free air, periappendiceal fluid, and appendicolith. Of the 284 patients, 150 had a score of 6 points or less, of whom eight (5.3 %) had complicated appendicitis, giving a negative predictive value (NPV) of 94.7 %. Herein, we report another simple scoring system predicting the complicated appendicitis.

To better identify preoperative predictive factors of complicated appendicitis, we conducted a retrospective and a prospective study to determine the validity of three potential factors (body temperature ≥37.4 °C, CRP ≥4.7 mg/dl, and fluid collection surrounding the appendix on CT) [5]. We performed a receiver operating characteristic (ROC) analysis to identify the most sensitive cut-off level and used multivariate logistic regression analysis to investigate these three predictive values for clinical events in the retrospective study [5]. In the prospective study, we were able to exclude all cases of uncomplicated appendicitis using these predictive factors. Similarly, we could exclude all cases of complicated appendicitis by selecting cases with no predictive factors, giving an NPV of 100 %. In these latter cases, indicated procedures could be postponed to avoid surgeries at night or over holidays. Moreover, a short, in-hospital delay for uncomplicated appendicitis indicated for surgery has proved to be a safe procedure. However, the discrimination of cases with only one or two predictive factors remains controversial, and further prospective study is needed to support decisions regarding emergency surgery in such cases.

After adopting our scoring system, we observed an increase in the frequency of complicated appendicitis, and we expected that the number of patients treated successfully with antibiotics also increased. Non-operative management would be an alternative for uncomplicated appendicitis if cases of complicated appendicitis can be excluded prior to surgery. However, we also recognized some bias in this study, as we excluded patients who were treated successfully with antibiotics from the trial, because we have no way to know their actual pathology. We observed a statistically significant reduction in the frequency of immediate surgery among cases admitted at night or on holidays from 83 % to 58 % after this scoring system was adopted, indicating an effective reduction in the burden placed on surgeons and medical staff. Recently, the strategy of short, in-hospital delay for uncomplicated appendicitis indicated for surgery has been recommended in the World Society of Emergency Surgery Jerusalem guidelines for diagnosis and treatment of acute appendicitis [1].

Conclusions

In conclusion, the three factors, body temperature ≥37.4 °C, C-reactive protein ≥4.7 mg/dl, and fluid collection surrounding the appendix on CT, are useful in predicting cases of complicated appendicitis preoperatively and can thus facilitate decisions regarding emergency surgery. The scoring system can avoid emergency surgery at night or on a holiday and lead to non-operative management.

Abbreviations
AIR: Appendicitis inflammatory response; CRP: C-reactive protein; CT: Computed tomography; NPV: Negative predictive value; ROC: Receiver operating characteristic

Acknowledgments
Not applicable.

Funding
This research received no specific grant from any funding agency, commercial, or not-for-profit sectors.

Authors' contributions
Y.I. and T.I. performed the research/study, analyzed the data, and wrote the manuscript. Y.T., T.S., S.I., and T.U. performed the research/study and analyzed the data. T.I. designed the study and interpreted the results. All authors read and approved the final manuscript.

Competing interests
The authors declare that they have no competing interests.

References
1. Saverio S, Birindelli A, Kelly MD, Catena F, Weber DG, Sartelli M, et al. WSES Jerusalem guidelines for diagnosis and treatment of acute appendicitis. World J Emerg Surg. 2016;11:34.
2. Varadhan KK, Neal KR, Lobo DN. Safety and efficacy of antibiotics compared with appendicectomy for treatment of uncomplicated acute appendicitis: meta-analysis of randomised controlled trials. BMJ. 2012;344:e2156.
3. Anderson PA. Nonsurgical treatment of patients with thoracolumbar fractures. Instr Course Lect. 1995;44:57–65.
4. Styrud J, Eriksson S, Nilsson I, Ahlberg G, Haapaniemi S, Neovius G, et al. Appendectomy versus antibiotic treatment in acute appendicitis. a prospective multicenter randomized controlled trial. World J Surg. 2006;30:1033–7.
5. Imaoka Y, Urushihara T, Ohhara M, Itamoto T. A study of preoperative predictive factors of appendicitis requiring rapid emergency operation (in Japanese with English abstract). Nihon Rinshogeka Gakkaizasshi (J Jpn Surg Assoc). 2015;76:1–5.
6. Alvarado A. A practical score for the early diagnosis of acute appendicitis. Ann Emerg Med. 1986;15:557–64.
7. Andersson M, Andersson RE. The appendicitis inflammatory response score: a tool for the diagnosis of acute appendicitis that outperforms the Alvarado score. World J Surg. 2008;32:1843–9.
8. Di Saverio S, Sibilio A, Giorgini E, Biscardi A, Villani S, Coccolini F, et al. The NOTA Study (Non Operative Treatment for Acute Appendicitis): prospective study on the efficacy and safety of antibiotics (amoxicillin and clavulanic acid) for treating patients with right lower quadrant abdominal pain and long-term follow-up of conservatively treated suspected appendicitis. Ann Surg. 2014;260:109–17.
9. Sartelli M, Weber DG, Ruppé E, Bassetti M, Wright BJ, Ansaloni L, et al. Antimicrobials: a global alliance for optimizing their rational use in intra-abdominal infections (AGORA). World J Emerg Surg. 2016;11:33.
10. Eriksson S, Granstrom L. Randomized controlled trial of appendicectomy versus antibiotic therapy for acute appendicitis. Br J Surg. 1995;82:166–9.
11. Hansson J, Korner U, Khorram-Manesh A, Solberg A, Lundholm K. Randomized clinical trial of antibiotic therapy versus appendicectomy as primary treatment of acute appendicitis in unselected patients. Br J Surg. 2009;96:473–81.
12. Malik AA, Bari SU. Conservative management of acute appendicitis. J Gastrointest Surg. 2009;13:966–70.
13. Temple CL, Huchcroft SA, Temple WJ. The natural history of appendicitis in adults. A prospective study. Ann Surg. 1995;221:278–81.
14. Schwerk WB, Wichtrup B, Rothmund M, Ruschoff J. Ultrasonography in the diagnosis of acute appendicitis: a prospective study. Gastroenterology. 1989;97:630–9.
15. Deakin DE, Ahmed I. Interval appendicectomy after resolution of adult inflammatory appendix mass – is it necessary? Surgeon. 2007;5:45–50.
16. de Castro SM, Unlu C, Steller EP, van Wagensveld BA, Vrouenraets BC. Evaluation of the appendicitis inflammatory response score for patients with acute appendicitis. World J Surg. 2012;36:1540–5.
17. Wu JY, Chen HC, Lee SH, Chan RC, Lee CC, Chang SS. Diagnostic role of procalcitonin in patients with suspected appendicitis. World J Surg. 2012;36:1744–9.
18. Andersson RE. Meta-analysis of the clinical and laboratory diagnosis of appendicitis. Br J Surg. 2004;91:28–37.
19. Atema JJ, van Rossem CC, Leeuwenburgh MM, Stoker J, Boermeester MA. Scoring system to distinguish uncomplicated from complicated acute appendicitis. Br J Surg. 2015;102:979–90.

A combination of SOFA score and biomarkers gives a better prediction of septic AKI and in-hospital mortality in critically ill surgical patients

Chao-Wei Lee[1,2,3], Hao-wei Kou[1], Hong-Shiue Chou[1], Hsu-huan Chou[1], Song-Fong Huang[1], Chih-Hsiang Chang[4], Chun-Hsing Wu[3], Ming-Chin Yu[1,2] and Hsin-I Tsai[3,5*]

Abstract

Background: Sepsis is a syndrome characterized by a constellation of clinical manifestations and a significantly high mortality rate in the surgical intensive care unit (ICU). It is frequently complicated by acute kidney injury (AKI), which, in turn, increases the risk of mortality. Therefore, it is of paramount importance to identify those septic patients at risk for the development of AKI and mortality. The objective of this pilot study was to evaluate several different biomarkers, including NGAL, calprotectin, KIM-1, cystatin C, and GDF-15, along with SOFA scores, in predicting the development of septic AKI and associated in-hospital mortality in critically ill surgical patients.

Methods: Patients admitted to the surgical ICU were prospectively enrolled, having given signed informed consent. Their blood and urine samples were obtained and subjected to enzyme-linked immunosorbent assay (ELISA) to determine the levels of various novel biomarkers. The clinical data and survival outcome were recorded and analyzed.

Results: A total of 33 patients were enrolled in the study. Most patients received surgery prior to ICU admission, with abdominal surgery being the most common type of procedure (27 patients (81.8%)). In the study, 22 patients had a diagnosis of sepsis with varying degrees of AKI, while the remaining 11 were free of sepsis. Statistical analysis demonstrated that in patients with septic AKI versus those without, the following were significantly higher: serum NGAL (447.5 ± 35.7 ng/mL vs. 256.5 ± 31.8 ng/mL, P value 0.001), calprotectin (1030.3 ± 298.6 pg/mL vs. 248.1 ± 210.7 pg/mL, P value 0.049), urinary NGAL (434.2 ± 31.5 ng/mL vs. 208.3 ± 39.5 ng/mL, P value < 0.001), and SOFA score (11.5 ± 1.2 vs. 4.4 ± 0.5, P value < 0.001). On the other hand, serum NGAL (428.2 ± 32.3 ng/mL vs. 300.4 ± 44.3 ng/mL, P value 0.029) and urinary NGAL (422.3 ± 33.7 ng/mL vs. 230.8 ± 42.2 ng/mL, P value 0.001), together with SOFA scores (10.6 ± 1.4 vs. 5.6 ± 0.8, P value 0.003), were statistically higher in cases of in-hospital mortality. A combination of serum NGAL, urinary NGAL, and SOFA scores could predict in-hospital mortality with an AUROC of 0.911.

Conclusions: This pilot study demonstrated a promising panel that allows an early diagnosis, high sensitivity, and specificity and a prognostic value for septic AKI and in-hospital mortality in surgical ICU. Further study is warranted to validate our findings.

Keywords: Sepsis, Acute kidney injury, AKI, Mortality, SOFA score, NGAL, Calprotectin, Critically ill patients, Intensive care unit, Surgical ICU

* Correspondence: alanlee@adm.cgmh.org.tw
[3]Graduate Institute of Clinical Medical Sciences, Chang Gung University, Guishan, Taoyuan, Taiwan, Republic of China
[5]Department of Anesthesiology, Chang Gung Memorial Hospital, Linkou, Taiwan, Republic of China
Full list of author information is available at the end of the article

Background

Recently, the Third International Consensus Definitions Task Force (Sepsis-3) has proposed new criteria defining sepsis as the presence of infection and an increase in the Sequential Organ Failure Assessment (SOFA) score greater than or equal to 2, which has been associated with an in-hospital mortality as high as 10% [1]. A change in the SOFA score has been found to have high predictive validity and prognostic accuracy for in-hospital mortality in the intensive care unit setting [2, 3]. Sepsis is a known major contributing factor to the development of acute kidney injury (AKI), and the incidence of AKI among critically ill patients can be as high as 67% [4–6]. AKI is a continuum of clinical manifestations ranging from mild, reversible injury to severe, irreversible damage leading to permanent loss of renal function. Sepsis-associated acute kidney injury (or septic AKI) should, therefore, describe a syndrome characterized by Sepsis-3, in addition to the presence of AKI.

Septic AKI arises in approximately 51–64% of patients with sepsis, with a six- to eightfold increase in the risk of in-hospital mortality [7]. The diagnosis of AKI has been made based on the changes of two parameters, serum creatinine (SCr), and urine output. The Acute Dialysis Quality Initiative (ADQI) working party published the RIFLE criteria in 2004, which differentiated three levels of AKI severity (risk, injury, failure) and two outcome stages (loss and end-stage renal disease) [8]. However, such a diagnosis based solely on SCr or on the detection of oliguria may be inadequate, as it may take up to 48 h before a sufficient change in SCr levels becomes detectable [9, 10]. Of late, new biomarkers related to the underlying pathogenesis of AKI, such as neutrophil gelatinase-associated lipocalin (NGAL) [11] and cystatin C [12] have been studied extensively in the diagnosis and prognosis of septic AKI. Calprotectin, composed of two monomers S100A8 and S100A9, is another novel biomarker. It is produced mainly from neutrophils and monocytes in response to ischemic reperfusion injury [13]. Urine calprotectin appeared to have high diagnostic accuracy in differentiating prerenal from intrinsic AKI [14, 15].

Since sepsis and associated conditions represent a significant proportion of complications in the surgical intensive care unit (ICU), it is mandatory to identify those septic patients at risk for the development of AKI and mortality. The objective of the present study was thus to evaluate several different biomarkers, including NGAL, calprotectin, KIM-1, cystatin C, and GDF-15, along with SOFA scores with regard to predicting the development of septic AKI and associated in-hospital mortality in critically ill surgical patients.

Methods

Study population

This study was a prospective cohort study performed in a surgical intensive care unit (ICU) of a 3500-bed tertiary center in Taiwan. The surgical ICU is a 10-bed closed unit managed by a surgeon who is also certified to care for ICU patients. The study was approved by the Institutional Review Board of Chang Gung Memorial Hospital (IRB103-2722A3) and conducted according to the guidelines established by the Declaration of Helsinki. Written informed consent was obtained from all participants. The admission criteria to our surgical ICU include the following: (1) major postoperative complications requiring further invasive intervention; (2) complicated gastrointestinal disorders such as life-threatening gastrointestinal bleeding, fulminant hepatic failure, or severe pancreatitis; (3) hepatic failure complicated with multi-organ dysfunction related to liver transplantation; (4) acute postoperative respiratory distress; (5) cardiovascular instability such as shock of any cause; and (6) other clinical presentations deemed acceptable for ICU admission by the attending physician. We have consecutively recruited all patients admitted to the surgical ICU for 7 months spanning from November 2014 to June 2015. On ICU admission, the patients were initially excluded if they were less than 20 years of age and had a history of chronic kidney disease (CKD) for more than 3 months, inflammatory bowel disease, renal transplantation, or a need for a routine dialysis program. Applying the Sepsis-3 criteria or the identification of an infection site and an increase of greater than or equal to two points in the Sequential Organ Failure Assessment (SOFA) score [1], the patients were allocated into a non-septic group and a septic group. A baseline SOFA score of 0 was assumed for all patients. Among the septic group, some patients were further excluded if no consent form was obtained from the patient or next-of-kin, blood/urine specimens were not collected within the first 24 h of the ICU admission, or patients were transferred to our ICU with the initial treatments started in another ICU. The non-septic group was defined as those patients who had no clinical or laboratory evidence of infection. As this was a pilot study, it was predetermined that patients would be assigned to the septic or non-septic groups in a 2:1 ratio.

Upon admission, patients' demographic information, comorbidities, type of surgery, use of vasopressors, the Acute Physiology and Chronic Health Evaluation (APACHE II), and the Sequential Organ Failure Assessment (SOFA) scores were recorded. SOFA was calculated sequentially based on the worst value of the parameters including partial pressure of oxygen (PaO_2), fraction of inspired oxygen (FiO_2), platelet count, bilirubin, mean arterial blood pressure (MAP), Glasgow Coma Scale (GCS), creatinine, and urine output over the preceding 24 h. The status of AKI was also documented and defined according to the risk, injury, failure, loss of kidney function, and end-stage kidney disease (RIFLE) criteria [8], as follows: a percentage decrease of > 25% in the glomerular filtration rate (GFR) or an increase of ≥ 1.5 times in serum creatinine (SCr) level is defined as risk; a > 50% decrease in GFR or ≥ 2 times increase in SCr is defined as injury; a > 75% decrease in GFR or ≥ 3 times increase in SCr is defined as failure; persistent acute renal failure more than 4 weeks is defined as loss; and complete loss of renal function for more than 3 months is considered end-stage renal disease (ESRD). The patients were followed throughout their ICU stay. CKD was defined as a GFR lower than 60 ml/min/1.73m^2 using the baseline creatinine and the CKD Epidemiology Collaboration equation [16].

Blood sampling and assays

Blood and urine samples were obtained as soon as possible after patients were admitted to the ICU. Blood samples were centrifuged at 1500g for 10 min, while urine samples were centrifuged at 500g for 10 min; both were aliquoted and stored at − 80 °C for batch analysis. Serum and urinary gelatinase-associated lipocalin (NGAL), calprotectin, KIM-1, cystatin C, and GDF-15 were measured using an enzyme-linked immunosorbent assay (ELISA) kit (DuoSet ELISA, R&D Systems; Minneapolis, MN, USA) [17–23]. The dilution ratios for NGAL, calprotectin, KIM-1, cystatin C, and GDF-15

were 1:100, 1:1, 1:100, 1:400, and 1:100, respectively. Albumin, creatinine, procalcitonin, lactate, and C-reactive protein (CRP) were analyzed using enzymatic methods on an automated chemical analyzer in the central laboratory of Chang Gung Memorial Hospital.

Statistical analysis

The continuous variable data were tested for normality distribution using Kolmogorov-Smirnov and Shapiro-Wilk tests and presented as the mean ± standard error of mean (SEM). The independent sample t test and the Mann–Whitney U test were used for comparison of the study groups. Categorical variables were compared using Fisher's test or Pearson's chi-square test and presented as absolute frequency and percentages. Receiver operating characteristic (ROC) curve analysis was performed to determine the performance of biomarker concentration in the prediction of septic AKI and in-hospital mortality. Data analysis was performed using SPSS version 13 (SPSS Inc., Chicago, IL, USA). P values less than 0.05 were considered statistically significant.

Results

Study population

Over the 7-month study period, a total of 315 patients were admitted to the surgical ICU, and after applying exclusion criteria, 83 patients were allocated to the septic group, as depicted in Fig. 1. Of the 83 patients with sepsis, 61 were further excluded from the study due to a refusal to participate ($N = 42$), an absence of next-of-kin to

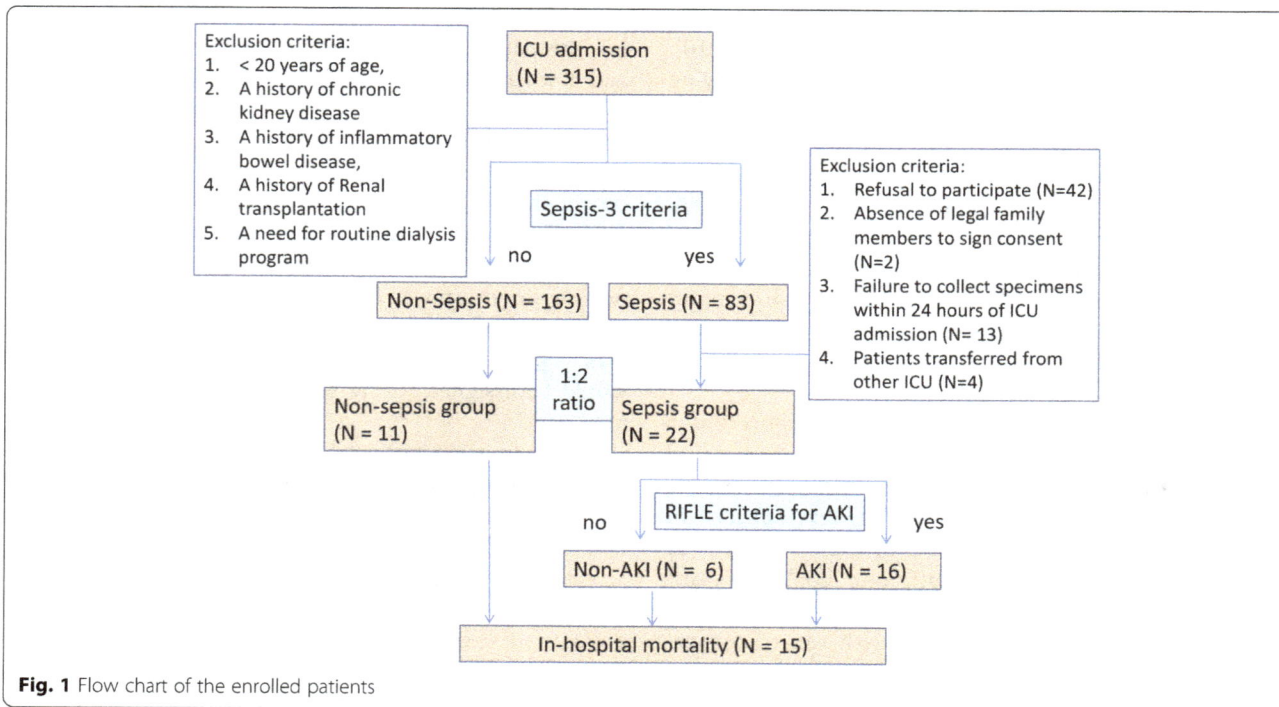

Fig. 1 Flow chart of the enrolled patients

consent ($N = 2$), a failure to collect blood/urine specimens within 24 h of ICU admission ($N = 13$), and a transfer from another ICU where initial treatments had been started ($N = 4$). The baseline demographics and clinical characteristics of the 33 patients are shown in Tables 1 and 2. A majority of the patients were males (60.6%) and over 65 years of age (63.6%), with a mean age of 66.3 years. Among these 33 patients, 22 had a diagnosis of sepsis with varying degrees of AKI, while the remaining 11 were free of sepsis. In 15 (45.6%) patients, intra-abdominal infection was the sepsis etiology, 2 patients (6.1%) had pneumonia, 2 (6.1%) had Fournier's gangrene identified as soft tissue infection, 1 (3.0%) had a urinary tract infection, while 2 (6.1%) had sepsis of unknown origin. Of the 16 patients finally diagnosed with AKI, 14 (42.4%) had a status of R, I, or F, according to the RIFLE criteria, while the other two had a status of L. As depicted in Tables 1 and 2, although 60% of the patients were not on vasopressors, 84.8% of patients required the assistance of mechanical ventilation, with an average of 8.9 ± 20.3 days before successful endotracheal extubation. The length of hospital stay ranged from 2 to 114 days (mean 39.1 ± 25.1 days), with a mean ICU stay of 12.6 ± 25.3 days.

Analysis of biomarkers and clinical parameters

Serum and urinary levels of calprotectin, NGAL, and cystatin C, in addition to the SOFA and APACHE II scores, were measured in septic AKI patients and represented as scatter dot plots in Fig. 2. Serum and urinary levels of GDF-15 and KIM-1 are depicted in the Additional file 1: Figure S1. Similar scatter dot plots representing in-hospital mortality are shown in Fig. 3 and in the Additional file 2: Figure S2.

Sepsis

The mean levels of the five different biomarkers, namely, NGAL, calprotectin, KIM-1, cystatin C, and GDF-15, in the serum and urine samples were compared, as shown in the Sepsis column of Table 3. Patients with sepsis had significantly higher levels of both serum and urinary NGAL (both P values < 0.001). Serum and urinary cystatin C (P value 0.016 and P value 0.046, respectively) levels were also significantly higher in septic patients. Other biochemical parameters showing statistical significance included serum albumin, creatinine, and CRP (P values 0.025, 0.004, and < 0.001, respectively). Septic patients also had statistically higher SOFA (P value 0.001) and APACHE II (P value 0.001) scores upon ICU admission.

Septic AKI

As shown in the Septic AKI column of Table 3, the levels of serum and urinary NGAL (P values 0.001 and < 0.001, respectively) were significantly higher in patients

Table 1 Demographic characteristics at ICU admission (categorical variable)

Variables		No.	(%)
Age (years)	≥ 65	21	63.6
	< 65	12	36.4
Gender	Male	20	60.6
	Female	13	39.4
BMI (kg/m2)	< 18.5	4	12.1
	18.5–24.9	16	48.5
	25–29.9	12	36.4
	30–34.9	1	3.0
Comorbidity	Diabetes mellitus	5	15.1
	Hypertension	10	30.3
	Cerebrovascular disease	3	9.1
	Cardiovascular disease	5	15.2
	Chronic lung disease	3	9.1
	Liver cirrhosis	4	12.1
	Malignancy	18	54.5
Type of surgery	Hepatobiliary surgery	6	18.2
	Gastrointestinal surgery	21	63.6
	Others	2	6.1
	Without surgery	4	12.1
Sepsis	Yes	22	66.7
	No	11	33.3
Sepsis etiology	IAI	15	45.6
	Pneumonia	2	6.1
	Soft tissue infection	2	6.1
	Urinary tract infection	1	3.0
	Unknown	2	6.1
SOFA score	0–1	1	3.0
	2–7	17	51.5
	8–11	7	21.2
	> 11	8	24.2
Kidney dysfunction (RIFLE criteria)	Normal	17	51.5
	R, I, F	14	42.4
	L, E	2	6.1
Albumin (g/dL)	≥ 3.5	3	9.1
	< 3.5	30	90.9
Use of vasopressors	Yes	13	39.4
	No	20	60.6
Use of MV	Yes	28	84.8
	No	5	15.2

ICU intensive care unit, *BMI* body mass index, *SOFA* Sequential Organ Failure Assessment, *IAI* intra-abdominal infection, *UTI* urinary tract infection, *MV* mechanical ventilator

Table 2 Demographic characteristics at ICU admission (continuous variable)

Variables	Mean ± SD	Range
Age (years)	66.3 ± 14.7	30–87
BMI (kg/m²)	23.6 ± 3.6	16.6–30.9
SOFA score	7.9 ± 5.0	1–21
APACHE II score	17.4 ± 8.0	7–38
ICU stay (days)	12.6 ± 25.3	1–103
Hospital stay (days)	39.1 ± 25.1	2–114
Duration of MV (days)	8.9 ± 20.3	1–103
Glasgow Coma Scale	11.6 ± 2.7	3–15
Survival time for expired patients (days)	35.1 ± 33.9	1–103
Albumin (g/dL)	2.7 ± 0.57	1.7–4.2
CRP (mg/L)	123.3 ± 95.8	4.7–311.1
Procalcitonin (ng/mL)	33.8 ± 58.7	0.0–200.0
Lactate (mg/dL)	40.4 ± 40.2	10.0–179.7
Creatinine (mg/dL)	1.4 ± 1.7	0.4–9.7
eGFR (mL/min)	80.4 ± 51.3	5.3–192.0
Na (mEq/L)	138.0 ± 6.3	127.0–157.0
K (mEq/L)	4.0 ± 0.8	2.0–6.0
Bilirubin (mg/dL)	3.6 ± 5.9	0.1–31.0
INR	1.6 ± 0.6	1.1–3.3
Platelet count (103/uL)	166.1 ± 137.0	25.0–613.0

ICU intensive care unit, *SD* standard deviation, *BMI* body mass index, *SOFA* Sequential Organ Failure Assessment, *APACHE* Acute Physiology and Chronic Health Evaluation, *MV* mechanical ventilation, *CRP* C-reactive protein, *eGFR* estimated glomerular filtration rate, *INR* international normalized ratio

with septic AKI than in those without. Although serum calprotectin (*P* value 0.049) showed statistical significance, urinary calprotectin (*P* value 0.102) was not significantly elevated in patients with septic AKI. The levels of serum albumin, creatinine, CRP, SOFA score, and the APACHE II score (*P* values 0.007, < 0.001, 0.008, < 0.001, and 0.001, respectively) all showed significant elevation in the septic AKI group when compared to the non-septic AKI group.

In-hospital mortality

Patients with in-hospital mortality (*n* = 15) showed significantly higher levels of serum NGAL (*P* value 0.029) and urinary NGAL (*P* value 0.001) on ICU admission, as shown in the In-hospital Mortality column of Table 3. The SOFA and APACHE II scores, serum albumin, and creatinine also showed statistical significance (*P* values 0.003, 0.004, 0.003, and 0.027, respectively).

Performance of SOFA and biomarkers

Table 4 summarizes the area under the ROC curves (AUROC) of significant variables regarding septic AKI and in-hospital mortality. In predicting septic AKI,

serum and urinary NGAL showed an AUROC of 0.991 and 0.915, respectively. Serum calprotectin showed an AUROC of 0.889. Other parameters with statistical significance in predicting septic AKI included serum creatinine, CRP, SOFA, and APACHE II scores, with the exception of serum albumin.

In predicting in-hospital mortality, serum and urinary NGAL gave a statistical significant AUROC of 0.768 and 0.780, respectively. Similarly, the SOFA and APACHE II scores showed an AUROC of 0.774 and 0.762, respectively. Albumin also showed statistical significance in predicting in-hospital mortality, even though no statistical significance was observed in predicting septic AKI. Of great interest, a combination of serum NGAL, serum calprotectin, and SOFA score presented an AUROC of 1.000 (*P* value < 0.001) for septic AKI, while a combination of serum NGAL, urinary NGAL, and SOFA score gave an AUROC of 0.911 (*P* value < 0.001) for in-hospital mortality.

The ROC curves of individual plasma and urinary biomarkers along with the SOFA and APACHE II scores are shown in Fig. 4a, c, for the prediction of septic AKI and in-hospital mortality, and a combination of biomarkers and SOFA score is shown in Fig. 4b, d.

Further analysis was performed within the sepsis cohort, as shown in Additional file 3: Table S1. In predicting septic AKI, serum and urinary NGAL and serum calprotectin appeared to be statistically significant with an AUROC of 0.981, 0.885, and 0.962, respectively. A combination of serum NGAL, serum calprotectin, and SOFA score gave a high AUROC of 1.000 (*P* value 0.003). In predicting in-hospital mortality, similarly to what was demonstrated previously, a combination of serum NGAL, urinary NGAL, and SOFA score gave an AUROC of 0.963 (*P* value 0.001). The ROC curves of a combination of biomarkers and SOFA score in predicting septic AKI and in-hospital mortality are demonstrated in Additional file 4: Figure S3A and B.

Discussion

The incidence of sepsis remains high among critically ill patients. Septic patients tend to have longer ICU stays, hospital stays, and significantly higher ICU and in-hospital mortality than those in the general ICU population [24]. The new Sepsis-3 criteria include suspected or documented infection and a two-point increase in SOFA score. The first step to optimal treatment of sepsis is to promptly identify patients with sepsis. The SOFA score has been shown to have a high predictive validity and prognostic accuracy for in-hospital mortality, with an AUROC of 0.74 and 0.753, respectively [2, 3]. Because septic AKI is common during the first 24 h after ICU admission and is

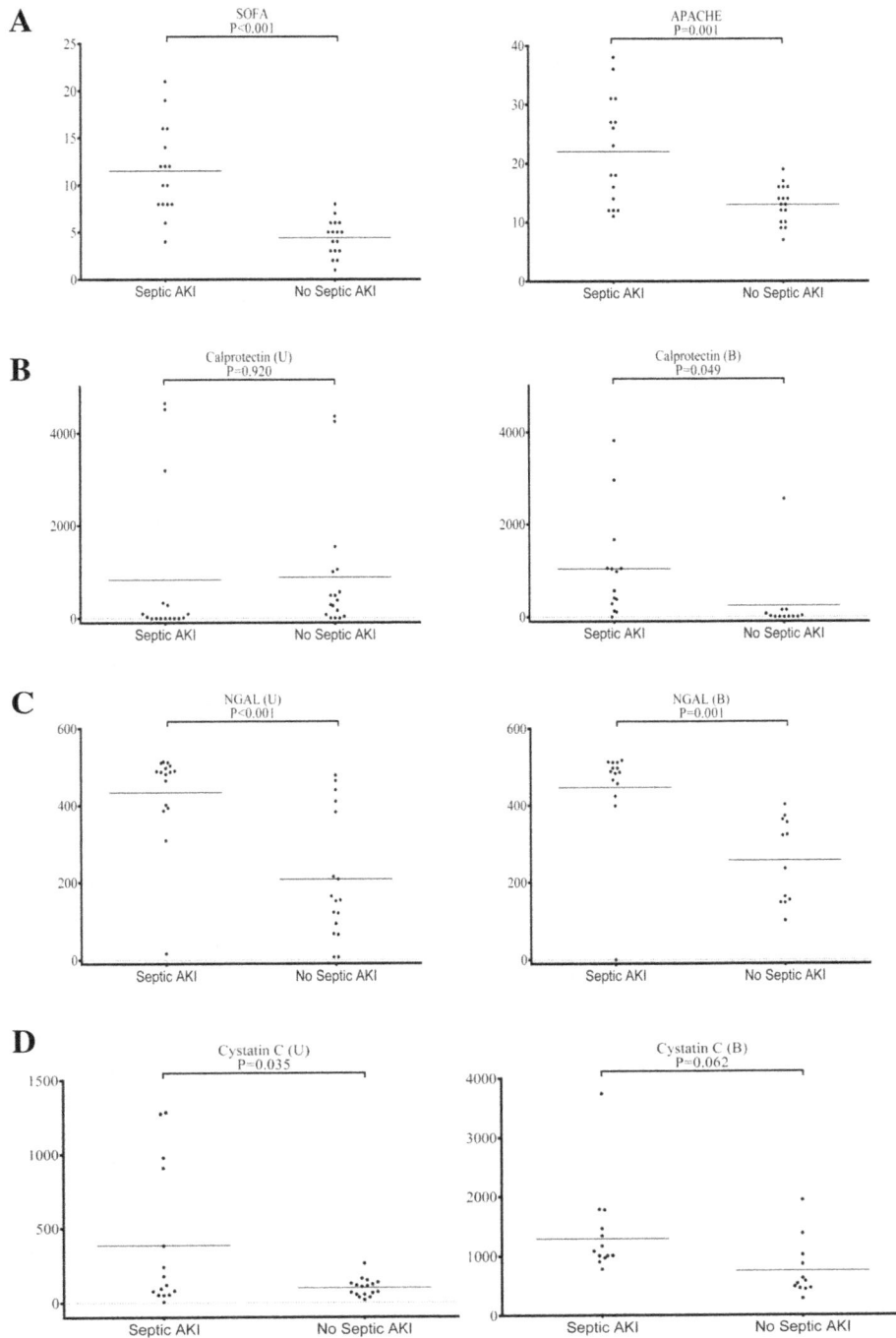

Fig. 2 a–d Septic AKI. SOFA and APACHE II scores and serum and urinary levels of calprotectin, NGAL, and cystatin C. SOFA and APACHE II scores (**a**), calprotectin (**b**), NGAL (**c**), and cystatin C (**d**). The serum and urinary levels are represented as scatter dot plots, and the medians are reported. The arithmetic means of the tested parameters are indicated by a line. SOFA Sequential Organ Failure Assessment, APACHE Acute Physiology and Chronic Health Evaluation, NGAL neutrophil gelatinase-associated lipocalin

associated with higher ICU and in-hospital mortality [25], studies on biomarkers have become of great interest. With the recent literature available on novel biomarkers identified in septic AKI, we have conducted a prospective study in a surgical intensive care unit, investigating the use of NGAL, calprotectin, KIM-1, cystatin-C, and GDF-15 in combination with SOFA to improve early recognition of such patients.

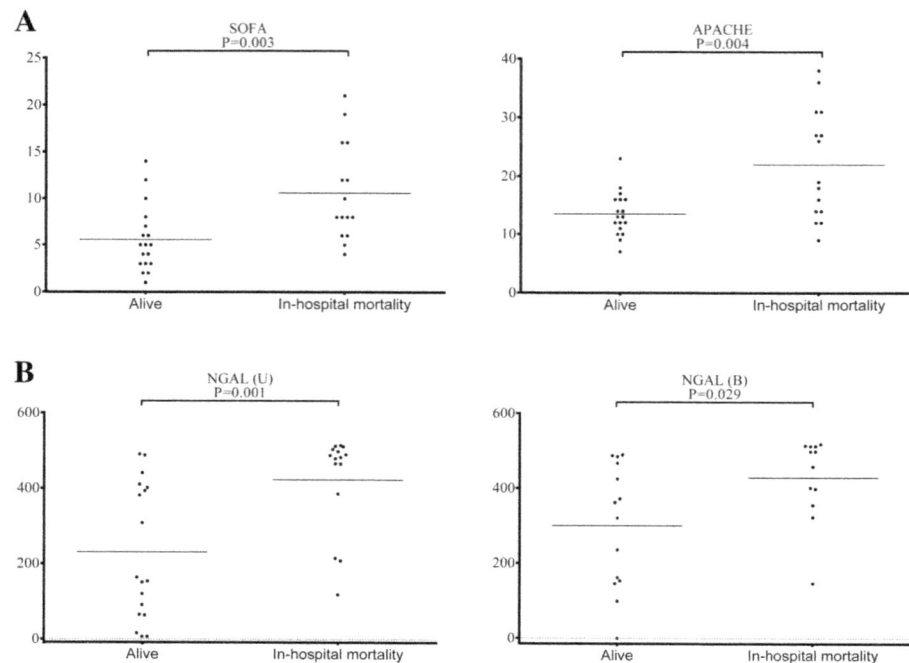

Fig. 3 a–b In-hospital mortality. SOFA and APACHE II scores and serum and urinary levels of NGAL. **a** SOFA and APACHE II scores. **b** NGAL. The serum and urinary levels are represented as scatter dot plots, and the medians are reported. The arithmetic means of the tested parameters are indicated by a line. SOFA Sequential Organ Failure Assessment, APACHE Acute Physiology and Chronic Health Evaluation, NGAL neutrophil gelatinase-associated lipocalin

NGAL has been proven to be a valuable biomarker for early identification of AKI [26]. Studies have been conducted investigating the predictive value of NGAL as a biomarker of septic AKI. Plasma NGAL has been shown to have an AUC of 0.86, indicating an adequate diagnostic accuracy [11]. Urine NGAL, similarly, showed an AUC of at least 0.84 in predicting septic AKI [27, 28]. NGAL also appears to be an independent predictor of 7-day and 28-day mortality in critically ill patients, with an AUROC of 0.883 and 0.723, respectively [29]. Supported by the literature, we have also demonstrated that plasma and urinary NGAL showed a comparable predictive value for septic AKI and in-hospital mortality in critically ill surgical patients. A combination of serum and urinary NGAL and SOFA score showed a high AUROC of 0.911, providing a better predictor of in-hospital mortality than any single parameter alone.

Calprotectin, a heterodimer complex of S100A8/A9 primarily released by neutrophils, monocytes, and macrophages, lately has been studied extensively [30]. Gao et al. [31] have shown that the level of calprotectin was correlated with the degree of sepsis severity, with an AUROC of 0.901 and a sensitivity and specificity of 83.1% and 88.5%, respectively. Similar to our study, they demonstrated that calprotectin levels were significantly higher in patients with septic AKI and in non-survivors at 28 days than in those not meeting these conditions.

We have also successfully revealed calprotectin to be a sensitive and specific biomarker in detecting septic AKI, with an AUROC as high as 0.889.

As sepsis is frequently complicated by AKI, which, in turn, is a major risk factor of mortality, a prompt diagnosis of sepsis is also crucial to establish timely treatment. The present study demonstrated that although the clinical practice scoring systems such as SOFA and APACHE showed good diagnostic and prognostic ability, a panel of serum/urinary NGAL and serum calprotectin and SOFA score raised the AUROC to 1.000 in diagnosing septic AKI and to 0.911 in predicting in-hospital mortality. Further analysis within the sepsis cohort demonstrated that such a panel likewise raised the AUROC to 1.000 in predicting septic AKI and to 0.963 in predicting in-hospital mortality. However, despite such promising results, some limitations apply. First, the sample size was limited, which may have led to patient selection bias. Second, although the results appear promising, only roughly 10% of the ICU patients were enrolled in the study, and the results should be extrapolated cautiously to other critically ill patients. Third, the temporal changes of biomarkers and clinical scores were not obtained. Last but not the least, the current study did not examine the relationship between intra-abdominal pressure and renal function. An elevation in intra-abdominal pressure or intra-abdominal hypertension (IAH) has long been recognized as a risk factor for the development of altered

Table 3 Analysis of various biomarkers and clinical parameters in surgical ICU regarding sepsis, septic AKI, and in-hospital mortality

Variables	Sepsis			Septic AKI			In-hospital mortality		
	Yes[a]	No[a]	P value	Yes[a]	No[a]	P value	Yes[a]	No[a]	P value
Serum									
NGAL (ng/mL)	428.1 ± 29.1	204.7 ± 34.2	<0.001	447.5 ± 35.7	256.5 ± 31.8	0.001	428.2 ± 32.3	300.4 ± 44.3	0.029
Calprotectin (pg/mL)	809.7 ± 251.2	353.3 ± 315.6	0.302	1030.3 ± 298.6	248.1 ± 210.7	0.049	1013.8 ± 354.8	373.9 ± 193.1	0.113
KIM-1 (pg/mL)	694.9 ± 398.8	142.9 ± 289.1	0.392	1150.5 ± 448.5	275.5 ± 135.1	0.081	838.1 ± 500.2	256.8 ± 329.9	0.329
Cystatin C (ng/ml)	1223.1 ± 186.8	640.5 ± 120.9	0.016	1290.4 ± 222.3	756.3 ± 138.9	0.062	1312.8 ± 260.4	813.3 ± 124.4	0.076
GDF-15 (ng/mL)	8.8 ± 2.7	9.5 ± 2.8	0.330	6.7 ± 2.7	10.8 ± 2.7	0.121	6.2 ± 1.9	11.5 ± 3.1	0.322
Urine									
NGAL (ng/mL)	393.2 ± 33.4	167.0 ± 41.9	<0.001	434.2 ± 31.5	208.3 ± 39.5	<0.001	422.3 ± 33.7	230.8 ± 42.2	0.001
Calprotectin (pg/mL)	933.4 ± 346.6	690.3 ± 367.5	0.462	825.1 ± 415.2	878.1 ± 328.8	0.102	646.2 ± 340.3	1024.2 ± 384.8	0.190
KIM-1 (pg/mL)	7149.0 ± 1491.0	9649.2 ± 2975.0	0.510	7377.5 ± 1970.0	8551.7 ± 2014.0	0.488	8765.3 ± 1949.0	7329.9 ± 2006.0	0.616
Cystatin C (ng/mL)	315.4 ± 89.9	79.5 ± 11.1	0.046	386.1 ± 121.5	100.4 ± 14.8	0.035	324.5 ± 115.6	154.7 ± 53.4	0.628
GDF-15 (ng/mL)	25.1 ± 3.2	34.0 ± 3.6	0.095	26.2 ± 3.6	29.8 ± 3.7	0.487	29.4 ± 3.8	26.9 ± 3.5	0.642
SOFA score	9.5 ± 1.1	4.6 ± 0.6	0.001	11.5 ± 1.2	4.4 ± 0.5	<0.001	10.6 ± 1.4	5.6 ± 0.8	0.003
APACHE II score	20.0 ± 1.8	12.1 ± 0.9	0.001	22.0 ± 2.3	13.0 ± 0.8	0.001	22.0 ± 2.4	13.5 ± 0.9	0.004
Albumin (g/dL)	2.6 ± 0.1	3.0 ± 0.1	0.025	2.5 ± 0.1	3.0 ± 0.1	0.007	2.4 ± 0.1	3.0 ± 0.1	0.003
Creatinine (mg/dL)	1.8 ± 0.4	0.7 ± 0.1	0.004	2.2 ± 0.6	0.7 ± 0.1	<0.001	2.1 ± 0.6	0.9 ± 0.1	0.027
Procalcitonin (ng/mL)[b]	28.8 ± 10.9	0.2	0.095	35.9 ± 14.2	6.2 ± 3.1	0.205	29.6 ± 13.2	25.1 ± 17.3	0.512
Lactate (mg/dL)[b]	40.4 ± 9.2	N.A.	N.A.	47.7 ± 11.9	19.8 ± 3.8	0.190	49.9 ± 15.4	27.3 ± 3.6	0.180
CRP (mg/L)	142.1 ± 20.4	40.9 ± 12.9	<0.001	163.9 ± 24.7	64.4 ± 15.8	0.008	132.6 ± 24.2	113.3 ± 28.8	0.610
Age (year)	63.1 ± 3.4	72.8 ± 2.8	0.072	64.1 ± 3.9	68.5 ± 3.4	0.397	63.9 ± 4.2	68.3 ± 3.2	0.400
BMI (kg/m²)	23.0 ± 0.7	24.7 ± 1.1	0.228	23.0 ± 0.9	24.2 ± 0.8	0.350	22.3 ± 0.9	24.6 ± 0.8	0.066

AKI acute kidney injury, *NGAL* neutrophil gelatinase-associated lipocalin, *GDF-15* growth differentiation factor 15, *KIM-1* kidney injury molecule-1, *SOFA* Sequential Organ Failure Assessment, *APACHE* Acute Physiology and Chronic Health Evaluation, *BMI* body mass index, *N.A.* not applicable

[a]Expressed as mean ± standard error of mean (SEM)

[b]Not routinely checked in patients without sepsis

Table 4 Area under the ROC curve (AUROC) of significant variables regarding septic AKI and in-hospital mortality

Variables	Septic AKI				In-hospital mortality			
	AUROC	P value	Cutoff value	Sensitivity/specificity (%)	AUROC	P value	Cutoff value	Sensitivity/specificity (%)
Serum NGAL	0.991	< 0.001	413.2	92.3/100	0.768	0.021	385.3	75.0/64.3
Urinary NGAL	0.915	0.001	383.7	92.3/77.8	0.780	0.016	383.7	75.0/64.3
Serum calprotectin	0.889	0.002	219.8	84.6/88.9				
Serum KIM-1	0.752	0.049	17.2	69.2/77.8				
Urinary Cystatin C	0.641	0.271	118.9	53.8/66.7				
Albumin	0.269	0.071	2.6	38.5/33.3	0.232	0.021	2.5	41.7/35.7
Creatinine	0.966	< 0.001	0.9	100.0/88.9	0.676	0.129	0.9	75.0/57.1
CRP	0.795	0.021	82.4	76.9/77.8				
SOFA score	0.957	< 0.001	7.5	92.3/88.9	0.774	0.018	7.5	75.0/71.4
APACHE II Score	0.842	0.008	13.5	76.9/77.8	0.762	0.024	15.0	66.7/71.4
Serum NGAL+ Serum Calprotectin + SOFA score	1.000	< 0.001						
Serum NGAL + urinary NGAL + SOFA score					0.911	< 0.001		

AKI acute kidney injury, *NGAL* neutrophil gelatinase-associated lipocalin, *SOFA* Sequential Organ Failure Assessment, *APACHE* Acute Physiology and Chronic Health Evaluation

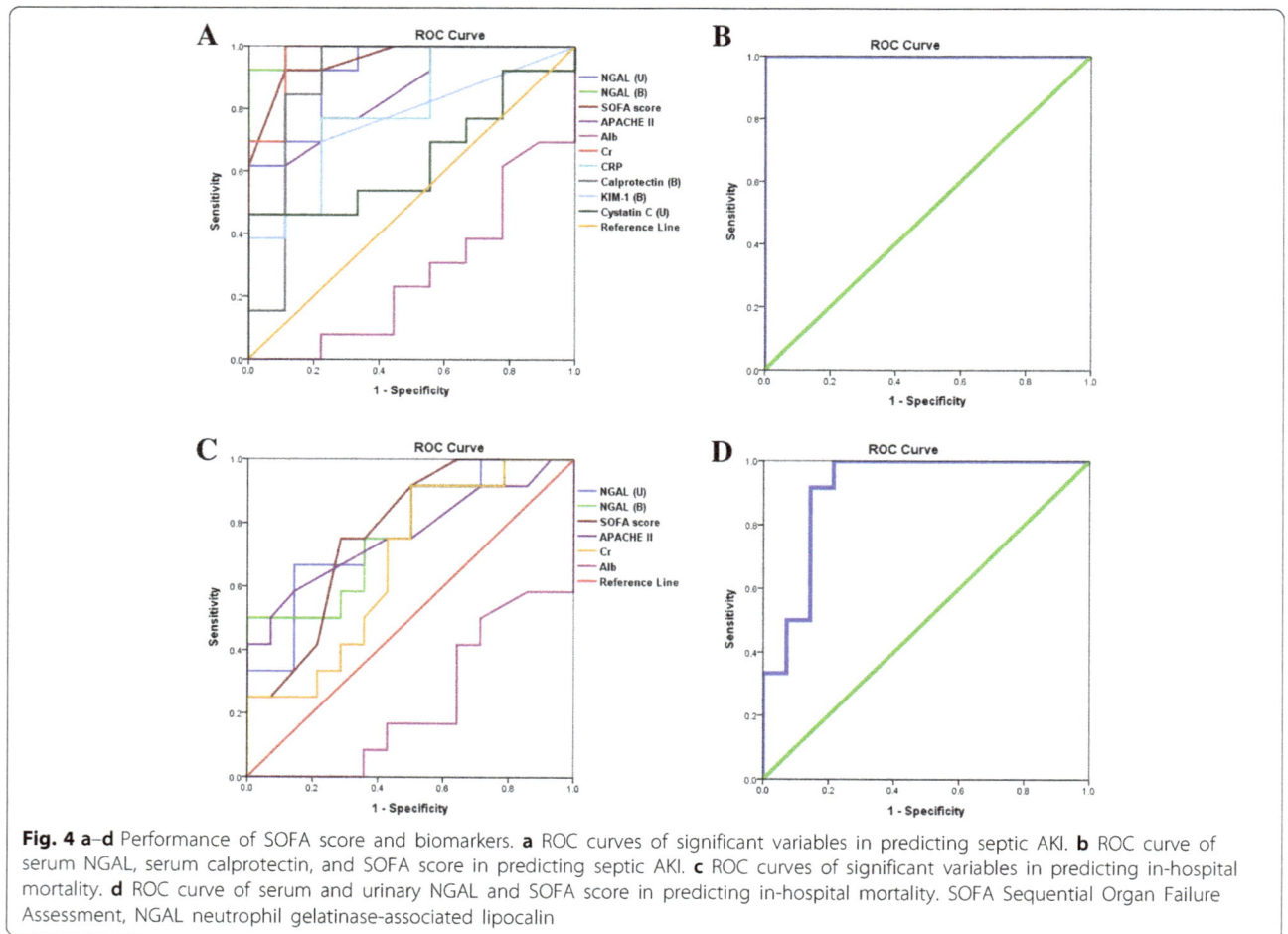

Fig. 4 a–d Performance of SOFA score and biomarkers. **a** ROC curves of significant variables in predicting septic AKI. **b** ROC curve of serum NGAL, serum calprotectin, and SOFA score in predicting septic AKI. **c** ROC curves of significant variables in predicting in-hospital mortality. **d** ROC curve of serum and urinary NGAL and SOFA score in predicting in-hospital mortality. SOFA Sequential Organ Failure Assessment, NGAL neutrophil gelatinase-associated lipocalin

renal function among critically ill patients [32, 33]. IAH has been reported to occur in 51–76% of patients with septic shock and in 33–41% of patients after emergency abdominal surgery and is associated with AKI and mortality [34, 35]. In addition to timely recognition and management of IAH to lower IAP, novel biomarkers may be utilized to predict prognosis in patients with established AKI [36]. As a result, future studies with a larger population size incorporating dynamic changes of biomarkers and intra-abdominal pressure may be warranted. Even though we have shown favorable results using biomarkers and the SOFA score in predicting the development of septic AKI and in-hospital mortality, in daily practice, other more immediate parameters and clinical judgment may be useful in the early assessment of these critically ill patients.

Conclusions

Septic AKI arises in more than 50% of patients with sepsis, with a six- to eightfold increase in the risk of in-hospital mortality. Thus far, no single scoring system appears sufficiently sensitive and specific in predicting the development of septic AKI and in-hospital mortality for critically ill patients. In this pilot study, we have established a panel incorporating serum biomarkers and the SOFA score that appears promising in the early detection of septic AKI, which, in turn, opens a window for prompt treatment in the clinical setting. Furthermore, the panel presents with a great prognostic value for in-hospital mortality among patients in surgical intensive care units. That said, further, larger well-designed studies are warranted.

Additional files

Additional file 1: Figure S1. (A–B) Septic AKI. Serum and urinary levels of GDF-15 and KIM-1 measured by ELISA in patients with or without septic AKI. The serum and urinary levels are represented as scatter dot plots, and the medians are reported. The arithmetic means of the tested parameters are indicated by a line. (A) GDF-15; (B) KIM-1. B in parenthesis indicates blood samples; U in parenthesis indicates urine samples. GDF-15 growth differentiation factor 15, KIM-1 Kidney Injury Molecule-1. (TIF 77 kb)

Additional file 2: Figure S2. (A–D) In-hospital mortality. Serum and urinary levels of calprotectin, Cystatin C, GDF-15, and KIM-1 measured by ELISA in patients with or without in-hospital mortality. The serum and urinary levels are represented as scatter dot plots, and the medians are reported. The arithmetic means of the tested parameters are indicated by a line. (A) Calprotectin, (B) cystatin C, (C) GDF-15, and (D) KIM-1. B in parenthesis indicates blood samples; U in parenthesis indicates urine samples. GDF-15 growth differentiation factor 15, KIM-1, Kidney Injury Molecule-1. (TIF 149 kb)

Additional file 3: Table S1. Area under the ROC curve (AUROC) of various variables regarding septic AKI and in-hospital mortality within the septic cohort. (DOCX 19 kb)

Additional file 4: Figure S3. (A–B). Performance of SOFA score and biomarkers within the septic cohort. (A) ROC curve of serum NGAL, calprotectin, and SOFA score in predicting septic AKI. (B) ROC curve of serum and urinary NGAL and SOFA score in predicting in-hospital

mortality. SOFA Sequential Organ Failure Assessment, NGAL neutrophil gelatinase-associated lipocalin. (TIF 1447 kb)

Abbreviations
ADQI: Acute Dialysis Quality Initiative; AKI: Acute kidney injury; APACHE: Acute Physiology and Chronic Health Evaluation; AUROC: Area under the ROC curve; BMI: Body mass index; CKD: Chronic kidney disease; CRP: C-Reactive protein; eGFR: Estimated glomerular filtration rate; ELISA: Enzyme-linked immunosorbent assay; ESRD: End-stage renal disease; FiO_2: Fraction of inspired oxygen; GCS: Glasgow Coma Scale; GDF-15: Growth differentiation factor 15; GFR: Glomerular filtration rate; IAI: Intra-abdominal infection; ICU: Intensive care unit; INR: International normalized ratio; IRB: Institutional review board; KIM-1: Kidney injury molecule-1; MAP: Mean arterial blood pressure; MV: Mechanical ventilation; NGAL: Neutrophil gelatinase-associated lipocalin; PaO_2: Partial pressure of oxygen; RIFLE: Risk, Injury, Failure, Loss, and End-Stage Renal Disease; ROC Curve: Receiver operating characteristic curve; sCr: Serum creatinine; SD: Standard deviation; SOFA: Sequential Organ Failure Assessment; UTI: Urinary tract infection

Acknowledgements
We are grateful to all our colleagues in the GSICU1, Chang Gung Memorial Hospital, Linkou and Graduate Institute of Clinical Medical Sciences, Chang Gung University, for their technical assistance.

Funding
This study was supported by Chang Gung Memorial Hospital (CMRPG3D1621 and CMRPG3G1301) and by the Ministry of Science and Technology, Taiwan, R.O.C. (MOST 106-2314-B-182A-018-).

Authors' contributions
CWL designed the study and drafted the manuscript. HWK, HSC, and HHC collected patient samples and revised the manuscript. SFH and CHC analyzed the clinical data and performed the statistics. CHW and MCY performed the ELISA assays and revised the manuscript. HIT collected the clinical data, coordinated the study, and drafted the manuscript. All authors read and approved the final manuscript.

Competing interests
The authors declare that they have no competing interests.

Author details
[1]Department of Surgery, Chang Gung Memorial Hospital, Linkou, Taiwan, Republic of China. [2]College of Medicine, Chang Gung University, Guishan, Taoyuan, Taiwan, Republic of China. [3]Graduate Institute of Clinical Medical Sciences, Chang Gung University, Guishan, Taoyuan, Taiwan, Republic of China. [4]Division of Nephrology, Kidney Research Center, Chang Gung Memorial Hospital, Linkou, Taiwan, Republic of China. [5]Department of Anesthesiology, Chang Gung Memorial Hospital, Linkou, Taiwan, Republic of China.

References

1. Singer M, Deutschman CS, Seymour CW, et al. The third international consensus definitions for sepsis and septic shock (Sepsis-3). JAMA. 2016; 315(8):801–10.

2. Seymour CW, Liu VX, Iwashyna TJ, et al. Assessment of clinical criteria for sepsis: for the Third International Consensus Definitions for Sepsis and Septic Shock (Sepsis-3). JAMA. 2016;315(8):762–74.

3. Raith EP, Udy AA, Bailey M, et al. Prognostic accuracy of the SOFA score, SIRS criteria, and qSOFA score for in-hospital mortality among adults with suspected infection admitted to the intensive care unit. JAMA. 2017;317(3):290–300.

4. Hoste EA, Clermont G, Kersten A, et al. RIFLE criteria for acute kidney injury are associated with hospital mortality in critically ill patients: a cohort analysis. Critical care (London, England). 2006;10(3):R73.

5. Srisawat N, Sileanu FE, Murugan R, et al. Variation in risk and mortality of acute kidney injury in critically ill patients: a multicenter study. Am J Nephrol. 2015;41(1):81–8.

6. Thakar CV, Christianson A, Freyberg R, Almenoff P, Render ML. Incidence and outcomes of acute kidney injury in intensive care units: a Veterans Administration study. Crit Care Med. 2009;37(9):2552–8.

7. Gomez H, Kellum JA. Sepsis-induced acute kidney injury. Curr Opin Crit Care. 2016;22(6):546–53.

8. Bellomo R, Ronco C, Kellum JA, Mehta RL, Palevsky P. Acute renal failure—definition, outcome measures, animal models, fluid therapy and information technology needs: the Second International Consensus Conference of the Acute Dialysis Quality Initiative (ADQI) Group. Critical care (London, England). 2004;8(4):R204–12.

9. Nejat M, Pickering JW, Walker RJ, Endre ZH. Rapid detection of acute kidney injury by plasma cystatin C in the intensive care unit. Nephrol Dial Transplant. 2010;25(10):3283–9.

10. Aydogdu M, Gursel G, Sancak B, et al. The use of plasma and urine neutrophil gelatinase associated lipocalin (NGAL) and cystatin C in early diagnosis of septic acute kidney injury in critically ill patients. Dis Markers. 2013;34(4):237–46.

11. Zhang A, Cai Y, Wang PF, et al. Diagnosis and prognosis of neutrophil gelatinase-associated lipocalin for acute kidney injury with sepsis: a systematic review and meta-analysis. Critical Care (London, England). 2016; 20:41.

12. Leem AY, Park MS, Park BH, et al. Value of serum cystatin C measurement in the diagnosis of Sepsis-induced kidney injury and prediction of renal function recovery. Yonsei Med J. 2017;58(3):604–12.

13. Dessing MC, Tammaro A, Pulskens WP, et al. The calcium-binding protein complex S100A8/A9 has a crucial role in controlling macrophage-mediated renal repair following ischemia/reperfusion. Kidney Int. 2015;87(1):85–94.

14. Heller F, Frischmann S, Grunbaum M, Zidek W, Westhoff TH. Urinary calprotectin and the distinction between prerenal and intrinsic acute kidney injury. Clin J Am Soc Nephrol. 2011;6(10):2347–55.

15. Seibert FS, Pagonas N, Arndt R, et al. Calprotectin and neutrophil gelatinase-associated lipocalin in the differentiation of pre-renal and intrinsic acute kidney injury. Acta Physiologica (Oxford, England). 2013;207(4):700–8.

16. Levey AS, Stevens LA, Schmid CH, et al. A new equation to estimate glomerular filtration rate. Ann Intern Med. 2009;150(9):604–12.

17. Ali H, Hussain N, Naim M, et al. A novel PKD1 variant demonstrates a disease-modifying role in trans with a truncating PKD1 mutation in patients with autosomal dominant polycystic kidney disease. BMC Nephrol. 2015;16:26.

18. Basu RK, Kaddourah A, Terrell T, et al. Assessment of Worldwide Acute Kidney Injury, Renal Angina and Epidemiology in critically ill children (AWARE): study protocol for a prospective observational study. BMC Nephrol. 2015;16:24.

19. Conroy AL, Hawkes MT, Elphinstone R, et al. Chitinase-3-like 1 is a biomarker of acute kidney injury and mortality in paediatric severe malaria. Malar J. 2018;17(1):82.

20. Gruda MC, Ruggeberg KG, O'Sullivan P, et al. Broad adsorption of sepsis-related PAMP and DAMP molecules, mycotoxins, and cytokines from whole blood using CytoSorb(R) sorbent porous polymer beads. PLoS One. 2018; 13(1):e0191676.

21. Liu X, Chi X, Gong Q, et al. Association of serum level of growth differentiation factor 15 with liver cirrhosis and hepatocellular carcinoma. PLoS One. 2015;10(5):e0127518.

22. Zackular JP, Moore JL, Jordan AT, et al. Dietary zinc alters the microbiota and decreases resistance to Clostridium difficile infection. Nat Med. 2016; 22(11):1330–4.

23. Zager RA, Johnson AC, Frostad KB. Rapid renal alpha-1 antitrypsin gene induction in experimental and clinical acute kidney injury. PLoS One. 2014; 9(5):e98380.

24. Vincent JL, Marshall JC, Namendys-Silva SA, et al. Assessment of the worldwide burden of critical illness: the intensive care over nations (ICON) audit. Lancet Respir Med. 2014;2(5):380–6.

25. Bagshaw SM, George C, Bellomo R. Early acute kidney injury and sepsis: a multicentre evaluation. Critical Care (London, England). 2008;12(2):R47.

26. Martensson J, Martling CR, Bell M. Novel biomarkers of acute kidney injury and failure: clinical applicability. Br J Anaesth. 2012;109(6):843–50.

27. Dai X, Zeng Z, Fu C, Zhang S, Cai Y, Chen Z. Diagnostic value of neutrophil gelatinase-associated lipocalin, cystatin C, and soluble triggering receptor expressed on myeloid cells-1 in critically ill patients with sepsis-associated acute kidney injury. Critical Care (London, England). 2015;19:223.

28. Yamashita T, Doi K, Hamasaki Y, et al. Evaluation of urinary tissue inhibitor of metalloproteinase-2 in acute kidney injury: a prospective observational study. Critical Care (London, England). 2014;18(6):716.

29. Hang CC, Yang J, Wang S, Li CS, Tang ZR. Evaluation of serum neutrophil gelatinase-associated lipocalin in predicting acute kidney injury in critically ill patients. J Int Med Res. 2017;45(3):1231–44.

30. Ulas T, Pirr S, Fehlhaber B, et al. S100-alarmin-induced innate immune programming protects newborn infants from sepsis. Nat Immunol. 2017; 18(6):622–32.

31. Gao S, Yang Y, Fu Y, Guo W, Liu G. Diagnostic and prognostic value of myeloid-related protein complex 8/14 for sepsis. Am J Emerg Med. 2015; 33(9):1278–82.

32. Patel DM, Connor MJ Jr. Intra-abdominal hypertension and abdominal compartment syndrome: an underappreciated cause of acute kidney injury. Adv Chronic Kidney Dis. 2016;23(3):160–6.

33. Villa G, Samoni S, De Rosa S, Ronco C. The pathophysiological hypothesis of kidney damage during intra-abdominal hypertension. Front Physiol. 2016;7:55.

34. De Waele JJ, De Laet I, Kirkpatrick AW, Hoste E. Intra-abdominal hypertension and abdominal compartment syndrome. Am J Kidney Dis. 2011;57(1):159–69.

35. Kirkpatrick AW, Roberts DJ, De Waele J. High versus low blood-pressure target in septic shock. N Engl J Med. 2014;371(3):282–3.

36. Chang HJ, Yang J, Kim SC, et al. Intra-abdominal hypertension does not predict renal recovery or in-hospital mortality in critically ill patients with acute kidney injury. Kidney Res Clin Pract. 2015;34(2):103–8.

19

A novel method for multiple bowel injuries: a pilot canine experiment

Jun Ke[1†], Weihang Wu[2†], Nan Lin[2], Weijin Yang[2], Zhicong Cai[2], Wei Wu[2], Dongsheng Chen[3*] and Yu Wang[2*]

Abstract

Background: Intestinal ligation is the cornerstone for damage control in abdominal emergency, yet it may lead to bowel ischemia. Although intestinal ligation avoids further peritoneal cavity pollution, it may lead to an increased pressure within the bowel segments and rapid bacterial translocation. In this study, we showed that severed intestine could be readily reconnected by using silicon tubes and be secured by using rubber bands in a canine model.

Methods: Adult Beagle dogs, subject to multiple intestinal transections and hemorrhagic shock by exsanguination, randomly received conventional ligation vs. silicon tubes reconnecting ($n = 5$ per group). Intestinal transections were carried out under general anesthesia after 24-h fasting. The abdomen was opened with a midline incision. The small intestine was severed at 50, 100, and 150 cm below the Treitz ligament. Hemorrhagic shock was established by streaming blood from the left carotid artery until the mean arterial pressure reached 40 mmHg in 20 min. Fluid resuscitation and surgery began 30 min after the establishment of hemorrhagic shock. Severed intestines were ligated or connected with silicon tubes. Definitive repair was conducted in subjects surviving for at least 48 h.

Results: Operation time was comparable between the two groups (39.6 ± 8.9 vs. 36.6 ± 7.8 min in ligation and reconnecting groups, respectively; $p = 0.56$). The time spent in managing each resection was also comparable (4.6 ± 1.1 vs. 3.8 ± 0.84 min; $p = 0.24$). Blood loss (341.2 ± 28.6 vs. 333.8 ± 34.6 ml; $p = 0.48$), and fluid resuscitation within the first 24 h (1676 ± 200.6 vs. 1594 ± 156.5 ml; $p = 0.46$) were similar. One subject in the ligation group was sacrificed at 36-h due to severe vomiting that led to aspiration. Four remaining dogs in the ligation group received definitive surgery, but two out of four had to be sacrificed at 24-h after definitive repair due to imminent death. All five dogs in the reconnecting group survived for at least a week. Radiographic examination confirmed the integrity of the GI tract in the reconnecting group. In both groups, plasma endotoxin concentration increased after damage control surgery, but the increase was much more pronounced in the ligation group. Microscopic examination of the involved segment of the intestine revealed much more severe pathology in the ligation group.

Conclusion: The current study showed that the reconnecting resected intestine by using silicon tubes is feasible under emergency. Such a method could decrease short-term mortality and minimize endotoxin translocation.

Keywords: Intestinal injury, Ligation, Reconnecting, Endotoxin translocation

Background

In critically injured patients, primary repair of gastrointestinal (GI) tract injuries is often not feasible due to hemodynamic instability, coagulopathy, and metabolic acidosis [1–3]. In such cases, management of the GI tract injury is limited to the control of sepsis and hemorrhage [4–8]. Damaged intestines are excised, and the ends are simply ligated to prevent further contamination of the peritoneal cavity. Intestinal continuity is restored in subsequent definitive surgeries.

As the pressure inside the GI tract increases upon ligation, the intestinal wall becomes damaged, and the bacteria translocate into the systemic circulation [9]. Increased pressure also impedes blood supply to the intestine and aggravates the already existing damage [10]. In this study, we examined the effects of home-made

* Correspondence: cdsheng315@sohu.com; flyfishwang@hotmail.com
†Equal contributors
3Department of Anesthesiology, Dongfang Hospital, Xiamen University, Fuzhou, Fujian 350025, China
2Department of General Surgery, Dongfang Hospital, Xiamen University, Fuzhou, Fujian 350025, China
Full list of author information is available at the end of the article

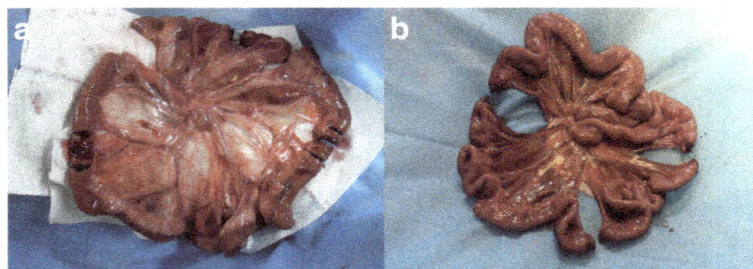

Fig. 1 Representative small intestine segments after ligation (**a**) and reconnecting (**b**)

silicon tubes to allow rapid damage control and to restore intestinal continuity in a Beagle dog model of multiple transection of small intestine and hemodynamic shock, with promising preliminary results.

Methods

Experimental design

Adult male Beagle dogs (n = 10.13–15 kg; Dasuo Biotech, Chengdu, China) were housed individually at 22–26 °C with 45–65% humidity. After 24-h fasting, dogs were anesthetized with ketamine (10 mg/kg; im). Induction was conducted with bolus i.v. pentobarbital injection (12–15 mg/kg) and was maintained at a speed of 1 mg/kg h. A central venous catheter was placed through the left external jugular vein for maintaining anesthesia and blood sampling. A catheter was placed in the right common carotid artery to monitor arterial pressure and heart rate.

The abdomen was opened with a midline incision. The small intestine was severed at 50, 100, and 150 cm below the ligament of Treitz. Then the abdominal cavity was temporarily closed with towel forceps. Hemorrhagic shock was induced with bleeding from the jugular artery to maintain mean arterial pressure (MAP) at 40 mmHg in 20 min. Fluid resuscitation with Ringer's solution was initiated 30 min after the hemorrhagic shock. Severed intestine was managed with conventional ligation or reconnection using a silicon tube (Xiangshu, Shanghai, China) (n = 5 for each, Fig. 1). The tube was inserted 2–3 cm into the edge of resection and was secured with rubber bands. A gastrostomy catheter (16 F) was placed for nutritional support later.

Definitive surgery was carried out at 48 h in dogs that survived beyond 48 h. Prior to definitive operation, the upper digestive tract was examined using imaging analysis of Meglumine Diatrizoate. 24 h after definitive surgery, the remaining animals in both groups were given nutritional support through a gastrostomy catheter (250 cal/day, in 250 ml volume).

Outcome assessment

Plasma endotoxin concentration was determined by an enzyme-linked immunosorbent assay (ELISA) kits from Jinshanchuan (Beijing, China). Tissues were fixed in 10% formalin for 24 h and embedded in paraffin, and were processed for light microscopy with hematoxylin and eosin staining. For transmission electron microscopy (TME), tissues (at 50-cm distal to ligament of Treitz) were fixed in 4% glutaraldehyde and 1% paraformaldehyde, dehydrated, and embedded in Spurr resin. Ultrathin sections (2–3 mm) were stained with citrate. Photographs were obtained with a Philips EM208S transmission electron microscope (Philips; Eindhoven, Netherlands). The magnification of images was 10×1000.

Statistical methods

Continuous variables are presented as means ± standard deviation and analyzed with Student's t test or analysis of variance (ANOVA) of repeated measure with Statistical Package (SPSS 20.0 for windows, SPSS Inc., Illinois, USA). A probability of less than 0.05 was accepted as significant.

The Ethics Committee of Dongfang Hospital approved the study.

Results

The current study showed practically zero short-term mortality in dogs receiving reconnecting after multiple

Table 1 Plasma endotoxin concentration after ligation and reconnecting

	0 h	2 h	4 h	8 h	24 h
Reconnecting	3.95 ± 0.75	25.19 ± 21.50	39.43 ± 22.86	55.55 ± 23.72	46.50 ± 19.22
Ligation	3.98 ± 0.60	51.78 ± 23.81	85.26 ± 26.89	96.89 ± 19.82	102.27 ± 20.03
P value	0.94	0.10	0.02*	0.01*	< 0.01*

Note: values were expressed as mean ± SD; * refers to the p value between two groups was statistically significant, ANOVA of repeated measures

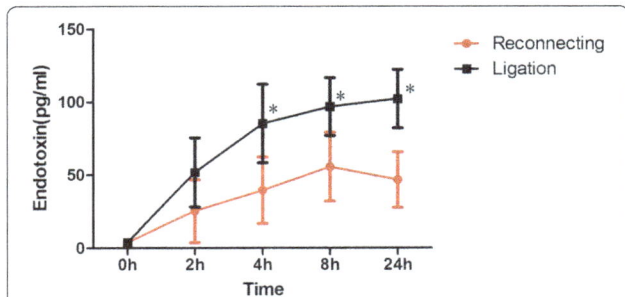

Fig. 2 Plasma endotoxin concentration after ligation and reconnecting.* refers to the p value between two groups was statistically significant

transections of the small intestine, as well as much lower plasma endotoxin concentration.

Operation time of the damage control operation was comparable between the two groups (39.6 ± 8.9 vs. 36.6 ± 7.80 min in the ligation and reconnecting groups, respectively; $p = 0.56$). The time spent in managing each resection was comparable (4.6 ± 1.1 vs. 3.8 ± 0.8 min; $p = 0.24$). Blood loss (341.2 ± 28.6 vs. 333.8 ± 34.6 ml; $p = 0.48$) and fluid resuscitation within the first 24 h (1676 ± 200.6 vs. 1594 ± 156.5 ml; $p = 0.46$) were similar between the two groups.

Plasma endotoxin concentration increased after the surgery in both groups, but was much more pronounced in the ligation group (Table 1; Fig. 2). One dog in the ligation group was sacrificed after 36 h due to severe vomiting that led to aspiration. The remaining four dogs in the ligation groups received definitive operation, but two had to be sacrificed within 24 h after definitive repair due to imminent death. Post-mortem analysis revealed large amount of ascites in abdominal cavity. All five dogs in the reconnecting group survived for at least a week after the definitive operation.

Microscopic examination of the involved intestine revealed much more severe damage, including sloughing of surface epithelium, massive intraepithelial neutrophil infiltration and necrosis, in the ligation group vs. the reconnecting group (light microscopy in Fig. 3; TEM in

Fig. 4). Radiographic examination of the upper digestive tract at 48 h in the reconnecting group showed the contrast medium flowed through the intestine (Fig. 5).

Discussion

Patients with severe multiple enteric injuries often had severe comorbid conditions (such as hemodynamic shock). Currently, damage control surgery is to carry out ligation of severed/injuried GI tract [4, 7, 8]. Aggravated abdominal cavity contamination and bleeding can be easily controlled; however, continuing loss of fluids from the vascular compartment to the interstitial and third spaces leads to hemodynamic imbalance [11]. The ligations also elevate pressure within the bowel segments left in discontinuity and facilitate the development of pressure-related complications, such as bacterial translocation [12–14]. Consistent with a previous study [15], we observed rapid endotoxin translocation in the current study. Attempts have been made by previous studies to address the issue, such as an intraluminal drainage system to reduce intraluminal pressure [16]. Procedures required, however, are complex and time consuming.

In this study, we showed feasibility of reconnecting severed small intestine with silicon tubes. The method allowed rapid re-establishment of GI tract continuity. Comparison with ligation indicated that reconnecting could reduce bacteria translocation and tissue damage to small intestine in the involved segments. More importantly, short-term mortality (within a week after definitive surgery) is reduced to practically zero.

Time is of essence in definitive surgery; physicians must weigh risks vs. benefits [6, 17]. Ligation is considered a gold standard that could stabilize the physiological conditions of most patients. Definitive surgery, however, must be performed within a short period of time. Otherwise, patient's condition will deteriorate [13, 18]. In the current series, we could complete the procedure within a very short period of time, without failure of this simple device (such as slipping-out of the tubes).

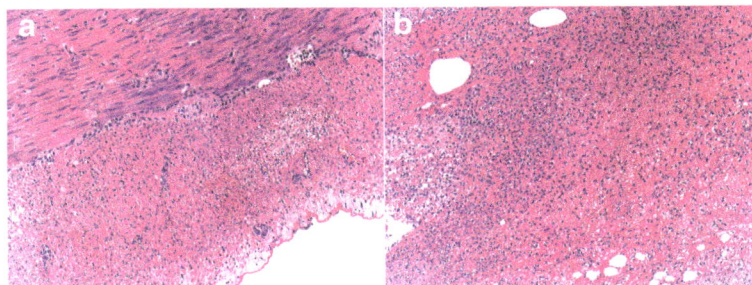

Fig. 3 Intestinal mucosa (at 50-cm distal to ligament of Treitz) in dogs subjected to ligation (**a**) and reconnecting (**b**), at 48 h under light microspcopy (× 100)

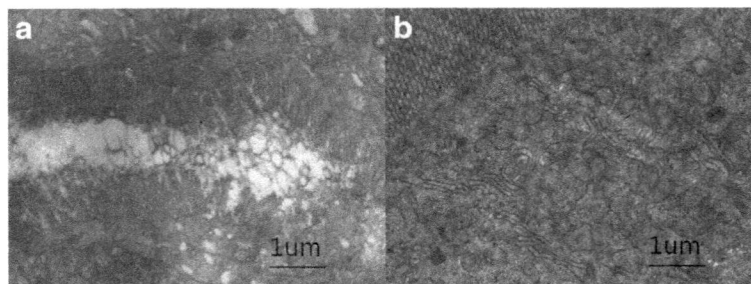

Fig. 4 Transmission electron microscopy examination of the bowel (at 50-cm distal to ligament of Treitz) in dogs subjected to ligation (**a**) and reconnecting (**b**) at 48 h(10 × 1000)

Another critical issue in the management of severe abdominal trauma is preserving the function of the gastrointestinal tract. Primary anastomosis could be hazardous because of the prolonged operation time and compromised hemodynamic conditions [4–7]. In this regard, temporally reconnecting transected intestines restored the continuity and the function of the GI tract, as evidenced by radiographic examination at 48 h after the reconnection.

We suspect in the future, this tubes system will be applied to patients with bowels ruptured, who be allowed for damage control surgical conditions. However,

injuries in clinical settings are typically far more complex than those modeled in the current study. Clearly, the current study is a proof-of-concept in nature and requires further studies in animal studies before applying to human subjects.

Conclusions
Reconnecting transected small intestine with silicon tubes and tuber bands is a viable method of damage control. Further studies are required to validate the results of this preliminary study.

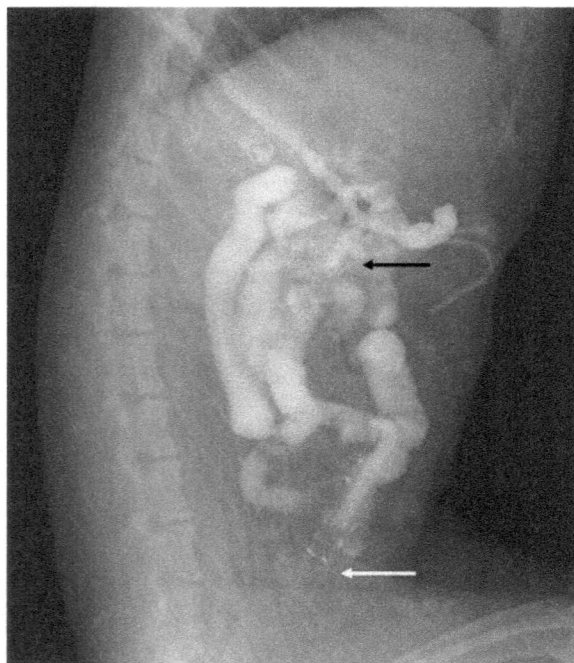

Fig. 5 Radiographic examination of the upper digestive tract in a dog subjected to reconnecting at 48 h showed the contrast medium flowed smoothly through the intestine. There were no sign of air fluid level and swollen or obstructed intestines. Note: black arrow refers to proximal intestines; white arrow refers to distal intestines

Abbreviations
GI: Gastrointestinal; MAP: Mean arterial pressure; TME: Transmission electron microscopy

Acknowledgements
The authors thank the Animal Experimental Center and the Department of Pathology at Dongfang Hospital for technical assistance.

Funding
This study was supported by the Key Project of Nanjing Command (14ZX25), Key Medicine Project of PLA (CNJ15J004), Cooperate Project of Fujian Province (2015I0013), and Key Project of Nanjing Command (15DX024).

Authors' contributions
YW and DC designed this study. JK, NL, WY, ZC, and WWH performed the experiments. WWH, ZC, and WW collected and analyzed the data. YW and DC provided additional support, including review of the manuscript. JK and WWH wrote the manuscript, which was critically reviewed and revised by YW and DC. All of the authors read and approved the final manuscript.

Competing interests
The authors declare that they have no competing interests.

Author details
¹Department of Gastroenterology, Dongfang Hospital, Xiamen University, Fuzhou, Fujian 350025, China. ²Department of General Surgery, Dongfang Hospital, Xiamen University, Fuzhou, Fujian 350025, China. ³Department of Anesthesiology, Dongfang Hospital, Xiamen University, Fuzhou, Fujian 350025, China.

References
1. Smith IM, Beech ZK, Lundy JB, Bowley DM. A prospective observational study of abdominal injury management in contemporary military operations: damage control laparotomy is associated with high survivability and low rates of fecal diversion. Ann Surg. 2015;261:765–73.
2. Burch J, Ortiz VB, Richardson RJ, Martin RR, Mattox KL, Jordan GL Jr. Abbreviated laparotomy and planned reoperation for critically injured patients. Ann Surg. 1992;215:476.
3. Lier H, Krep H, Schroeder S, Stuber F. Preconditions of hemostasis in trauma. A review. The influence of acidosis, hypocalcemia, anemia, and hypothermia on functional hemostasis in trauma. J Trauma Acute Care. 2008;65:951–60.
4. Olofsson P, Vikström T, Nagelkerke N, Wang J, Abu-Zidan F. Multiple small bowel ligation compared to conventional primary repair after abdominal gunshot wound with haemorrhagic shock. Scand J Surg. 2009;98:41–7.
5. Chovanes J, Cannon JW, Nunez TC. The evolution of damage control surgery. Surg Clin N Am. 2012;92:859–75.
6. Waibel BH, Rotondo MM. Damage control surgery: it's evolution over the last 20 years. Rev Col Bras Cir. 2012;39:314–21.
7. Weber D, Bendinelli C, Balogh Z. Damage control surgery for abdominal emergencies. Brit J Surg. 2014;101:e109–18.
8. Rotondo MF, Schwab CW, McGonigal MD, Phillips GR, Fruchterman TM, Kauder DR, et al. 'Damage control': an approach for improved survival in exsanguinating penetrating abdominal injury. J Trauma Acute Care. 1993;35:375–83.
9. Wang P, Wei X, Li Y, Li J. Influences of intestinal ligation on bacterial translocation and inflammatory response in rats with hemorrhagic shock: implications for damage control surgery. J Investig Surg. 2008;21:244–54.
10. Wu J, Ding W, Liu X, Kao X, Xu X, Li N, et al. Intraintestinal drainage as a damage control surgery adjunct in a hypothermic traumatic shock swine model with multiple bowel perforations. J Surg Res. 2014;192:170–6.
11. Plante GE, Chakir M, Ettaouil K, Lehoux S, Sirois P. Consequences of alteration in capillary permeability. Can J Physiol Pharm. 1996;74:824–33.
12. Zanoni FL, Benabou S, Greco KV, Moreno ACR, Cruz JWMC, Filgueira FP, et al. Mesenteric microcirculatory dysfunctions and translocation of indigenous bacteria in a rat model of strangulated small bowel obstruction. Clinics. 2009;64:911–9.
13. Raeburn CD, Moore EE, Biffl WL, Johnson JL, Meldrum DR, Offner PJ, et al. The abdominal compartment syndrome is a morbid complication of postinjury damage control surgery. Am J Surg. 2001;182:542–6.
14. Baker JW, Deitch EA, Li M, Berg RD, Specian RD. Hemorrhagic shock induces bacterial translocation from the gut. J Trauma Acute Care. 1988;28:896–913.
15. Deitch EA, Berg R, Specian R. Endotoxin promotes the translocation of bacteria from the gut. Arch Surg. 1987;122:185–90.
16. Ji W, Ding W, Liu X, Kao X, Xu X, Li N, et al. Intraintestinal drainage as a damage control surgery adjunct in a hypothermic traumatic shock swine model with multiple bowel perforations. J Surg Res. 2014;192:170–6.
17. Faria GR, Almeida AB, Moreira H, Barbosa E, Correia-da-Silva P, Costa-Maia J. Prognostic factors for traumatic bowel injuries: killing time. World J Surg. 2012;36:807–12.
18. Enochsson L, Nylander G, Öhman U. Effects of intraluminal pressure on regional blood flow in obstructed and unobstructed small intestines in the rat. Am J Surg. 1982;144:558–61.

20

A contemporary case series of Fournier's gangrene at a Swiss tertiary care center—can scoring systems accurately predict mortality and morbidity?

C. Wetterauer[1]* (ID), J. Ebbing[1], A. Halla[1], R. Kuehl[2], S. Erb[2], A. Egli[3,4], D. J. Schaefer[5] and H. H. Seifert[1]

Abstract

Background: Fournier's gangrene (FG) is a life-threatening infection of the genital, perineal, and perianal regions with a morbidity range between 3 and 67%. Our aim is to report our experience in treatment of FG and to assess whether three different scoring systems can accurately predict mortality and morbidity in FG patients.

Methods: All patients that were treated for FG at the Department of Urology of the University Hospital Basel between June 2012 and March 2017 were included and assessed retrospectively by chart review. Furthermore, we calculated Fournier's Gangrene Severity Index (FGSI), the Laboratory Risk Indicator for Necrotizing Fasciitis (LRINEC), and the neutrophil–lymphocyte ratio (NLR) in every patient and assessed whether those scores correlate with the patients' morbidity and mortality.

Results: Twenty patients were included, with a median (IQR) age of 66 (46–73) years. Fifteen of twenty (75%) patients required treatment on an intensive care unit, and three died (mortality rate: 15%). The mean FGSI, LRINEC, and NLR scores were 13.0, 9.3, and 45.3 for non-survivors and 7.7, 6.5, and 26 for survivors, respectively. None of the risk scores correlated significantly with mortality; however, all three significantly correlated with infection- and surgically-induced morbidity.

Conclusions: In our series, Fournier's gangrene was associated with a mortality rate of 15% despite maximum multidisciplinary therapy at a specialized center. All risk scores were able to predict the morbidity of the disease in terms of local extent and the required surgical measures.

Keywords: Fournier's gangrene, Morbidity, Mortality, FGSI, LRINEC, NLR

Background

Fournier's gangrene (FG) is a life-threatening infection of the genital, perineal, and perianal regions first described by Fournier in 1883 [1]. The male to female ratio is reported as 10:1 [2], with an incidence of 1:7500 to 1:750,000 [3]. Conditions leading to decreased host immunity and thus rapid spread of infection are considered predisposing factors [3]. FG is a polymicrobial aerobic and anaerobic infection caused by three or more pathogens and therefore classified as type 1 necrotizing tissue infection [4]. *Bacteroides fragilis* is the most commonly isolated anaerobic bacterial pathogen [5, 6], while *Escherichia coli* and *Enterococcus faecalis* represent the most commonly isolated aerobic pathogens [7]. In patients with diabetes mellitus, *Streptococcus* spp., *Staphylococcus* spp., and aerobic flora are regularly detected [8]. The combination of aerobic and anaerobic bacteria can lead to the production of several enzymes, such as collagenases and heparinases, which may result in tissue destruction and rapid progression of the infection. Thus, the combination of less pathogenic bacteria can develop high virulence in immunocompromised patients [2]. The FG diagnosis is based on clinical and laboratory findings. Patients usually present with classical

* Correspondence: Christian.wetterauer@usb.ch
[1]Department of Urology, University Hospital Basel, Spitalstr. 21, 4031 Basel, Switzerland
Full list of author information is available at the end of the article

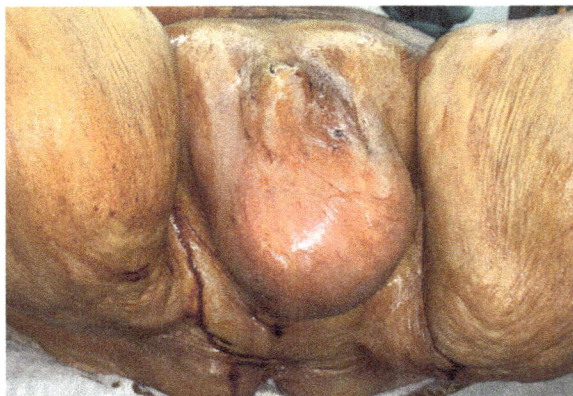

Fig. 1 Classic clinical presentation of Fournier's gangrene with scrotal/perineal swelling, tenderness on palpation, and poorly demarcated erythema, yet no visible necrosis of the skin

signs of soft tissue infections of the scrotum, perineum, and/or perianal areas (Fig. 1). Additionally, gangrenous or necrotic tissue and skin areas may be visible. Leukocyte and C-reactive protein levels are usually elevated. Imaging can be helpful if the diagnosis is uncertain. Early diagnosis is essential for the outcome, yet diagnosis is often delayed in this relatively rare disease, which in turn results in a delayed treatment start [9]. Optimal multimodal treatment consists of hemodynamic stabilization and supportive intensive care if necessary, broad spectrum antibiotic therapy, and extensive surgical debridement of the necrotic tissue [9]. Modern reconstructive techniques, such as skin grafting and flaps, provide reliable coverage of significant tissue defects and acceptable cosmetic results [10]. Despite the advancements in health care over the last decades, the mortality rates of FG still range between 3 and 67% even in developed countries [3]. Several risk scores, like Fournier's Gangrene Severity Index (FGSI), the Laboratory Risk Indicator for Necrotizing Fasciitis (LRINEC), and the neutrophil–lymphocyte ratio (NLR), have been developed to predict survival and prognosis in FG [11]. To the best of our knowledge, we are the first to report our experiences in treatment of FG in a Swiss tertiary care center and to assess the capability of three different scoring systems (FGSI, LRINEC, and NLR) to predict not only mortality, but also morbidity.

Methods

Twenty patients treated for FG at the Clinic for Urology of the University Hospital Basel during June 2012 and March 2017 were enrolled in this retrospective study, which was approved by the local IRB (EKNZ number 2017-01336). Patients were identified based on ICD10 coding, and the diagnosis was confirmed by surgical and clinical assessment. Demographic and clinical data, such

as age, sex, comorbidities, laboratory and microbiological findings, surgical and antibiotic treatment, supportive measures, reconstructive techniques, and outcomes, were extracted by chart review. Mortality was defined as disease-related death during hospital stay. FGSI [12] was calculated based on clinical (temperature, heart rate, and respiration rate) and laboratory parameters (serum sodium, serum potassium, serum creatinine, serum bicarbonate, hematocrit, and leukocyte count) upon admission. LRINEC [13] was obtained by combining the values for C-reactive protein, leukocyte count, hemoglobin, serum sodium, serum creatinine, and glucose. NLR [14] was calculated as neutrophil–lymphocyte count ratio at admission. We performed prompt radical surgical debridement in all patients and initiated immediate antibiotic treatment. In case of scrotectomy, testes were temporarily placed in medial thigh pockets. Sequential debridement was performed until healthy granulation tissue had developed. Reconstruction of large tissue defect was achieved with skin grafts or flaps. Empiric antibiotic treatment was adjusted according to antibiotic susceptibility testing of the recovered pathogens. Septic patients requiring intensive fluid resuscitation, vasopressors, or mechanical ventilation were treated in intensive care unit (ICU).

All data were analyzed with SPSS 19 (SPSS Inc., Chicago, Illinois, USA). Data on an ordinal or continuous level were analyzed using a non-parametric Mann-Whitney U test. Non-normality Spearman's correlation tests and simple logistic regression tests were performed to determine the association between different independent variables, the severity scores, and mortality. All tests were performed at a significance level of $\alpha = 0.05$.

Results

A total of 20 male patients were evaluated. Seventeen patients survived and three patients succumbed to the disease (mortality rate 15%). Median (IQR) age of the patients was 66 (46–73) years. Median (IQR) age of survivors and of non survivors was 64 (43–72) and 84 (67–94) years, respectively. Median (IQR) BMI was 28 (24.8–33.8) kg/m². Predisposing factors like diabetes mellitus, smoking, and renal insufficiency were present in 6/20 (30%), 9/20 (45%), and 9/20 (45%) patients, respectively. Chest X-ray was performed in 8/20 (40%) patients; abdominal CT scan and thoraco-abdominal CT scan were performed in 6/20 (30%) and 3/20 (15%) patients, respectively. For 5/20 (25%) patients, no imaging was performed and diagnosis was based solely on clinical findings. Fifteen (75%) patients required treatment on an ICU with a median (IQR) duration of ICU stay of 3 (2–5) days. None of these parameters correlated significantly with mortality. Nine patients (45%)

required mechanical ventilation, with a median (IQR) duration of 2 (1.5–3.5) days. Unilateral orchiectomy was performed in five (35.7%) patients, and one (5%) patient required bilateral orchiectomy. Penectomy was necessary in two (10%) patients due to complete necrosis (Fig. 2). Auxiliary procedures like cystostomy and colostomy were performed in three (15%) and five (25%) patients, respectively. The bacteria cultured from the wound mainly comprised a broad spectrum of aerobic and anaerobic pathogens. *Escherichia coli* was the most common pathogen, identified in 10 (50%) patients. Polymicrobial infections were causative in 18 (90%) patients. Blood cultures were positive in two (12.5%) out of 16 patients with detection of *Klebsiella species* and *Pseudomonas aeruginosa*, respectively. In 17 (85%) patients, the combination of carbapenem antibiotics and clindamycin was used as empiric antibiotic therapy and adjusted according to the cultured bacteria and antibiotic susceptibility testing. Median (IQR) duration of antibiotic treatment was 18 (15–23) days. Extensive and sequential debridements regularly resulted in significant tissue defects. Therefore, nine (45%) patients had to be treated with vacuum-assisted closure (VAC) and five (25%) patients eventually required reconstructive surgery with flaps or skin grafts. The median (IQR) number of required operations was 4 (2–6), and the median (IQR) time to restore the integrity of the body surface was 18 (14–39) days. The mean scores for FGSI, LRINEC, and NLR were 13.0, 9.3, and 45.3 for non-survivors and 7.7, 6.5, and 26.0 for survivors,

respectively. Detailed results of the scoring systems are displayed in Table 1. None of the risk scores correlated significantly with mortality, the need of ICU treatment, mechanical ventilation, or the time to restore the integrity of the body surface ($p > 0.05$). However, FGSI ($p = 0.01$), LRINEC ($p = 0.04$), and NLR ($p = 0.01$) correlated significantly with the necessity to perform orchiectomy. We also found a significant correlation for LRINEC ($p = 0.02$) and a borderline significant correlation for NLR ($p = 0.06$) in terms of the need to perform cystostomy but no correlation with the need to perform colostomy. Furthermore, FGSI ($p = 0.02$), LRINEC ($p = 0.04$), and NLR ($p = 0.03$) significantly correlated with the necessity to perform penectomy.

Discussion

Mortality rate in our series was 15%. Two recent reviews [3, 15] reported mortality rates of 3–67%, with higher rates in underdeveloped countries. The high mortality rate that occurs despite major advances in healthcare in general and the implementation of the most modern treatment options and resources at a Swiss tertiary care center reflects the severity of the disease. Yet, with a median age of 66 years (range 46–73), our patients were rather old, as compared to a recent review that reported a median age of 51.8 years (range 47–63 years) [16]. In our series, we could only demonstrate a borderline significance for the correlation of age and mortality, even though it is well known that increasing patient age is a strong independent predictor of mortality [15]. Interestingly, age is not part of the three scoring systems. As age as a variable is easy to assess, we would suggest to include age into scoring systems. Moreover, morbidity of FG is high [3]. Multiple debridements resulted in significant tissue defects (Fig. 3). Therefore, VAC was required in 45% of patients and five patients eventually required reconstructive surgery. Generally, polymicrobial infections comprising a broad spectrum of aerobic and anaerobic pathogen are causative for FG [3], as it was the case in our series. Therefore, the combination of carbapenems and clindamycin is used as standard empiric antibiotic regimen at our institution, adapted from the guidelines of the Infectious Diseases Society of America (IDSA), concerning skin and soft tissue infections [17].

Prediction of the course of the disease is always challenging for the physician. Prognostic indicators like FGSI [12], LRINEC [13], and NLR [14] have been used to determine severity and prognosis of FG (1). The LRINEC had initially been developed to differentiate necrotizing from other soft tissue infections, and the NLR was initially used as sepsis marker, yet both scores were shown to correlate with mortality as well [11]. In the original report, LRINEC scores >6 were shown to be

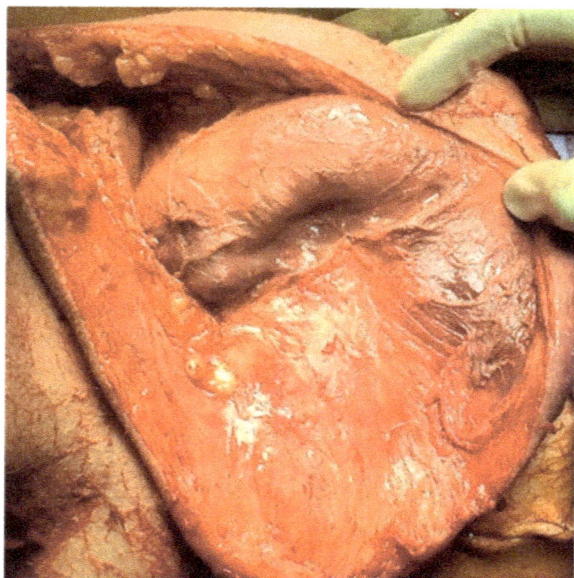

Fig. 2 Fournier's gangrene with complete penile necrosis. Scrotectomy and right orchiectomy already performed

Table 1 Risk scores, mortality, and surgical measures in Fournier's gangrene

Patient	Age	FGSI	LRINEC	NLR	Mortality	Orchiectomy	Penectomy	Reconstructive surgery
1	41	2	2	2.6	No	No	No	Yes
2	37	6	1	6.2	No	No	No	No
3	45	3	2	8.5	No	No	No	No
4	47	6	7	9.3	No	No	No	No
5	66	14	7	16.9	Yes	Yes	No	No
6	87	15	11	107.0	No	Yes	Yes	No
7	63	8	8	27.6	No	No	No	Yes
8	40	7	6	19.0	No	Yes[a]	No	No
9	52	11	11	24.1	No	Yes	No	Yes
10	75	10	8	2.3	No	No	No	No
11	66	10	11	85.2	No	Yes	No	No
12	89	11	9	n.c.	Yes	Yes	No	No
13	72	3	9	21.1	No	No	No	No
14	67	9	4	n.c	No	No	No	No
15	31	13	2	3.7	No	No	No	No
16	65	6	7	21.6	No	No	No	Yes
17	94	14	12	73.7	Yes	No	Yes	No
18	51	6	5	6.7	No	No	No	No
19	72	7	7	38.4	No	No	No	Yes
20	70	8	8	33.6	No	No	No	No

n.c. not calculable

[a]Bilateral

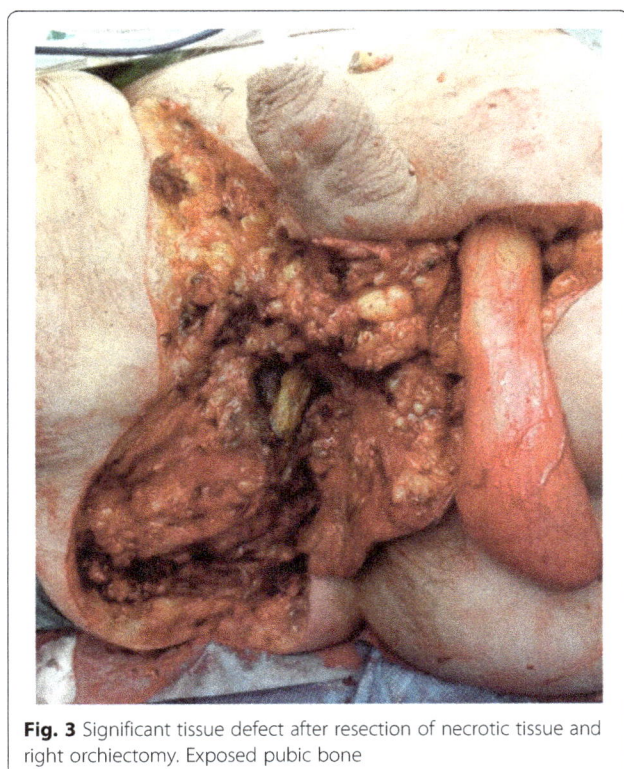

Fig. 3 Significant tissue defect after resection of necrotic tissue and right orchiectomy. Exposed pubic bone

associated with the likelihood to have necrotizing soft tissue infection [13]. Several reports demonstrated that patients with systemic infection and NLR scores > 10 had a more severe course of the disease [14, 18]. When applying the prognostic index FGSI [12], scores of ≥ 9 suggested a probability of 75% to succumb to the disease, while scores of < 9 were associated with 78% survival. We applied these risk scores on our temporary series, but we could not demonstrate a significant correlation with mortality for any of these prognostic indices, which is most likely due to the small sample size of our study. All non-survivors in our series had FGSI scores > 10. However, several studies have shown controversial results for the accuracy of this test [19–22]. We further assessed whether or not the prognostic indicators correlated with severity of the disease. Patients with a FGSI score ≥ 4 were more likely to require ICU treatment and eventually die than patients with FGSI scores < 4 [11]. We could not reproduce these findings in our cohort. However, we could demonstrate a significant correlation of all risk scores with morbidity in terms of local extent of the disease. Due to spread of necrotizing infection to testicles and penis, the radical and mutilating surgical procedures of orchiectomy ($n = 6$) and penectomy ($n = 2$) were performed to confine further spread of infection.

FGSI, LRINEC, and NLR proofed to be predictors for the extent of surgery required, as all of these risk score significantly correlated with orchiectomy, as well as with penectomy. Auxiliary measures like cystostomy or colostomy are regularly required in extensive disease. We found no correlation of the three risk scores with the need to perform colostomy in our cohort, but LRINEC significantly correlated ($p = 0.02$) with the need to perform cystostomy, while NLR showed borderline significance ($p = 0.06$).

To the best of our knowledge, our series is the first to report treatment outcomes of FG in Switzerland. Fournier's gangrene is a rare disease, which is displayed by our small sample size. In addition to the retrospective nature of the study, the small sample size represents the main limitation of this study. This might explain why we were not able to demonstrate the predictive ability of FGSI, LRINEC, and NLR for mortality. Nevertheless, our report is the first to demonstrate the predictive ability of the risk scores for the local extent of the disease and the required surgical methods in terms of orchiectomy and penectomy. Thus, the application of these risk scores can be a useful adjunct to clinical examination to aid diagnosis and can be helpful in predicting the course of disease. Furthermore, our results highlight that FG remains a potentially fatal disease despite most modern treatment at a Swiss tertiary care center.

Conclusions

In our series, Fournier's gangrene was associated with a mortality of 15% despite maximum multidisciplinary therapy at a specialized center. None of the risk score correlated with mortality, but all risk scores correlated with the morbidity of the disease in terms of local extent and the required surgical measures.

Acknowledgements
We thank Selina Ackermann from University Hospital Basel for the editorial assistance.

Authors' contributions
CW carried out the data collection or management, data analysis, manuscript writing/editing, and protocol/project development. JE was responsible for the data analysis. AH took part in the data collection or management. RK, SE, and AE carried out the data collection or management and manuscript writing/editing. DJS took part in the manuscript writing/editing. HHS took part in the protocol/project development and manuscript writing/editing. All authors read and approved the final manuscript.

Competing interests
The authors declare that they have no competing interests.

Author details
[1]Department of Urology, University Hospital Basel, Spitalstr. 21, 4031 Basel, Switzerland. [2]Division of Infectious Diseases and Hospital Epidemiology, University Hospital Basel, University Basel, Basel, Switzerland. [3]Division of Clinical Microbiology, University Hospital Basel, University Basel, Basel, Switzerland. [4]Applied Microbiology Research, Department of Biomedicine, University Basel, Basel, Switzerland. [5]Department of Plastic, Reconstructive, Aesthetic and Hand Surgery, University Hospital Basel, University Basel, Basel, Switzerland.

References
1. Fournier JA (1988) Jean-Alfred Fournier 1832-1914. Gangrene foudroyante de la verge (overwhelming gangrene) Sem Med 1883 Dis Colon Rectum 31 (12):984–988.
2. Wallner C, Behr B, Ring A, Mikhail BD, Lehnhardt M, Daigeler A. Reconstructive methods after Fournier gangrene. Urologe A. 2016;55(4):484–8. https://doi.org/10.1007/s00120-015-4001-2.
3. Shyam DC, Rapsang AG. Fournier's gangrene. Surgeon. 2013;11(4):222–32. https://doi.org/10.1016/j.surge.2013.02.001.
4. Voelzke BB, Hagedorn JC. Presentation and diagnosis of Fournier gangrene. Urology. 2017; https://doi.org/10.1016/j.urology.2017.10.031.
5. Efem SE. Recent advances in the management of Fournier's gangrene: preliminary observations. Surgery. 1993;113(2):200–4.
6. Paty R, Smith AD. Gangrene and Fournier's gangrene. Urol Clin North Am. 1992;19(1):149–62.
7. Morua AG, Lopez JA, Garcia JD, Montelongo RM, Guerra LS. Fournier's gangrene: our experience in 5 years, bibliographic review and assessment of the Fournier's gangrene severity index. Arch Esp Urol. 2009;62(7):532–40.
8. Nisbet AA, Thompson IM. Impact of diabetes mellitus on the presentation and outcomes of Fournier's gangrene. Urology. 2002;60(5):775–9.
9. Misiakos EP, Bagias G, Patapis P, Sotiropoulos D, Kanavidis P, Machairas A. Current concepts in the management of necrotizing fasciitis. Front Surg. 2014;1:36. https://doi.org/10.3389/fsurg.2014.00036.
10. Karian LS, Chung SY, Lee ES. Reconstruction of defects after Fournier gangrene: a systematic review. Eplasty. 2015;15:e18.
11. Bozkurt O, Sen V, Demir O, Esen A. Evaluation of the utility of different scoring systems (FGSI, LRINEC and NLR) in the management of Fournier's gangrene. Int Urol Nephrol. 2015;47(2):243–8. https://doi.org/10.1007/s11255-014-0897-5.
12. Laor E, Palmer LS, Tolia BM, Reid RE, Winter HI. Outcome prediction in patients with Fournier's gangrene. J Urol. 1995;154(1):89–92.
13. Wong CH, Khin LW, Heng KS, Tan KC, Low CO. The LRINEC (Laboratory Risk Indicator for Necrotizing Fasciitis) score: a tool for distinguishing necrotizing fasciitis from other soft tissue infections. Crit Care Med. 2004;32(7):1535–41.
14. Zahorec R. Ratio of neutrophil to lymphocyte counts—rapid and simple parameter of systemic inflammation and stress in critically ill. Bratisl Lek Listy. 2001;102(1):5–14.
15. Sorensen MD, Krieger JN. Fournier's gangrene: epidemiology and outcomes in the general US population. Urol Int. 2016;97(3):249–59. https://doi.org/10.1159/000445695.
16. Tang LM, Su YJ, Lai YC. The evaluation of microbiology and prognosis of Fournier's gangrene in past five years. Springerplus. 2015;4:14. https://doi.org/10.1186/s40064-014-0783-8.
17. Stevens DL, Bisno AL, Chambers HF, Dellinger EP, Goldstein EJC, Gorbach SL, Hirschmann JV, Kaplan SL, Montoya JG, Wade JC. Practice guidelines for the diagnosis and management of skin and soft tissue infections: 2014 Update by the Infectious Diseases Society of America. Clin Infect Dis. 2014; 59(2):147–59. https://doi.org/10.1093/cid/ciu444.
18. de Jager CP, van Wijk PT, Mathoera RB, de Jongh-Leuvenink J, van der Poll T, Wever PC. Lymphocytopenia and neutrophil-lymphocyte count ratio predict bacteremia better than conventional infection markers in an emergency care unit. Crit Care. 2010;14(5):R192. https://doi.org/10.1186/cc9309.
19. Kabay S, Yucel M, Yaylak F, Algin MC, Hacioglu A, Kabay B, Muslumanoglu AY. The clinical features of Fournier's gangrene and the predictivity of the Fournier's Gangrene Severity Index on the outcomes. Int Urol Nephrol. 2008;40(4):997–1004. https://doi.org/10.1007/s11255-008-9401-4.
20. Corcoran AT, Smaldone MC, Gibbons EP, Walsh TJ, Davies BJ. Validation of the Fournier's gangrene severity index in a large contemporary series. J Urol. 2008;180(3):944–8. https://doi.org/10.1016/j.juro.2008.05.021.

21

Emergency surgeons' perceptions and attitudes towards antibiotic prescribing and resistance

Francesco M. Labricciosa[1], Massimo Sartelli[2*], Sofia Correia[3,4], Lilian M. Abbo[5], Milton Severo[3,4], Luca Ansaloni[6], Federico Coccolini[6], Carlos Alves[7], Renato Bessa Melo[8], Gian Luca Baiocchi[9], José-Artur Paiva[10,11], Fausto Catena[12] and Ana Azevedo[3,4,13]

Abstract

Background: Antibiotic resistance (AMR) is a growing public health problem worldwide, in part related to inadequate antibiotic use. A better knowledge of physicians' motivations, attitudes and practice about AMR and prescribing should enable the design and implementation of effective antibiotic stewardship programs (ASPs). The objective of the study was to assess attitudes and perceptions concerning AMR and use of antibiotics among surgeons who regularly perform emergency or trauma surgery.

Methods: A cross-sectional web-based survey was conducted contacting 4904 individuals belonging to a mailing list provided by the World Society of Emergency Surgery. Participation was voluntary and anonymous. The survey was open for 5 weeks (from May 3, 2017, to June 6, 2017), within which two reminders were sent. The self-administered questionnaire was developed by a multidisciplinary team; reliability and validity were assessed.

Results: The overall response rate was 12.5%. Almost all participants considered AMR an important worldwide problem, but 45.6% of them underrated the problem in their own hospitals. Surgeons provided with periodic reports on local AMR demonstrated a lower underrating in their hospital. Only 66.3% of the surgeons stated to receive periodic reports on local AMR data, and among them, 56.2% had consulted them to select an antibiotic in the previous month. Availability of systematic reports about AMR, availability of guidelines for therapy of infections, and advice from an infectious diseases specialist were considered very helpful measures to improve antibiotic prescribing by 68.0, 65.7, and 64.9%, respectively. Persuasive and restrictive ASPs were both considered helpful measures by 64.5%. Moreover, 86.3% considered locally developed guidelines more useful than national ones. Only 21.9% received formal training in antibiotic prescribing in the previous year; among them, 86.6% declared to be interested in receiving more training.

Conclusions: Availability of periodic reports on local AMR data was considered an important tool to guide surgeons in choosing the correct antibiotic and to increase awareness of the problem of AMR. Local guidelines for therapy of infections should be implemented in every emergency surgery setting, and developed by a multidisciplinary team directly involving surgeons, infectious diseases specialists, and microbiologists, and formally established in an ASP.

Keywords: Cross-sectional survey, Emergency surgery, Antimicrobial stewardship, Antibiotic prescribing, Antibiotic resistance

* Correspondence: massimosartelli@gmail.com
[2]Department of Surgery, Macerata Hospital, Macerata, Italy
Full list of author information is available at the end of the article

Background

Antibiotic resistance (AMR) is a serious and growing public health problem in both hospital- and community-acquired infections worldwide [1], in part related to inadequate antibiotic use [2, 3]. Spreading of antibiotic-resistant bacteria has a negative impact on patient outcomes such as prolonged morbidity, hospital stay, and increased risk of death [4], resulting in increased health care costs and financial burden [5]. Development, namely through selection, of AMR is accelerated by inadequate antibiotic exposure [6]. Studies have estimated that between 20 and 50% of antibiotic use is either unnecessary or inappropriate and decreasing misuse is a necessary step of the strategy to curb antibiotic resistance [3, 7].

Antibiotics, unlike many other drugs, are utilized by virtually all doctors, across a wide spectrum of practices and various levels of training and knowledge [8–10]. In spite of the severe consequences and global spread of antibiotic resistance, effective dissemination of information to healthcare professionals about adverse outcomes associated with antibiotic misuse and assurance of an evidence-based approach in practice remain challenging [11].

Antimicrobial stewardship programs (ASPs) have emerged as a strategy to tackle the problem of AMR, as a systematic approach to improve and optimize the appropriate prescription of antibiotics through a variety of interventions and have been proven to be cost-effective [12]. ASPs should promote education, feedback, and effect changes in prescribing behaviors of healthcare providers [13]. In order to better plan these behavioral interventions, it is important to understand physicians' motivation, knowledge, attitude, and practice [14]. A multidisciplinary collaboration among various specialties within a healthcare institution is essential to ensure that antibiotic management maximizes patient clinical outcomes and minimizes emergence and selection of AMR. In this context, the direct involvement of surgeons in ASPs can be highly impactful [15].

Emergency surgical admissions account for approximately half of all surgical admissions [16]. Emergency operative procedures are associated with an increased risk for surgical site infections (SSIs) [17], since they do not allow for the standard preoperative preparation normally performed for an elective operation. Typically performed on critical patients, emergency operative procedures are often carried out on contaminated or dirty wounds which are clearly identified as a significant risk factor for SSIs [18, 19]. Therefore, the role of the emergency surgeon is paramount in prescribing antibiotics judiciously, both for therapeutic use and preoperative prophylaxis. The necessity of systematic approaches for the optimization of antibiotic therapy in surgical units has become increasingly urgent [20].

Previous surveys have been conducted in hospital settings to assess physicians' perceptions, attitudes, and knowledge about antibiotic use and resistance, including physicians from various specialties [13, 21–29]. Three surveys focused their investigation upon all physicians of targeted hospitals [30–32]. However, in these studies, mainly aggregated data were provided, without specifically analysing surgeons' perceptions, attitudes, and knowledge apart from other professionals. Therefore, to the best of our knowledge, no previous physician surveys have focused only on surgeons, and they are one of the most frequent prescribers of broad spectrum antibiotics. Thus, it seems important to better understand the perceptions and attitudes of this group of prescribers worldwide.

We surveyed junior and senior surgeons, belonging to all surgical specialties, performing regularly emergency or trauma surgery in their activities. The objective of our study was to assess their knowledge, attitudes, and perceptions concerning antibiotic resistance and prescribing, in order to gain a deeper understanding of these processes in different cultural contexts, so as to provide information to enable the design and implementation of more effective antibiotic stewardship interventions in emergency and trauma surgery settings.

Methods

We conducted a cross-sectional web-based survey evaluating emergency surgeons' perceptions, attitudes, and knowledge about antibiotic use and resistance. The study was promoted by the World Society of Emergency Surgery (WSES) and by the Global Alliance for Infections in Surgery (GAIS) [33].

The population target was represented by the surgeons who regularly perform emergency or trauma surgery. Participants were registered as WSES ordinary members or professionals who subscribed to the newsletter of the World Journal of Emergency Surgery (WJES). A total of 4904 individuals were contacted via e-mail with an invitation letter and a survey link (http://www.docs.google.com), using a mailing list provided by the WSES. Although all members were invited to participate, only surveys completed by surgeons regularly performing emergency or trauma surgery were included in the analysis. The survey was written in English, participation was voluntary and anonymous, and no incentives for participation were given. The survey was opened for 5 weeks between May 3, 2017, and June 6, 2017. Two reminders were sent: the first one after 14 days and the second one after 28 days.

The self-administered questionnaire was developed by a multidisciplinary team of investigators including epidemiologists, surgeons, infectious diseases physicians, pharmacologists, and a statistician, after searching the medical literature for comparable studies and adapting questions designed in other physicians' surveys previously carried out [34, 35]. The questionnaire (see Additional file 1) started with a characterization of the surgeons' professional profiles (country, sex, surgical speciality, years of experience) and working setting (type of hospital, hospital inpatient beds, existence of an antimicrobial stewardship team, implementation of local guidelines for therapy of infections, and availability of periodic reports on local antibiotic resistance data). It included questions about surgeons' perception regarding the importance and the causes of antibiotic resistance and attitudes towards antibiotic prescribing and about interventions designed to improve antimicrobial stewardship. Participants' attitudes during the antibiotic prescribing process, perceptions of the factors influencing that process, and perceptions of the helpfulness of potential interventions to improve it were surveyed.

Published recommendations for the development and implementation of web-based surveys were applied to the design of our questionnaire [36, 37]. Questions about attitudes and perceptions towards antibiotic prescribing and resistance were designed using the 4-point Likert scale with response options from very helpful/important/confident to very unhelpful/unimportant/unconfident.

Anonymous data were automatically entered in an Excel database (Microsoft Corporation, Redmond, Washington, USA). The study was approved by the Ethics Committee of the Institute of Public Health of the University of Porto (ISPUP), which waived the need for written informed consent from the participants considering the anonymous nature of the collected data.

Statistical analysis

To assess reliability and validity of the instrument, an online invitation letter was sent in May 2017 to 150 members randomly selected from the WSES mailing list, asking them to complete the questionnaire on a voluntary basis. Responses from 102 individuals were used to test content validity and reliability of the questionnaire (48 non-respondents). From those respondents, a sample of 31 individuals was used to test the reproducibility of the questionnaire.

We started assessing the dimensionality of the scale using principal component analysis with varimax rotation. The scree plot was used to define the number of dimensions, and the items whose factor loadings were greater than 0.4 were considered as being correlated with a specific principal component. The indirect reliability of the resulting domains was assessed using Cronbach's alpha, in the overall sample. Test-retest reliability was assessed using consistency two-way mixed single intraclass correlation coefficient (ICC). We hypothesized that most of the subtests would have good test-retest reliability (minimum ICC of 0.70). Items were classified from 1 to 4. In each domain, the final score was estimated as the sum of the classification in the included items. Two independent-sample t test and analysis of variance (ANOVA) were used to compare the mean of final scores according to participants' characteristics: sex, years of experience, type of hospital, availability of antimicrobial stewardship teams, local guidelines, and reports on AMR. In this process, statistical analysis was conducted using SPSS Statistical Package 21.0 (IBM Corporation, Armonk, NY, USA).

Descriptive analysis for categorical variables was presented in absolute frequency and percentage. Data obtained from questions concerning attitudes and perceptions and based on a 4-point Likert scale option were collapsed into two categories (very helpful/ important/confident and helpful/important/confident were collapsed into the first category; unhelpful/unimportant/unconfident and very unhelpful/unimportant/ unconfident were collapsed into the second category). The frequency of each category was compared by working setting and professional profile, existence of antimicrobial stewardship team, local guidelines, and reports using, as appropriate, chi-square or Fisher's exact tests.

We defined "underrating" if the participant ranked (in a 4-point Likert scale option) the problem of AMR in its own institution less important than worldwide and "overrating" if the participant ranked (in a 4-point Likert scale option) its colleague's prescriptions as more important contributing factor to AMR than its own.

All tests were two-sided; p values below 0.05 were considered statistically significant. Statistical calculations assessed on final data were performed using Stata 11 software package (StataCorp, College Station, TX, USA).

Results

Validity and reproducibility

Results are presented in Additional files 2, 3, 4, and 5. The principle component analysis (PCA) identified six principal components with eigenvalue higher than 1. The six principal components, hereafter referred to as domains, explained 58% of total variance. The Cronbach alpha was higher than 0.7 for domains 1, 2, 4, and 6, and only domains 3 and 5 had value lower than 0.7 (see Additional file 2). In the test-retest reliability analysis, the ICC ranged from 0.52 (score 1) to 0.82 (score 3) (see Additional file 3).

In the validation sample, we observed significant differences between sexes in scores 2 and 5, by years of experience in domain 2, and by type of hospital in domains 2 and 6 (see Additional file 4). In the final sample, we observed significant differences between sex in domains 1, 2, and 6; among years of experience in domain 4; among type of hospital in domains 2 and 6; and among local guidelines for therapy of infections in domains 2 and 5 (see Additional file 5).

Baseline data: coverage, response rate, working setting, and professional profile

Six hundred thirty-seven of the 4904 professionals invited by e-mail to participate in the survey returned a filled-in questionnaire. Twenty-five participants stated they did not perform emergency or trauma surgery regularly; therefore, 612 questionnaires were deemed appropriate for analysis, with a final overall response rate of 12.5%. Surveyed emergency surgeons' working setting and professional profile are described in Table 1.

Table 1 Surveyed surgeons' working setting and professional profile

Characteristics	N (%)
WHO region classification	
Africa Region	35 (5.7)
Region of the Americas	128 (20.9)
South-East Asia Region	18 (2.9)
European Region	372 (60.8)
Easter Mediterranean Region	36 (5.9)
Western Pacific Region	23 (3.8)
Gender	
Male	526 (85.9)
Female	86 (14.1)
Surgeries regularly performed*	
Abdominal	577 (94.3)
Cardiac surgery	10 (1.6)
Gynecologic	30 (4.9)
Neurosurgery	4 (0.7)
Orthopedic	32 (5.2)
Pediatric	73 (11.9)
Thoracic	143 (23.4)
Urological	41 (6.7)
Vascular	74 (12.1)
Other	58 (9.5)
Years of experience	
Less than 10 years	126 (20.6)
10–20 years	210 (34.3)
21–30 years	155 (25.3)
More than 30 years	121 (19.8)
Type of hospital	
University hospital	395 (64.5)
Community teaching hospital	133 (21.7)
Community hospital	68 (11.1)
Other	16 (2.6)
Hospital inpatient beds	
Less than 100	27 (4.4)
100–500	225 (36.8)
501–1000	247 (40.4)
More than 1000	107 (17.5)
Unsure	6 (1.0)
Hospital with antimicrobial stewardship team	
Yes	448 (73.2)
No	139 (22.7)
Unsure	25 (4.1)
Local GLs for therapy of infections implemented	
Yes	465 (76.0)
No	137 (22.4)

Table 1 Surveyed surgeons' working setting and professional profile (Continued)

Characteristics	N (%)
Unsure	10 (1.6)
Reports on local AMR data periodically received	
Yes	406 (66.3)
No	177 (28.9)
Unsure	29 (4.7)

WHO World Health Organization, GLs guidelines, AMR antibiotic resistance
*Sum of numbers is greater than the overall sample (n = 612) since the question was based on a multiple choice

Surgeons' importance of the problem of antibiotic resistance and perceptions of causes of antibiotic resistance

Almost all the surveyed surgeons strongly agreed (493, 80.6%) or agreed (117, 19.1%) that antibiotic resistance is a worldwide problem; only two (0.3%) strongly disagreed. While the majority strongly agreed (240, 39.2%) or agreed (317, 51.8%), a minority disagreed (53, 8.7%) or strongly disagreed (2, 0.3%) that this is a problem in their own hospital. Two hundred seventy-nine (45.6%) surgeons underrated the problem in their hospital. Surgeons provided with periodic reports on local antibiotic resistance data underrated the problem in their hospitals less than their colleagues who did not receive these reports (39.9% versus 56.8%, $p < 0.001$).

Perceptions of causes of AMR are reported in Fig. 1 and Table 2. Poor hand hygiene was more often considered an important cause of AMR by surgeons who declared to receive regularly report on resistance data than their colleagues who did not (85.7 versus 79.1%, $p = 0.038$). One hundred ninety-five (31.9%) surgeons overrated their colleagues' prescriptions. However, we observed that surgeons whose surgical unit or department had local guidelines for therapy of infections tended to overrate less their colleagues' prescriptions compared to surgeons who declared not to have them (28.2 versus 44.2%, $p < 0.001$). Overrating was similar throughout all other analysed characteristics.

Participants' attitudes during the antibiotic prescribing process

National guidelines for therapy of infections were used or consulted by 55.7% (341/612) of the surveyed surgeons, when considering an antibiotic for a patient in the previous month. Local guidelines for therapy of infections were used or consulted by 77.2% (359/465) of surgeons who stated to have them available in their surgical unit or department. Reports on local resistance data were personally consulted to define an antibiotic empiric therapy for a patient in the previous month by 56.2% (228/406) of the participants who declared to receive periodically these reports. No statistically significant differences in these three attitudes were found according to the working setting or professional profile.

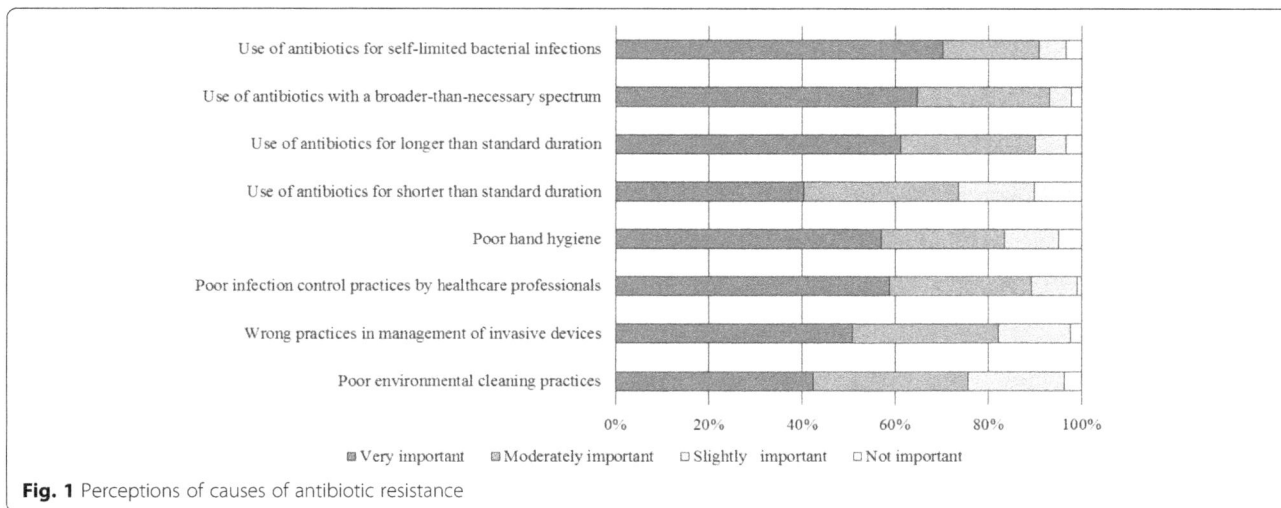

Fig. 1 Perceptions of causes of antibiotic resistance

Surveyed surgeons' confidence levels for seven scenarios during an antibiotic prescribing process are described in Fig. 2. Surgeons working in hospitals where local guidelines for therapy of infections are implemented showed to be more confident in deciding not to prescribe an antibiotic if not sure about the diagnosis (82.6 versus 70.7%, $p = 0.002$) than those working in hospitals with no guidelines available. Moreover, those who stated to have consulted the guidelines in the previous month seemed to be more confident in choosing the correct antibiotic (93.9 versus 86.6%, $p = 0.023$).

Perceptions of the factors influencing the antibiotic prescribing process

In the previous 12 months, 134 (21.9%) surgeons received formal training in antibiotic prescribing; among them, 116 (116/134, 86.6%) declared to be interested in receiving more training. On the contrary, 477 (77.9%) participants did not receive any training in antibiotic prescribing; among

them, 370 (370/477, 77.6%) stated to be interested in receiving more training.

Perceptions of the helpfulness of potential interventions to improve antibiotic prescribing

Surgeons' ratings of the helpfulness of potential interventions to improve antibiotic prescribing are reported in Fig. 3. The majority of surveyed surgeons (395, 64.5%) attributed the same value to both persuasive and restrictive ASPs, while 145 (23.7%) considered persuasive ASPs more helpful than restrictive ASPs, and 72 (11.8%) found restrictive ASPs more helpful than persuasive ASP.

Participants who stated to receive periodically reports on resistant data rated this measure as very helpful (285/406, 70.2%) or helpful (107/406, 26.4%). Participants regularly receiving reports on local antibiotic resistance data considered helpful the implementation of restrictive measures more than their colleagues who did not receive them (76.8 versus 68.0%, $p = 0.018$). The majority of surveyed surgeons declared that locally developed guidelines for antibiotic treatment are more useful than national ones (528, 86.3%).

Discussion

Our survey shows that surgeons of our sample are highly aware of and concerned about AMR, demonstrating awareness of a widespread issue that poses a threat for their patients. However, 45.6% of the surveyed surgeons underrated the problem in their own hospitals, perceiving the risk as more theoretical than real. These findings are consistent with other surveys previously published [21, 25, 28, 34]. However, it is noteworthy that surgeons provided with periodic reports on local antibiotic resistance data proved to have a lower underrating of the AMR issue in their hospital, probably demonstrating a better knowledge of local microbiology and consequently a higher awareness of the problem.

Table 2 Perceptions of causes of antibiotic resistance

Questions	Very likely	Likely	Unlikely	Very unlikely
Do you think that your antibiotic prescriptions contribute to the problem of antibiotic resistance?	103 (16.8)	307 (50.2)	185 (30.2)	17 (2.8)
Do you think that your colleagues' prescriptions contribute to the problem of antibiotic resistance?	155 (25.3)	381 (62.3)	72 (11.8)	4 (0.7)
Do you expect that antibiotic resistance will be a greater clinical problem for your patients in the future?	395 (64.5)	205 (33.5)	10 (1.6)	2 (0.3)
Do you expect that new antibiotics will be developed in the next 10 years will keep up with the problem of resistance?	88 (14.4)	230 (37.6)	262 (42.8)	32 (5.2)

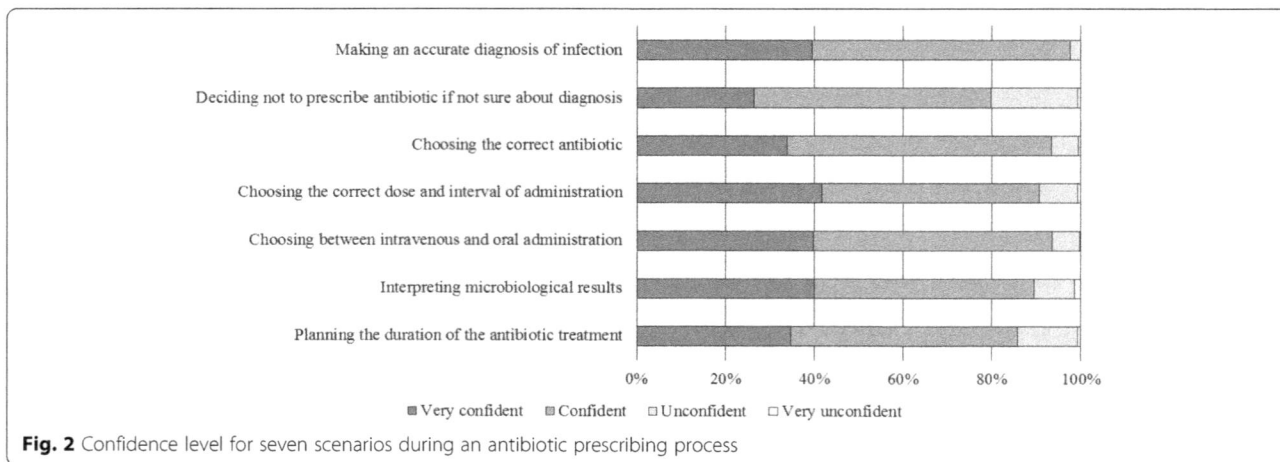

Fig. 2 Confidence level for seven scenarios during an antibiotic prescribing process

The availability of periodic reports on local rates of antibiotic resistance patterns is an essential component of the clinical decision-making process, since they can be used not only to evaluate trends of antibiotic resistance rates, but also to educate clinicians on optimal antibiotic use, and to assess the impact of interventions. Ideally, a microbiology service should provide analyses of AMR at least annually to both clinicians and antimicrobial stewardship committees, to inform local empirical therapy recommendations and formulary management [38]. This period should be adapted to every facility, taking into account human and financial resources required for its implementation and maintenance. Moreover, Infectious Diseases Society of America (IDSA) antimicrobial stewardship guidelines recommended to provide selective or cascade reporting to help guide appropriate antibiotic use [39], by taking into account both local susceptibility of the microorganisms and drug availability. In our study, just over half of the surveyed surgeons declaring to receive periodically reports on local resistance data had personally consulted

them to select an antibiotic empiric therapy in the previous month. Even so, 70% of them stated that availability of reports on local resistance data is a very helpful measure to improve antibiotic prescribing. Therefore, in order to increase the active consultation of these reports, it is paramount to establish a solid communication between microbiologists and emergency surgeons, for example, through the existence of privileged interlocutors and the participation of microbiologists in regular surgeons' meetings. This solution is likely to be welcomed by the emergency surgeons, since the vast majority of them considered helpful an advice from a microbiologist.

It is noteworthy that surgeons periodically provided with reports on local resistance data were more likely to consider poor hand hygiene an important cause of spread of AMR than their colleagues, highlighting again the importance of available reports in promoting the awareness of AMR. These findings should be emphasised, since both hand hygiene and infection control practices are effective preventive measures, stopping transmission of multidrug resistant organisms and

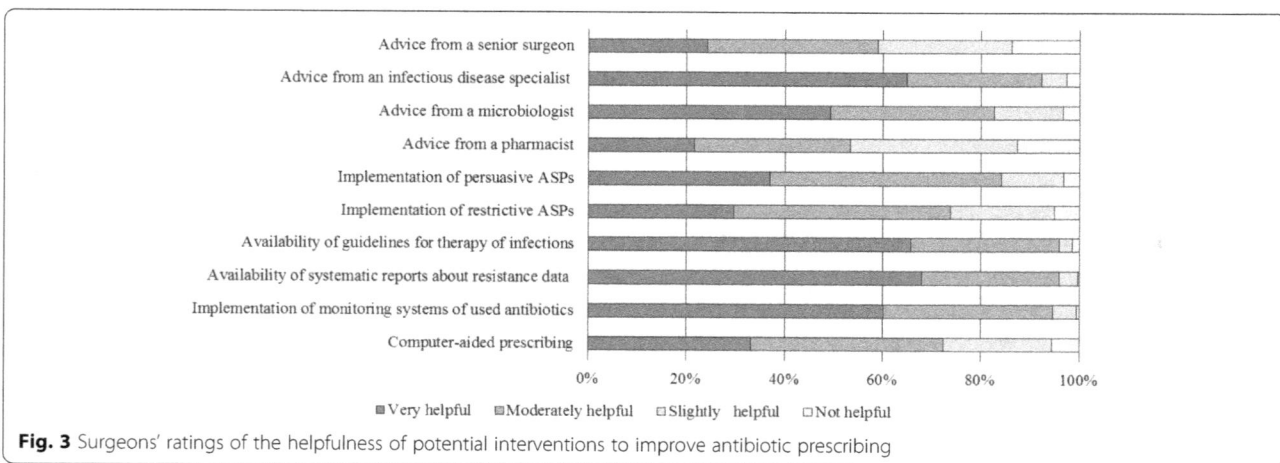

Fig. 3 Surgeons' ratings of the helpfulness of potential interventions to improve antibiotic prescribing

preventing surgical site infections [40, 41]. Once multidrug-resistant organism infection or carriage is detected in hospitalized patients, in order to reduce person-to-person spread and prevent hospital diffusion, it is recommended the immediate implementation of standard and contact precautions [42]. Infection control measures have to be quickly implemented not only to minimize cross-transmission, but also to enable timely antimicrobial optimization, which, in turn, may lead to decreased deaths, shortened hospital stay, and lower hospitalization costs.

In our survey, only a minority of participants ranked restrictive ASPs more helpful than persuasive ones. Restrictive ASP may be perceived by the surveyed surgeons as a deprivation of autonomy in antibiotic prescribing [38], and its impact on surgeon autonomy may also create barriers to collaboration and communication with other members of the ASP [12]. Therefore, when restrictive interventions are required—as in urgent situations—it is important to add persuasive components to the programs since the first phases of its implementation.

As the majority of surveyed surgeons found the advice from an infectious diseases specialist very helpful and such strategy has recognised effectiveness in reducing antibiotic consumption and resistance with no impairment on clinical outcomes [43], a close collaboration between these two clinicians should be encouraged and formally included in the ASP, for example, implementing systematic bedside infectious disease consultation. A successful ASP should focus on collaboration among various professionals within a healthcare institution including prescribing clinicians. The quality of professional relationships between experts and non-experts remains a key component to achieving a real change and improvement.

Almost all the surveyed surgeons perceived locally developed treatment guidelines as a tool to improve antibiotic prescription. Furthermore, the majority declared that locally developed guidelines are more useful than national ones, as observed in a previous survey in a hospital setting [35]. However, almost one in four surgeons did not use or consult local guidelines when considering an antibiotic for a patient in the previous month. The attitude of relying on personal knowledge and experience rather than on recommendations of guidelines and formal policy was already reported and described by other authors [26, 28, 44]. In order to achieve optimal adherence to local antibiotic guidelines, more efforts are needed by antibiotic policy makers, promoting and achieving consensus before implementation and facilitating situations to make them more applicable.

Our study has strengths and limitations. To the best of our knowledge, no previous physician surveys have been focused only on emergency surgeons, in a worldwide perspective. Antibiotic prescription practices are affected by socio-cultural factors that vary across countries [33, 45],

and we tried to address this issue extending the survey to surgeons from different countries all over the world. Moreover, the survey was conducted in a sample of surgeons with different working settings and professional profiles, supplying a wider framework in terms of surgical disciplines and years of experience. Furthermore, the study is methodologically robust, as the questionnaire underwent a formal statistical evaluation to ensure its validity and reliability. However, we selected the participants from a mailing list provided by a scientific society of emergency surgeons. Participants were not homogeneously distributed across all geographic regions of the world, and the majority of participants were from European countries, due to the difficulty in recruiting participants in some areas of the world. Participation rate was low which is in favor of some selection bias. However, participation might be underestimated because we were not able to define accurately the number of emergency or trauma surgeons among all the individuals invited to participate the survey. It is also possible that participation was more frequent among physicians with some interest or knowledge on the topic. Thus, generalizability may be impaired. Another potential limitation of any survey is the tendency of respondents to give socially desirable answers instead of revealing their true opinions. We tried to minimize this bias ensuring complete response anonymity with an online self-reported questionnaire.

Conclusions

This study, conducted and focused on emergency surgeons, showed that availability of periodic reports on local rates of antibiotic resistance data should be considered an important tool to increase awareness of the problem of AMR. Prompt implementation of standard and contact precautions is an essential measure to stop transmission of multidrug-resistant organisms and prevent surgical site infections. Therefore, the active consultation of these reports should be encouraged and promoted through a dynamic collaboration between microbiologists and emergency surgeons, formally established in an ASP. Moreover, locally developed treatment guidelines should be implemented in every emergency surgery setting. They should be developed by a multidisciplinary team directly involving a surgeon, and efforts are needed to make them more applicable, and to achieve optimal adherence to them. In this context, the direct involvement of surgeons with knowledge in surgical infections in ASPs can be highly impactful, since they are at the forefront in treating patients with infections. Managers and antibiotic stewardship teams could take into account information from our survey in designing more targeted interventions in emergency surgery settings.

Additional files

Additional file 1: Full-scale questionnaire. (DOCX 42 kb)

Additional file 2: Factor loadings from principal component analysis with varimax rotation and Cronbach alpha for each domain. (DOCX 18 kb)

Additional file 3: Test-retest of the domains: consistency two-way mixed single ICC. (DOCX 14 kb)

Additional file 4: Mean and standard deviation (SD) of each domain by surgeons' professional profile and working setting (validation sample). (DOCX 19 kb)

Additional file 5: Mean and standard deviation (SD) of each domain by surgeons' professional profile and working setting (final sample). (DOCX 18 kb)

Abbreviations

ANOVA: Analysis of variance; AMR: Antibiotic resistance; ASPs: Antimicrobial stewardship programs; GAIS: Global Alliance for Infections in Surgery; ICC: Intraclass correlation coefficient; ISPUP: Institute of Public Health of the University of Porto; PC: Principle component; PCA: Principle component analysis; SD: Standard deviation; SSIs: Surgical site infections; WJES: World Journal of Emergency Surgery; WSES: World Society of Emergency Surgery

Authors' contributions

LMA, AA, SC, FML, MSa, and MSe participated in building the full-scale questionnaire. AA, SC, FML, and MSe did the statistical analysis. FML wrote the first draft of the manuscript. All the authors reviewed the manuscript and approved the final draft.

Competing interests

The authors declare that they have no competing interests.

Author details

[1]Department of Biomedical Science and Public Health, School of Hygiene and Preventive Medicine, Faculty of Medicine and Surgery, Università Politecnica delle Marche, Ancona, Italy. [2]Department of Surgery, Macerata Hospital, Macerata, Italy. [3]Epidemiology Research Unit (EPIUnit), Instituto de Saúde Pública, Universidade do Porto (ISPUP), Porto, Portugal. [4]Departamento de Ciências da Saúde Pública e Forenses e Educação Médica, Faculdade de Medicina, Universidade do Porto, Porto, Portugal. [5]Infection Prevention and Antimicrobial Stewardship Jackson Health System, University of Miami Miller School of Medicine, Miami, FL, USA. [6]General Surgery Department, Papa Giovanni XXIII Hospital, Bergamo, Italy. [7]Unit of Prevention and Control of Infections and Antimicrobial Resistance (UPCIRA), Centro de Epidemiologia Hospitalar, Centro Hospitalar São João, Porto, Portugal. [8]Department of General Surgery, Centro Hospitalar São João, Porto, Portugal. [9]Department of Clinical and Experimental Sciences, University of Brescia, Brescia, Italy. [10]Department of Emergency and Intensive Care, Centro Hospitalar São João, Porto, Portugal. [11]Department of Medicine, Faculdade de Medicina, Universidade do Porto, Porto, Portugal. [12]Department of Emergency Surgery, Maggiore Hospital, Parma, Italy. [13]Centro de Epidemiologia Hospitalar, Centro Hospitalar São João, Porto, Portugal.

References

1. World Health Organization. In: Combat drug resistance. 2011. http://www.who.int/world-health-day/2011/en/. Accessed 14 Mar 2018.
2. Goldman DA, Weinstein RA, Wenzel RP, Tablan OC, Duma RJ, Gaynes RP, et al. Strategies to prevent and control the emergent and spreads of antimicrobial resistant microorganisms in hospitals. JAMA. 1996;275:234–40.
3. Dellit TH, Owens RC, McGowan JE Jr, Gerding DN, Weinstein RA, Burke JP, et al. Infectious Diseases Society of America and the Society for Healthcare Epidemiology of America guidelines for developing an institutional program to enhance antimicrobial stewardship. Clin Infect Dis. 2007;44:159–77.
4. Cosgrove SE. The relationship between antimicrobial resistance and patient outcomes: mortality, length of hospital stay, and health care costs. Clin Infect Dis. 2006;42(suppl 2):S82–9.
5. Coast J, Smith R, Miller M. Superbugs: should antimicrobial resistance be included as a cost in economic evaluation? Health Econ. 1996;5:217–26.
6. World Health Organization. In: Global strategy for the containment of antimicrobial resistance. 2001. http://www.who.int/drugresistance/WHO_Global_Strategy_English.pdf. Accessed 14 Mar 2018.
7. Pulcini C, Cua E, Lieutier F, Landraud L, Dellamonica P, Roger PM. Antibiotic misuse: a prospective clinical audit in a French university hospital. Eur J Clin Microbiol Infect Dis. 2007;26:277–80.
8. Roumie CL, Halasa NB, Edwards KM, Zhu Y, Dittus RS, Griffin MR. Differences in antibiotic prescribing among physicians, residents, and nonphysician clinicians. Am J Med. 2005;118:641–8.
9. Running A, Kipp C, Mercer V. Prescriptive patterns of nurse practitioners and physicians. J Am Acad Nurse Pract. 2006;18:228–33.
10. Edgar T, Boyd SD, Palame MJ. Sustainability for behaviour change in the fight against antibiotic resistance: a social marketing framework. J Antimicrob Chemother. 2009;63:230–7.
11. Charani E, Cooke J, Holmes A. Antibiotic stewardship programmes—what's missing? J Antimicrob Chemother. 2010;65:2275–7.
12. Davey P, Brown E, Fenelon L, Finch R, Gould I, Hartman G, et al. Interventions to improve antibiotic prescribing practices for hospital inpatients. Cochrane Database Syst Rev. 2005;(4):CD003543.
13. Abbo L, Sinkowitz-Cochran R, Smith L, Ariza-Heredia E, Gómez-Marín O, Srinivasan A, et al. Faculty and resident physicians' attitudes, perceptions and knowledge about antimicrobial use and resistance. Infect Control Hosp Epidemiol. 2011;32:714–28.
14. Cabana MD, Rand CS, Powe NR, Wu AW, Wilson MH, Abboud PA, et al. Why don't physicians follow clinical practice guidelines? A framework for improvement. JAMA. 1999;282:1458–65.
15. Cakmakci M. Antibiotic stewardship programmes and the surgeon's role. J Hosp Infect. 2015;89:264–6.
16. Mai-Phan TA, Patel B, Walsh M, Abraham AT, Kocher HM. Emergency room surgical workload in an inner city UK teaching hospital. World J Emerg Surg. 2008;3:19.
17. Malone DL, Genuit T, Tracy JK, Gannon C, Napolitano LM. Surgical site infections: reanalysis of risk factors. J Surg Res. 2002;103:89–95.
18. Cruse PJ, Foord R. The epidemiology of wound infection. A 10-year prospective study of 62,939 wounds. Surg Clin North Am. 1980;60:27–40.
19. Culver DH, Horan TC, Gaynes RP, Martone WJ, Jarvis WR, Emori TG, et al. Surgical wound infection rates by wound class, operative procedure, and patient risk index. National Nosocomial Infections Surveillance System. Am J Med. 1991;91(3B):152S–7S.
20. Sartelli M, Duane TM, Catena F, Tessier JM, Coccolini F, Kao LS, et al. Antimicrobial stewardship: a call to action for surgeons. Surg Infect. 2016;17:625–31.
21. Wester CW, Durairaj L, Evans AT, Schwartz DN, Husain S, Martinez E. Antibiotic resistance: a survey of physician perceptions. Arch Intern Med. 2002;162:2210–6.
22. Guerra CM, Pereira CA, Neves Neto AR, Cardo DM, Correa L. Physicians' perceptions, beliefs, attitudes and knowledge concerning antimicrobial resistance in a Brazilian teaching hospital. Infect Control Hosp Epidemiol. 2007;28:1411–4.
23. Tennant I, Nicholson A, Gordon-Strachan GM, Thoms C, Chin V, Didier MA. A survey of physicians' knowledge and attitudes regarding antimicrobial resistance and antibiotic prescribing practices at the University Hospital of the West Indies. West Indian Med J. 2010;59:165–70.

24. Garcia C, Llamocca LP, Garcia K, Jimenez A, Samalvides F, Gotuzzo E, et al. Knowledge, attitudes and practice survey about antimicrobial resistance and prescribing among physicians in a hospital setting in Lima, Peru. BMC Clin Pharmacol. 2011;11:18.

25. Navarro-San Francisco C, Del Toro MD, Cobo J, De Gea-García JH, Vañó-Galván S, Moreno-Ramos F, et al. Knowledge and perceptions of junior and senior Spanish resident doctors about antibiotic use and resistance: results of a multicenter survey. Enferm Infecc Microbiol Clin. 2013;31:199–204.

26. Thriemer K, Katuala Y, Batoko B, Alworonga JP, Devlier H, VanGeet C, et al. Antibiotic prescribing in DR Congo: a knowledge. Attitude and practice survey among medical doctors and students. PLoS One. 2013;8:e55495.

27. Abera B, Kibret M, Mulu W. Knowledge and beliefs on antimicrobial resistance among physicians and nurses in hospitals in Amhara Region, Ethiopia. BMC Pharmacol Toxicol. 2014;15:26.

28. Baadani AM, Baig K, Alfahad WA, Aldalbahi S, Omrani AS. Physicians' knowledge, perceptions, and attitudes toward antimicrobial prescribing in Riyadh, Saudi Arabia. Saudi Med J. 2015;36:613–9.

29. Alothman A, Algwizani A, Alsulaiman M, Alalwan A, Binsalih S, Knowledge BM. Attitude of physicians toward prescribing antibiotics and the risk of resistance in two reference hospitals. Infect Dis (Auckl). 2016;9:33–8.

30. Srinivasan A, Song X, Richard A, Sinkowitz-Cochran R, Cardo D, Rand C. A survey of knowledge, attitudes, and beliefs of house staff physicians from various specialties concerning antimicrobial use and resistance. Arch Intern Med 2004;164:1451–1456.

31. Lucet JC, Nicolas-Chanoine MH, Roy C, Riveros-Palacios O, Diamantis S, Le Grand J, et al. Antibiotic use: knowledge and perceptions in two university hospitals. J Antimicrob Chemother. 2011;66:936–40.

32. Kheder SI. Physcians knowledge and perception of antimicrobial resistance: a survey in Khartoum Stata Hospital settings. Br J Pharmaceut Res. 2013;3:347–62.

33. Global Alliance for Infections in Surgery. https://infectionsinsurgery.org. Accessed 3 May 2018.

34. Pulcini C, Williams F, Molinari N, Davey P, Nathwani D. Junior doctors' knowledge and perceptions of antibiotic resistance and prescribing: a survey in France and Scotland. Clin Microbiol Infect. 2011;17:80–7.

35. Abbo LM, Cosgrove SE, Pottinger PS, Pereyra M, Sinkowitz-Cochran R, Srinivasan A, et al. Medical students' perceptions and knowledge about antimicrobial stewardship: how are we educating our future prescribers? Clin Infect Dis. 2013;57:631–8.

36. Eysenbach G, Wyatt J. Using the Internet for surveys and health research. J Med Internet Res. 2002;4:E13.

37. Kelley K, Clark B, Brown V, Sitzia J. Good practice in the conduct and reporting of survey research. Int J Qual Health Care. 2003;15:261–6.

38. MacDougall C, Polk RE. Antimicrobial stewardship programs in health care systems. Clin Microbiol Rev. 2005;18:638–56.

39. Barlam TF, Cosgrove SE, Abbo LM, MacDougall C, Schuetz AN, Septimus EJ, et al. Implementing an Antibiotic Stewardship Program: guidelines by the Infectious Diseases Society of America and the Society for Healthcare Epidemiology of America. Clin Infect Dis. 2016;62:e51–77.

40. Siegel JD, Rhinehart E, Jackson M, Chiarello L, Health Care Infection Control Practices Advisory Committee. 2007 guideline for isolation precautions: preventing transmission of infectious agents in health care settings. Am J Infect Control. 2007;35:S65–164.

41. Siegel JD, Rhinehart E, Jackson M, Chiarello L; Healthcare Infection Control Practices Advisory Committee. Management of multidrug-resistant organisms in health care settings, 2006. Am J Infect Control 2007;35:S165–S193.

42. Tacconelli E, Cataldo MA, Dancer SJ, De Angelis G, Falcone M, Frank U, et al. ESCMID guidelines for the management of the infection control measures to reduce transmission of multidrug-resistant Gram-negative bacteria in hospitalized patients. Clin Microbiol Infect. 2014;20(Suppl 1):1–55.

43. Tedeschi S, Trapani F, Giannella M, Cristini F, Tumietto F, Bartoletti M, et al. An antimicrobial stewardship program based on systematic infectious disease consultation in a rehabilitation facility. Infect Control Hosp Epidemiol. 2017;38:76–82.

44. Charani E, Castro-Sánchez E, Holmes A. The role of behavior change in antimicrobial stewardship. Infect Dis Clin N Am. 2014;28:169–75.

45. Harbarth S, Albrich W, Brun-Buisson C. Outpatient antibiotic use and prevalence of antibiotic-resistant pneumococci in France and Germany: a sociocultural perspective. Emerg Infect Dis. 2002;8:1460–7.

22

An investigation of bedside laparoscopy in the ICU for cases of non-occlusive mesenteric ischemia

G. Cocorullo[1], A. Mirabella[2], N. Falco[1]* ⓘ, T. Fontana[1], R. Tutino[1], L. Licari[1], G. Salamone[1], G. Scerrino[1] and G. Gulotta[1]

Abstract

Background: Acute mesenteric ischemia is a rare affection with high related mortality. NOMI presents the most important diagnostic problems and is related with the higher risk of white laparotomy. This study wants to give a contribution for the validation of laparoscopic approach in case of NOMI.

Methods: Thirty-two consecutive patients were admitted in last 10 years in ICU of Paolo Giaccone University Hospital of Palermo for AMI. Diagnosis was obtained by multislice CT and selective angiography was done if clinical conditions were permissive. If necrosis was already present or suspected, surgical approach was done. Endovascular or surgical embolectomy was performed when necessary. Twenty NOMI patients underwent medical treatment performing laparoscopy 24 h later to verify the evolution of AMI. A three-port technique was used. In all patients we performed a bed side procedure 48–72 h later in both non-resected and resected group.

Results: In 14 up 20 case of NOMI the disease was extended throughout the splanchnic district, in 6 patients it involved the ileum and the colon; after a first look, only 6 patients underwent resection. One patient died 35 h after diagnosis of NOMI. The second look, 48 h later, demonstrated 4 infarction recurrences in the group of resected patients and onset signs of necrosis in 5 patients of non-resected group. A total of 15 resections were performed on 11 patients. Mortality rate was 6/20–30% but it was much higher in resected group (5/11–45,5%). Non-therapeutic laparotomy was avoided in 9/20 patients and in this group mortality rate was 1/9–11%. No morbidity was recorded related to laparoscopic procedure.

Conclusions: Laparoscopy could be a feasible and safety surgical approach for management of patient with NOMI. Our retrospective study demonstrates that laparoscopy don't increase morbidity, reduce mortality avoiding non-therapeutic laparotomy.

Keywords: Acute mesenteric ischemia, NOMI, Laparoscopy, Surgery, Intensive care

Background

Acute mesenteric ischemia is a rare affection with high related mortality. It accounts 1:1000 acute hospital admissions in Europe and the USA [1] and presents a very high mortality with a range from 50 to 69% [2–5] of cases.

The affection consists in an acute arterial occlusion due to embolism (EAMI), or thrombosis (TAMI), in a venous thrombosis (VAMI) or, at last, in an non-occlusive mesenteric ischemia (NOMI).

Pathophysiology is different in each type as risk factors. Different are also comorbidities and clinical findings. In all cases diagnosis is very difficult because there aren't specific laboratory tests.

EAMI is often related to hearth disease (atrial fibrillation, myocardial infarction, etc.) and causes acute symptoms as diarrhoea, vomiting, acute abdominal pain; TAMI is characterized by more indolent onset with post-prandial pain and weight loss in patients with history of atherosclerosis, hypertension, diabetes; VAMI occurs in 10% of cases in patients with hypercoagulable disorders, malignancies, hepatitis, pancreatitis, and other affections causing slow blood flow. NOMI occurs mostly

* Correspondence: nicola.falco87@libero.it
[1]General and Emergency Surgery–Policlinico P. Giaccone, University of Palermo, Via Liborio Giuffrè, 5, Palermo, Italy
Full list of author information is available at the end of the article

in critically ill patients with hypovolemia, hypotension, recent treatment with beta blockers or alpha adrenergic. Usually these are patients with endotracheal tube and symptoms can start in acute or gradual way.

Nowadays the gold standard for diagnosis is CT, which offers a good accuracy in AMI detection with high values of sensitivity and specificity [6], but it is well known that these values are not similar in each etiological type.

NOMI is an exclusion diagnosis. It presents the most important diagnostic problems due to lack of specific radiological features on CT, which usually shows a normal bowel wall and a high variability of its contrast enhancement ranging from absent or diminished to increased [7]. So, in the suspicious of NOMI an anamnesis of low arterial flow or low cardiac output (recent cardiac failure, prolonged cardio-pulmonary resuscitation, cardiac surgery, severe cardiac failure, aortic dissection and aneurism, recent aortic vascular surgery etc..), biochemical findings (>TGO/>TGP;> LDL, >CPK, >Bilirubin), signs of Acute Kidney Failure (altered level of creatinine, urea and electrolytes, reduced urine output). When possible a selective angiography or an angio-CT should be performed [8] to confirm diagnosis, exclude other form of AMI and to start the medical treatment (fluid infusion, prostaglandins, etc.) (Fig. 1).

Then NOMI needs a very close follow-up to obtain an early detection of mesenteric infarction which imposes bowel resection. Early diagnosis and prompt intervention are the goals of modern treatment. It can stop the fatal progression of sepsis that is responsible of the high mortality rate [9].

Also, the treatment is different in each type of AMI [10]: resolution of embolism in open surgery (especially if bowel necrosis is present) or in endovascular way is the choice treatment in patients with EAMI or TAMI. In case of VAMI the first choice is anticoagulation and finally in patients with NOMI the first step is the infusion of fluids and vasodilators; the last mentioned are administered directly via Superior Mesenteric Artery (SMA) when possible. If bowel necrosis is present, resection is necessary at the same time [10].

Although CT consents a differential diagnosis in patients with doubtful abdominal presentation and for these reason is the first diagnostic step for these patient, there isn't any diagnostic test which can early indicate the onset of bowel necrosis. The aim of this study is to show our results of systematic use of laparoscopy in bowel infarction detection in critical ill patients.

Methods

A retrospective study was carried out on 32 consecutive patients recovered in last 10 years (1st January 2006–31st December 2015) in ICU of Paolo Giaccone University Hospital of Palermo. The patients' age, clinical symptoms, biochemistry and radiological findings were considered.

In all patients, AMI was diagnosed by multislice CT (Fig. 2); selective angiography was done if clinical conditions were permissive.

If necrosis was already present or suspected, surgical approach was done. Moreover, endovascular or surgical embolectomy was performed in cases with EAMI or TAMI whilst VAMI and NOMI patients underwent

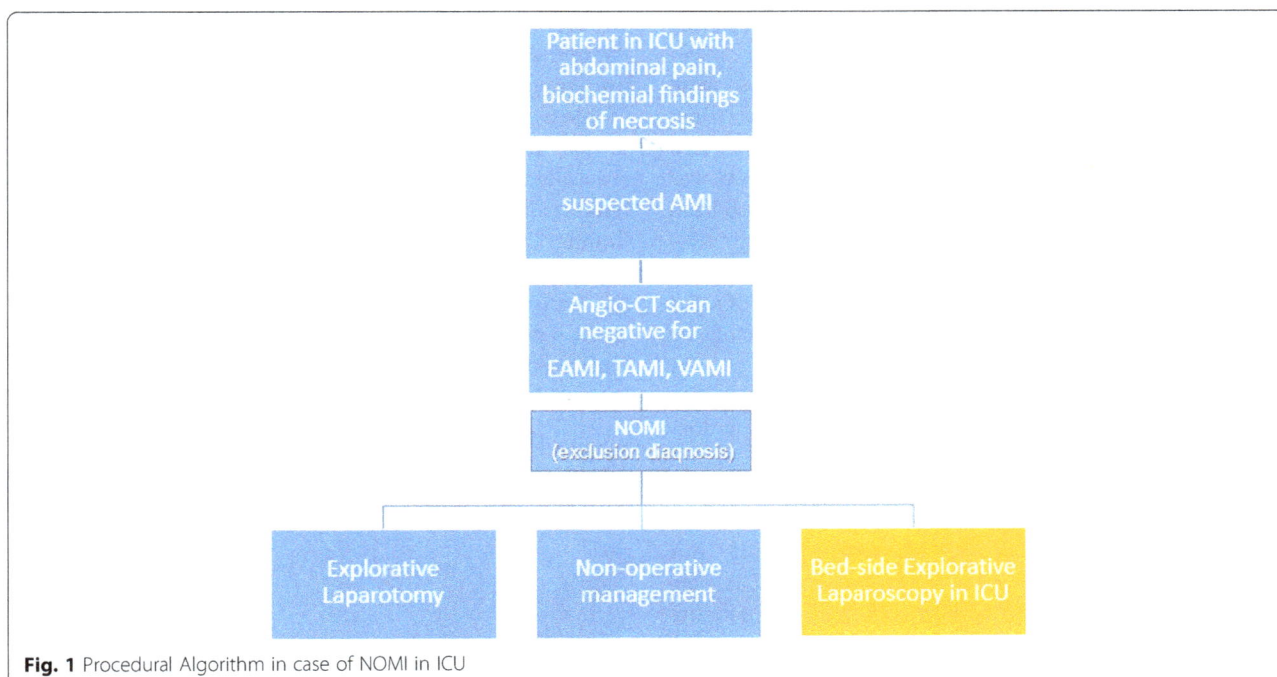

Fig. 1 Procedural Algorithm in case of NOMI in ICU

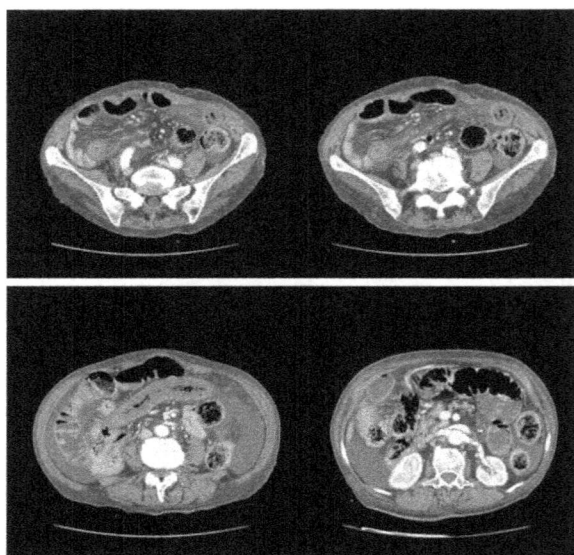

Fig 2 Angio-CT, a case of NOMI: Radiologic Science Department–AOUP Palermo

medical treatment performing laparoscopy 24 h later to verify the evolution of AMI.

A three-port technique was used [11, 12]: a 10-mm camera-port was positioned through the umbilical scar. After a first exploration of the abdomen, other two 5 mm operative-trocars were put in the left hypochondrium and in the left iliac fossa. In this way, as in right laparoscopic colectomy, an accurate exploration of entire small bowel was possible starting from the ileocecal junction and going back up to the Treitz ligament. Colon was entirely explored. Only in 4 patients a fourth 5 mm port in right flank was needed.

The bowel aspect and the ischemia extension were evaluated; all patients showed widespread intestinal pallor therefore, the first suffering loop was searched (intense pallor, necrosis signs) and the necrotic bowel was resected when present. The involved bowel was mobilized and after vessels ligation it was externalized through a 5–6 cm laparotomy. After resection, no anastomosis was done and an ostomy was performed. The absence of signs of necrosis is not to be underestimated because of the rapid precipitation of NOMI clinical features.

Therefore, in all patient medical therapy was continued and EBPM was administered using prophylactic dosages, the procedure was repeated 48–72 h later (Second Look) in both non-resected and resected group, looking for new necrotic areas.

Due the organization of our Hospital in nearly but separated departments, a bed-side laparoscopy was performed to avoid the transfer of the critically ill patients to the department of radiology or to operation room that often can leads to serious difficulties especially

when the transfers are multiple. A laparoscopic column and a centralized CO_2 distribution system are available in ICU and allow the execution of bed side laparoscopy. The availability of mobilizable beds in ICU support the surgeon to perform explorative laparoscopy with low Co_2 flow and pressure (8–10 mmHg). Only two surgeons need to perform the procedure and the second or further looks are performed through the same sites used before. A 10-mm optic and two laparoscopic forceps or an ultrasound dissector allow the exploration and the dissection of bowel needs resection (Table 1). In case of re-resection the bowel was extracted trough the same previous incision and after a distal ligation of vessels, resection was performed with linear stapler. Moreover, in all cases ostomy and mucous fistula was is performed.

Safety and efficacy of the procedure was evaluated in terms of mortality, diagnosed infarctions and avoided non-therapeutic laparotomy. Postoperative morbidity was an outcome not reliable due to multiple comorbidity already present in our patients.

Results

Among 32 critical ill patients with CT report of AMI, 6 presented EAMI, 3 TAMI, 1 VAMI and 20 NOMI (Table 2).

Main biochemical and CT findings of NOMI patients are collected in Table 3. In all NOMI cases (20) an intense pallor of bowel wall was the main laparoscopic finding. In 14 cases, it was extended throughout the splanchnic district, whilst in 6 patients it involved mainly the ileum and the colon (right colon 2 cases; left colon 3 cases; entire colon 1 case); every patient in last group underwent resection to prevent bowel necrosis and peritonitis in 5 cases, whilst in 1 patient bowel resection was

Table 1 Necessary equipment for bed-side laparoscopy

Laparoscopic Column including: CO2 insufflator, HD camera, light source, HD monitor
Optic 10 mm
N° 2 laparoscopic forceps
Ultrasound dissector with disposable device
N° 3 Trocars (10 mm, 5 mm, 5 mm)
Surgical drapes
Basic Surgical Kit

Table 2 ICU patients with AMI

ICU patients with AMI (1st January 2006–31 December 2015)	
Type of AMI	N° of cases
EAMI	6
TAMI	3
VAMI	1
NOMI	20

Table 3 Laboratory and CT findings

Patients	Age	GOT (U/L) nv: 0–31	GPT (U/L) nv: 0–31	LDH (U/L) nv: 240–480	CPK (U/L) nv: 26–192	CREATININE mg/dl nv: 0,51–0,95	WBC vn 4–11 10^3 uL	CT FINDINGS
1	66	520	489	3125	1223	5.1	26,28	negative for SMA obstruction, bowel infarction, peritoneal collections
2	79	610	498	1225	251	1,3	22,3	negative for SMA obstruction, paralytic ileum signs
3	75	426	286	1316	680	1,4	23,6	negative for SMA obstruction, paralytic ileum signs
4	54	838	778	1198	889	1,3	24,68	negative for SMA obstruction, right colon and ileum thickening
5	81	650	568	2218	1001	3,2	17,42	negative for SMA obstruction, diffuse colon and bowel infarction, peritoneal collections
6	82	466	598	1589	996	1,9	15,69	negative for SMA obstruction, paralytic ileum signs
7	61	835	687	1286	754	1,75	22,65	negative for SMA obstruction, right colon and ileum thickening
8	90	589	410	1857	1028	2,6	14,8	negative for SMA obstruction, left colon and ileum thickening
9	78	380	520	1635	987	2,4	15,1	negative for SMA obstruction, peritoneal collections
10	76	489	475	856	385	1,9	23,2	negative for SMA obstruction, bowel infarction
11	71	554	598	758	235	2,4	20,1	negative for SMA obstruction, bowel infarction, peritoneal collections
12	61	665	689	1105	624	1,4	18,7	negative for SMA obstruction, paralytic ileum signs
13	78	811	799	658	201	1,2	14,8	negative for SMA obstruction, bowel infarction
14	69	715	684	2890	1425	3,3	18,4	negative for SMA obstruction, left colon and ileum thickening
15	82	542	396	1687	1215	2,7	17,5	negative for SMA obstruction, paralytic ileum signs
16	69	496	389	1420	893	2,6	18,84	negative for SMA obstruction, bowel infarction, peritoneal collections
17	78	675	497	752	358	1,5	26,3	negative for SMA obstruction, paralytic ileum signs
18	87	742	694	3869	1845	4,8	24.3	negative for SMA obstruction, left colon and ileum thickening
19	78	868	688	1012	854	2,7	16,4	negative for SMA obstruction, paralytic ileum signs
20	72	308	258	1536	1088	3,7	37,26	negative for SMA obstruction, peritoneal collections

necessary to remove a necrotic segment. After a first look only 6 patients underwent bowel resection and its extension was since 15 up to 175 cm. After resection in each patient a stoma and a mucous fistula were performed on the proximal and the distal stump respectively (Table 4).

Only one non-resected patient died 35 h after diagnosis of NOMI and before the second look for cardiac failure.

The second look, 48 h later, demonstrated 4 infarction recurrences in the group of resected patients and the onset of necrosis in 5 patients of non-resected group. A total of 15 resections were performed on 11 patients (Table 5).

Table 4 Extension of ischemic tract in NOMI patients

Extension of Ischemia In NOMI patients		
Bowel site	N° of cases	1st look resection cases
Small Bowel and other splancnic organs	14	0
Ileum and right colon	2	2
Left colon	3	3
Entire colon	1	1

Table 5 Recurrent necrosis after second look

Second look evaluation (48 h later)	N° of recurrent necrosis
Resected group	4
Non-resected group	5

Mortality rate was 6/20 (30%) but it was much higher in resected group (5/11–45,5%). Non-therapeutic laparotomy was avoided in 9/20 patients (45%) and in this group mortality rate was 1/9 (11,1%). No morbidity was recorded related to laparoscopic procedure (Tables 6 and 7).

Discussion

NOMI is an infrequent type of AMI and accounts 20% of cases. It is more frequent in critically ill patients and depends on combination of two distinct factors; low cardiac output and vasoconstrictive agents.

In literature, there are no high evidences about clinical findings, diagnosis and therapy of AMI and even less about NOMI. It is possible to found some case-series recording the experience of single centres and in this way, the present report is a contribution about diagnostic and therapeutic pathway in critically ill patients with suspicious NOMI.

It is well known that decreased mortality for AMI in last years is related to more aggressive therapeutic approach in occlusive shapes like surgical or non-surgical blood flow restoration, resection of necrotic bowel, supportive intensive care. Moreover, the precocity of the treatment is highly related with its success.

But if in patients with occlusive forms the operative (surgical or not-surgical) approach ever follows diagnosis of AMI, in NOMI patients the treatment consists of pharmacological therapy with the need of continuous monitoring of ischemia. Only the onset of necrosis will require surgery. Because of the absence of tests that consent a determination of further bowel viability, laparoscopy can represent a diagnostic technique with high potential therapeutic options. We used it in NOMI patients both at the first and the second look to detect and remove dead bowel avoiding certain general and access-related risks associated with laparotomy [13].

Moreover, it is well known how the surgical stress could be life-threatening in these patients, and so to avoid a non-therapeutic laparotomy could be a very important step in their clinical course.

Table 6 Outcome of NOMI patients after treatment

Outcome of NOMI patients after treatment	N° of cases	Resected group	Non resected group
Mortality	6/20 (30%)	5/11 (45,5%)	1/9 (11,1%)
Morbidity related to laparoscopy	0	0	0

Table 7 Mortality rate

Mortality	Cases/TOT	Percent
First and second look negative	1/9	11,1
1 st look positivity	3/6	50
2 nd look positivity only	2/5	40

In our centre, it was started 10 years ago, routinely use of laparoscopy in critical ill patients presenting clinical and radiological findings suggesting AMI. Laparoscopy was utilized like the last diagnostic procedure and the first therapeutic step.

Explorative laparoscopy allowed to avoid 9/20 (45%) non-therapeutic laparotomies and at the same time it showed in 11 cases the presence of bowel necrosis; In 6 patients at the first look and in 9 patients at the second look. Four of second look resected patients had been already resected at the first look. The routinely execution of the second look 48 h after the first exploration of the abdomen is strongly suggested because of pathophysiology of NOMI [14]. The possible occurrence of low cardiac output due to surgical procedures (i.e. blood loss, ECC, etc.), in fact, can cause bowel ischemia but only in a variable percentage of cases necrosis will occur.

Then in our experience laparoscopy was positively used in patients with CT-scan diagnosed NOMI both for the first and the second look to detect the eventual onset of bowel necrosis. Its advantages were the possibility of bed-side performing without the surgical stress of laparotomic access.

Conclusions

NOMI represents a frequent type of AMI diagnosis. CT scan represent the golden standard in diagnosis of AMI but has a lower power in defining NOMI forms. Laparoscopy could be a feasible and safety surgical approach for diagnosis of ischaemic tract of bowel and to removing it. Our retrospective study demonstrate that laparoscopy don't increase morbidity and reduce mortality probably avoiding non-therapeutic laparotomy.

Abbreviations
AMI: Acute mesenteric ischemia; CT: Computed tomography; EAMI: Embolic acute mesenteric ischemia; ICU: Intensive care unit; NOMI: Non-occlusive mesenteric ischemia; SMA: superior mesenteric artery; TAMI: Thrombotic acute mesenteric ischemia; VAMI: Venous thrombosis acute mesenteric ischemia

Acknowledgements
Not applicable.

Funding
The authors declare that they have no funding.

Authors' contributions

GC and AM contributed performing the operation and providing their casuistry from where this case series was extracted. NF, contributed as corresponding author to the elaboration of the data and production of the manuscript. TF, RT and LL contributed to the elaboration of data, production of tables and to the revision of language. GSa and GSc contributed to the work providing the discussion section. GG contribute as supervisor to the validation of data and to the conclusions. All authors read and approved the final manuscript.

Competing interests

The authors declare that they have no competing interests.

Author details
[1]General and Emergency Surgery–Policlinico P. Giaccone, University of Palermo, Via Liborio Giuffrè, 5, Palermo, Italy. [2]General and Emergency Surgery–Villa Sofia Hospita, Palermo, Italy.

References

1. Stoney RJ, Cunningham CG. Acute mesenteric ischemia. Surgery. 1993; 114(3):489–90.
2. Aouini F, Bouhaffa A, Baazaoui J, Khelifi S, Ben Maamer A, Houas N, Cherif A. Acute mesenteric ischemia: study of predictive factors of mortality. Tunis Med. 2012;90(7):533–6. French.
3. Haghighi PH, Lankarani KB, Taghavi SA, Marvasti VE. Acute mesenteric ischemia: causes and mortality rates over sixteen years in southern Iran. Indian J Gastroenterol. 2008;27(6):236–8.
4. Wadman M, Syk I, Elmstahl S. Survival after operations for ischemic bowel disease. Eur J Surg. 2000;166:872–7.
5. Tsai M-S, Lin C-L, Chen H-P, Lee P-H, Sung F-C, Kao C-H. Long-term risk of mesenteric ischemia in patients with inflammatory bowel disease: A 13-year nationwide cohort study in an Asian population. Am J Surg. 2015;210(1):80–6.
6. Yikilmaz A, Karahan OI, Senol S, Tuna IS, Akyildiz HY. Value of multislice computed tomography in the diagnosis of acute mesenteric ischemia. Eur J Radiol. 2011;80(2):297–302.
7. Furukawa A, Kanasaki S, Kono N, Wakamiya M, Tanaka T, Takahashi M, Murata K. CT diagnosis of acute mesenteric ischemia from various causes. Am J Roentgenol. 2009;192(2):408–16.
8. Acosta S, Bjorck M. Modern treatment of acute mesenteric ischaemia. Br J Surg. 2014;101:e100–8.
9. Sartelli M, Abu-Zidan FM, Catena F, Griffiths EA, Di Saverio S, Coimbra R, Ordoñez CA, Leppaniemi A, Fraga GP, Coccolini F, Agresta F, Abbas A, Abdel Kader S, Agboola J, Amhed A, Ajibade A, Akkucuk S, Alharthi B, Anyfantakis D, Augustin G, Baiocchi G, Bala M, Baraket O, Bayrak S, Bellanova G, Beltràn MA, Bini R, Boal M, Borodach AV, Bouliaris K, Branger F, Brunelli D, Catani M, Che Jusoh A, Chichom-Mefire A, Cocorullo G, Colak E, Costa D, Costa S, Cui Y, Curca GL, Curry T, Das K, Delibegovic S, Demetrashvili Z, Di Carlo I, Drozdova N, El Zalabany T, Enani MA, Faro M, Gachabayov M, Giménez Maurel T, Gkiokas G, Gomes CA, Gonsaga RA, Guercioni G, Guner A, Gupta S, Gutierrez S, Hutan M, Ioannidis O, Isik A, Izawa Y, Jain SA, Jokubauskas M, Karamarkovic A, Kauhanen S, Kaushik R, Kenig J, Khokha V, Kim JI, Kong V, Koshy R, Krasniqi A, Kshirsagar A, Kuliesius Z, Lasithiotakis K, Leão P, Lee JG, Leon M, Lizarazu Pérez A, Lohsiriwat V, López-Tomassetti Fernandez E, Lostoridis E, Mn R, Major P, Marinis A, Marrelli D, Martinez-Perez A, Marwah S, McFarlane M, Melo RB, Mesina C, Michalopoulos N, Moldovanu R, Mouaqit O, Munyika A, Negoi I, Nikolopoulos I, Nita GE, Olaoye I, Omari A, Ossa PR, Ozkan Z, Padmakumar R, Pata F, Pereira Junior GA, Pereira J, Pintar T, Pouggouras K, Prabhu V, Rausei S, Rems M, Rios-Cruz D, Sakakushev B, Sánchez de Molina ML, Seretis C, Shelat V, Simões RL, Sinibaldi G, Skrovina M, Smirnov D, Spyropoulos C, Tepp J, Tezcaner T, Tolonen M, Torba M, Ulrych J, Uzunoglu MY, van Dellen D, van Ramshorst GH, Vasquez G, Venara A, Vereczkei A,

Vettoretto N, Vlad N, Yadav SK, Yilmaz TU, Yuan KC, Zachariah SK, Zida M, Zilinskas J, Ansaloni L. Global validation of the WSES Sepsis Severity Score for patients with complicated intra-abdominal infections: a prospective multicentre study (WISS Study). World J Emerg Surg. 2015;10:61. doi:10.1186/s13017-015-0055-0. eCollection 2015.
10. Tilsed JVT, et al. ESTES guidelines: Acute Mesenteric Ischaemia. Eur J Trauma Emerg Surg. 2016 Jan 28. Epub ahead of print.
11. Agrusa A, et al. Laparoscopic, SILS and three post cholecistectomy: a retrospective study. G Chir. 2013;34(9–10):249–53.
12. Cocorullo G, Tutino R, Falco N, Salamone G, Gulotta G. Three-port colectomy: reduced port laparoscopy for general surgeons. A single center experience. Ann Ital Chir. 2016;87:350–5.
13. Nassau AH, et al. The abdominal drain. A convenient port for second look laparoscopy. Surg Endosc. 1996;10:1114–5.
14. Yanar H, et al. Planned second look laparoscopy in te management of acute mesenteric ischemia. World J Gastroenterol. 2007;13(24):3350–3.

23

Impact of initial temporary abdominal closure in damage control surgery

Parker Hu[1,2]* , Rindi Uhlich[3], Frank Gleason[3], Jeffrey Kerby[1] and Patrick Bosarge[1]

Abstract

Background: Damage control surgery has revolutionized trauma surgery. Use of damage control surgery allows for resuscitation and reversal of coagulopathy at the risk of loss of abdominal domain and intra-abdominal complications. Temporary abdominal closure is possible with multiple techniques, the choice of which may affect ability to achieve primary fascial closure and further complication.

Methods: A retrospective analysis of all trauma patients requiring damage control laparotomy upon admission to an ACS-verified level one trauma center from 2011 to 2016 was performed. Demographic and clinical data including ability and time to attain primary fascial closure, as well as complication rates, were recorded. The primary outcome measure was ability to achieve primary fascial closure during initial hospitalization.

Results: Two hundred and thirty-nine patients met criteria for inclusion. Primary skin closure (57.7%), ABThera™ VAC system (ABT) (15.1%), Bogota bag (BB) (25.1%), or a modified Barker's vacuum-packing (BVP) (2.1%) were used in the initial laparotomy. Patients receiving skin-only closure had significantly higher rates of primary fascial closure and lower hospital mortality, but also significantly lower mean lactate, base deficit, and requirement for massive transfusion. Between ABT or BB, use of ABT was associated with increased rates of fascial closure. Multivariate regression revealed primary skin closure to be significantly associated with primary fascial closure while BB was associated with failure to achieve fascial closure.

Conclusions: Primary skin closure is a viable option in the initial management of the open abdomen, although these patients demonstrated less injury burden in our study. Use of vacuum-assisted dressings continues to be the preferred method for temporary abdominal closure in damage control surgery for trauma.

Keywords: Damage control surgery, Temporary abdominal closure, Loss of domain, ABThera, Bogota bag, Vacuum packing

Background

Injury claims the lives of approximately 200,000 individuals in the USA annually, with hemorrhage and subsequent coagulopathy serving as the leading causes of preventable death [1–4]. Many surgical advancements have been achieved in recent times, but the development of damage control surgery (DCS) has revolutionized trauma care and led to a drastic reduction in mortality related to hemorrhagic shock. First named in the literature by Rotondo in 1993, DCS has proven to be the most effective means of limiting ongoing hemorrhage and reducing traumatic coagulopathy utilized today [5]. The employment of DCS and temporary abdominal closure (TAC) techniques began to staunchly reduce the mortality attributed to hemorrhagic shock, though with this decline came the increased recognition of complications associated with the open abdomen.

The initial techniques described for TAC consisted of primary skin closure (PSC) with either suture or towel clips [6, 7], followed by improvised plastic silos or sterilized IV bags sewn to the skin, named by Mattox as

* Correspondence: phu@uabmc.edu

Presentation: This study was presented as a quick-shot presentation at the 8th World Congress of the Abdominal Compartment Society in Banff, Alberta, Canada, in 2017.

[1]Division of Acute Care Surgery, Department of Surgery, University of Alabama at Birmingham, Birmingham, AL, USA

[2]Division of Acute Care Surgery, Department of Surgery, University of Alabama at Birmingham, 701 19th Street South, 112 Lyons-Harrison Research Building, Birmingham, AL 35294, USA

Full list of author information is available at the end of the article

Bogotá bags (BB) [8]. While these measures were simple and cost effective, both focused simply on the containment of viscera and abdominal packings without providing a means for effective drainage of intraperitoneal fluid or visceral expansion caused by ongoing resuscitation. As a result, patients demonstrated elevated rates of abdominal compartment syndrome [6, 9]. The concept of negative pressure wound therapy was incorporated to address these issues. Known as Barker's vacuum-packing (BVP), these dressings have now become widely accepted and many modifications have since been described [10, 11]. At its core, BVP consists of a perforated, plastic sheet placed over the viscera that is then covered by either towels or GranuFoam sponge, before an occlusive dressing and negative pressure device are applied. The success of these rudimentary vacuum dressings inspired development of commercial products, such as the ABThera™ VAC system (ABT; KCI USA, San Antonia, TX). Improved outcomes with the ABT over BVP have been reported, with one prospective observational study reporting significant increases in overall rates of primary fascial closure (PFC) and 30-day mortality in a mixed surgical cohort. However, this observation did not persist in the trauma subpopulation [12].

Even with ongoing innovation, inability to re-approximate the fascial edges in the midline continues to be among the most feared complications of TAC. Failure to achieve PFC results in a large ventral hernia and loss of abdominal domain (LOD). The causes of LOD are multifactorial, but are primarily attributed to fascial retraction and increased intraabdominal pressure. PSC and BB do not prevent fascial retraction or adhesion of the bowel to the abdominal wall and have historically been associated with an increased risk of LOD and complications associated with an open abdominal wound [13]. Vacuum-mediated closure methods have generally been regarded as superior due to their ability to drain peritoneal effluent while also providing continuous fascial traction toward the midline. As a result, many current management algorithms advocate for the use of some form of negative pressure wound therapy for initial management of the open abdomen [14–16].

The initial method for TAC may influence rates of LOD and clinical outcomes [17–20]. Success with primary fascial approximation during the initial hospitalization varies widely in the literature, with rates of PFC of 29–100% reported for vacuum-assisted dressings [6, 11, 21–24] compared to 40–75% for PSC [6, 25] and 12–82% for BB [6, 26–28]. Widespread acceptance of vacuum dressings, in particular commercial devices such as ABT, as the standard of care for TAC has led to cheaper and more readily available methods such as BB and PSC to be abandoned despite few comparative studies existing to appropriately guide therapy [14]. Additionally, most available data on the subject predates the era of damage control resuscitation (DCR), which may limit

visceral edema and potentially negate previous complications experienced with TAC [29]. We sought to evaluate the role of initial TAC on eventual PFC and prevention of LOD.

Methods

We performed a retrospective review of all trauma patients admitted to the University of Alabama at Birmingham Medical Center (UABMC) from 2011 to 2016. UABMC is an American College of Surgeons (ACS)-verified level 1 trauma center that serves as a tertiary referral center for the state of Alabama, with approximately 3500 trauma admissions per year. A registry of all trauma patients containing demographics, injuries, and injury severity is maintained by the trauma service.

All patients ≥ 18 years old admitted to the trauma service undergoing exploratory laparotomy at the time of admission were eligible for inclusion. Those patients undergoing DCS, defined as laparotomy with TAC following injury, were included for analysis. Patients receiving PFC at their initial operation or suffering a traumatic hernia preventing eventual PFC were excluded. The primary outcome of interest was the ability to achieve PFC based on initial closure technique during the index hospitalization. Secondary outcomes of interest were complications related to DCS and an open abdominal wound (fistula, ongoing bleeding, fascial dehiscence, abdominal abscess) as well as hospital mortality. PFC was defined as primary approximation of the fascia with suture repair. Fistula and dehiscence were identified clinically, with fistula defined as persistent communication between abdominal viscera and either the atmosphere or through the abdominal wall. Dehiscence was defined as any clinically apparent disruption of fascial closure. Ongoing significant bleeding was defined by bleeding requiring unplanned abdominal re-exploration. Abscess was identified intraoperatively or following percutaneous drainage with positive culture results.

Demographic and operative data were obtained from the electronic medical record. Operative reports were reviewed to determine the method of TAC. Four different types of abdominal closure were identified at the initial operations during the defined study period: PSC (all with running, monofilament suture); ABT, an improvised non-occlusive vacuum dressing using a modified BVP with GranuFoam rather than the standard towel; or a BB fashioned with a sterilized 3-L I.V. fluid bag. Patients were stratified into cohorts by the type of initial TAC for analysis.

Values were expressed as mean ± standard deviation or proportion (percentage). Categorical variables were compared using Pearson's χ^2 test, while continuous variables were compared using one-way ANOVA. Pairwise comparisons were performed post hoc with pairwise χ^2 testing or by Tukey's method in the event of significance.

Multivariate logistic regression was used to determine the association of abdominal closure technique with PFC, adjusting for the preselected potentially confounding covariates of age, gender, mechanism of injury, injury severity score (ISS), and massive transfusion requirement (≥ 10 units pRBC/24 h). An a priori p value ≤ 0.05 was set to identify statistical significance. Similar adjusted regression analysis was further performed for hospital mortality and complications identified as significant on univariate analysis.

Results

Two-hundred and thirty-nine patients were identified during the study period and included for analysis. Patients shared similar demographics among the cohorts (Table 1). Overall, patients were predominately male (82%) and were more likely to suffer penetrating injury (55.2%). PSC was the most commonly used method for TAC (57.7%), followed by BB (25.1%), ABT (15.1%), and then BVP (2.1%). Injury patterns among the different cohorts were similar except for an increased proportion of pancreatic wounds in the PSC vs ABT cohorts ($p = 0.009$).

Markers of injury severity were not significantly different among patients with ABT, BB, or BVP (Table 1). Patients, managed with PSC though, demonstrated significantly lower mean lactate than patients with BB closure ($p < 0.001$) and lower base excess ($p < 0.001$) than patients managed with either BB or ABT. Further, patients managed with PSC were significantly less likely to require massive transfusion ($p < 0.001$) and required significantly less average units of pRBCs ($p < 0.001$) or total blood products ($p < 0.001$) over the first 24 h compared with patients managed with BB or ABT.

Rates of PFC were highest among patients managed with PSC at initial operation, which was significantly higher than patients managed with BB ($p = 0.001$). Comparing patients managed with ABT versus BB, there were no significant differences in rates of PFC (94.4 vs 83.3%, $p = 0.11$). Among patients able to undergo PFC, rates of fascial dehiscence were lowest among patients with ABT or BVP, although not significant. There was no difference in hospital mortality between patients with initial ABT or BB closure ($p = 0.88$), although both were significantly elevated compared to PSC ($p = 0.004$). With regard to other hospital complications, the only significant difference among the cohorts was ongoing bleeding among patients with BB compared to PSC ($p = 0.044$) (Table 2).

On multivariate evaluation with logistic regression, management with BB was significantly associated with failure to gain PFC (OR 0.24; 95% CI 0.08–0.74), as well as increased hospital mortality (OR 3.81; 95% CI 1.25–11.57). Patients with PSC conversely were significantly more likely to attain PFC (OR 4.14; 95% CI 1.25–13.69)

and less likely to die while hospitalized (OR 0.23; 95% CI 0.07–0.74) (Tables 3 and 4).

Discussion

Our objective was to evaluate outcomes following DCS based on the role of initial TAC, with the primary outcome of PFC during the index hospitalization and prevention of LOD. We identified that patients undergoing PSC were able to undergo PFC at significantly higher rates than patients managed with other methods of initial TAC on both univariate and multivariate analyses. These patients though had significantly lower admission lactate, base excess, and transfusion requirements when compared to patients in the ABT and BB cohorts, who were matched in terms of demographics and injury severity. We did not identify a difference in rates of PFC between ABT and BB. However, when adjusting for potential confounding covariates, BB was significantly associated with LOD as well as increased hospital mortality whereas ABT was associated with increased ability to achieve PFC and increased hospital mortality, although not significant.

Patients managed with PSC historically suffered from increased rates of abdominal compartment syndrome given the inability of the re-approximated skin to comply with increasing visceral edema [9, 30, 31]. Such patients suffered from greatly elevated rates of LOD and mortality, and PSC was largely abandoned in spite of the ease with which it may be performed. However within the present cohort, use of PSC was significantly more likely to result in PFC, despite adjustment for potential confounding variables. The improvement in our outcomes is likely twofold.

Patients managed with PSC suffered less injury burden, as demonstrated by the significantly lower levels of admission lactate, base deficit, and transfusion requirements. At our institution, the decision for DCS and the type of TAC is based on the clinical judgment of the operative surgeon. Nationally, there is wide variability in the frequency of and indication for use of DCS, and our institution is no different [32]. Given this, the improved outcomes may simply result from selection bias. However, PSC continued to demonstrate improved outcomes when adjusting for confounders such as ISS and massive transfusion requirement. With this in mind, additional factors must be responsible for our improvement in outcomes. It is likely that significant bowel edema had not developed in this patient group to preclude PSC as a means to close the abdomen. Over the last 15 years, resuscitation strategies have evolved to complement DCS. The focus of DCR places an emphasis on blood product over crystalloid in the treatment of hemorrhagic shock, thus limiting the severe edema previously seen with massive IV fluid resuscitation [33–35]. Thus, PSC may still be utilized with success in patients undergoing DCS. However, caution must be taken with this interpretation

Table 1 Comparison of demographic and clinical data by initial closure technique

	Overall (n = 239)	Skin Only (n = 138)	ABThera System (n = 36)	Bogotá Bag (n = 60)	Barker's vacuum packing (n = 5)	p value
Demographics						
Age (years)	38.12 ± 14.70	37.85 ± 14.44	41.75 ± 15.62	36.26 ± 13.94	41.71 ± 22.95	0.32
Gender (%)						
Male	196 (82.0)	107 (77.5)	33 (91.7)	51 (85.0)	5 (100)	0.13
Female	43 (18.0)	31 (22.5)	3 (8.3)	9 (15.0)	0 (0)	
Body mass index (kg/m²)	29.73 ± 6.72	29.69 ± 6.71	30.20 ± 6.47	29.00 ± 6.65	35.86 ± 8.04	0.17
Mechanism of injury (%)						
Blunt	107 (44.8)	59 (42.8)	19 (52.8)	29 (48.3)	0 (0)	0.14
Penetrating	132 (55.2)	79 (57.2)	17 (47.2)	31 (51.7)	5 (100)	
Ethnicity (%)						
Caucasian	111 (46.4)	65 (47.1)	16 (44.4)	28 (46.7)	2 (40.0)	0.72
African American	121 (50.6)	70 (50.7)	18 (50.0)	30 (50.0)	3 (60.0)	
Latin American	6 (2.5)	3 (2.2)	1 (2.8)	2 (3.3)	0 (0)	
Asian American	1 (0.4)	0 (0)	1 (2.8)	0 (0)	0 (0)	
Injury						
Injury Pattern (%)						
Major vascular	29 (12.1)	10 (7.2)	7 (19.4)	12 (20.0)	0 (0)	0.09
Pelvic	21 (8.8)	9 (6.5)	7 (19.4)	5 (8.3)	0 (0)	0.09
Splenic	71 (29.7)	35 (25.4)	14 (38.9)	20 (33.3)	2 (40.0)	0.34
Hepatic	72 (30.1)	42 (30.4)	10 (27.8)	18 (30.0)	2 (40.0)	0.95
Renal	12 (5.0)	6 (4.3)	2 (5.6)	4 (6.7)	0 (0)	0.86
Pancreatic	21 (8.8)	6 (4.3)	6 (16.7)	7 (11.7)	2 (40.0)	0.005
Gastric	28 (11.7)	15 (10.9)	5 (13.9)	6 (10.0)	2 (40.0)	0.23
Small bowel	88 (36.8)	48 (34.8)	13 (36.1)	25 (41.7)	2 (40.0)	0.83
Colorectal	91 (38.1)	52 (37.7)	15 (41.7)	22 (36.7)	2 (40.0)	0.97
Clinical						
Injury Severity Score	25.68 ± 13.77	25.14 ± 14.20	29.53 ± 14.37	24.83 ± 12.42	22.80 ± 10.99	0.33
Admission lactate (mMol/L)	5.66 ± 3.887	4.79 ± 2.95	6.18 ± 3.49	7.27 ± 5.31	6.58 ± 3.26	<0.001
Admission base excess (mMol/L)	−8.18 ± 5.69	−6.89 ± 4.95	−9.78 ± 5.46	−9.92 ± 6.65	−12.04 ± 5.76	<0.001
Massive transfusion (%)	82 (34.3)	27 (19.6)	21 (58.3)	33 (55.0)	1 (20.0)	<0.001
Units PRBC transfused first 24 h	9.27 ± 11.01	5.35 ± 4.98	13.78 ± 13.30	15.53 ± 15.35	9.80 ± 5.85	<0.001
Units total blood products transfused first 24 h	19.49 ± 22.29	11.67 ± 11.44	29.17 ± 29.97	31.38 ± 28.48	22.80 ± 12.95	<0.001

*Values displayed as mean ± SD unless otherwise specified. Estimates from χ² and one-way ANOVA for categorical and continuous variables, respectively

Table 2 Comparison of clinical outcomes by initial closure technique

Outcomes	Overall (n = 239)	Skin Only (n = 138)	ABThera System (n = 36)	Bogotá Bag (n = 60)	Barker's vacuum packing (n = 5)	p value
Length of stay (days)	28.70 ± 20.96	25.47 ± 16.94	35.67 ± 29.45	32.23 ± 22.38	25.20 ± 18.43	0.027
ICU length of stay (days)	22.04 ± 17.72	19.43 ± 15.07	28.58 ± 23.10	24.12 ± 18.80	18.80 ± 13.29	0.033
Number of abdominal operations	3.12 ± 1.77	2.75 ± 1.42	3.22 ± 1.48	3.80 ± 2.23	5.80 ± 8.01	0.001
Time to abdominal closure (days)	4.19 ± 4.25	3.35 ± 3.21	4.69 ± 3.89	5.70 ± 5.59	5.80 ± 8.01	0.002
Hospital mortality (%)	19 (7.9)	5 (3.6)	5 (13.9)	9 (15.0)	0 (0)	0.021
Achieve primary fascial closure	221 (92.5)	133 (96.4)	34 (94.4)	50 (83.3)	4 (80.0)	0.009
Loss of abdominal domain (%)	18 (7.5)	5 (3.6)	2 (5.6)	10 (16.7)	1 (20)	0.009
Fascial dehiscence	12 (5.0)	8 (5.8)	0 (0)	4 (6.7)	0 (0)	0.44
Repeat bleeding	19 (7.9)	7 (5.1)	2 (5.6)	8 (13.3)	2 (40.0)	0.011
Enterocutaneous fistula	12 (5.0)	4 (2.9)	2 (5.6)	6 (10.0)	0 (0)	0.19
Anastomotic leak	15 (6.3)	8 (5.8)	1 (2.8)	6 (10.0)	0 (0)	0.47
Early bowel obstruction	10 (4.2)	6 (4.3)	2 (5.6)	2 (3.3)	0 (0)	0.92
Intra-abdominal abscess	81 (33.9)	45 (32.6)	10 (27.8)	24 (40.0)	2 (40.0)	0.62
Wound infection	37 (15.5)	22 (15.9)	2 (5.6)	13 (21.7)	0 (0)	0.15

*Values displayed as mean ± SD unless otherwise specified. Estimates from χ² and one-way ANOVA for categorical and continuous variables, respectively

Table 3 Odds ratios (ORs) and associated 95% confidence intervals (CIs) for the association between initial abdominal closure technique and complications

	N (%)	Odds ratio	95% confidence interval	
			Lower	Upper
Fascial closure				
Skin only	133 (96.4)	4.14	1.25	13.69
ABThera	34 (94.4)	1.52	0.31	7.32
Bogotá bag	50 (83.3)	0.24	0.08	0.74
Barker's vacuum packing	4 (80.0)	0.26	0.02	2.73
Hospital mortality				
Skin only	5 (3.6)	0.23	0.07	0.74
ABThera	5 (13.9)	1.48	0.45	4.85
Bogotá bag	9 (15.0)	3.81	1.25	11.57
Barker's vacuum packing	0 (0)	1.00	–	–
Repeat bleeding				
Skin only	7 (5.1)	0.55	0.19	1.59
ABThera	2 (5.6)	0.39	0.08	1.87
Bogotá bag	8 (13.3)	1.96	0.69	5.55
Barker's vacuum packing	2 (40.0)	18.32	2.29	146.92

*Multivariate logistic regression adjusted for age, gender, Injury Severity Score, mechanism, and massive transfusion requirement (> 10 units RBC/24 h)

given the increased risk of complications with delayed abdominal closure [36].

Patients managed initially with BB demonstrated significantly worse outcomes, despite lower ISS, similar levels of admission lactate and base excess, and requirement for blood product transfusion compared with patients managed initially with ABT. The complications we identified associated with BB are likely inherent in its design, as LOD remains a problem with BB despite the same changes in resuscitation strategies that may allow PSC to be a viable option. Fixation of IV bags to the skin does not allow drainage of intra-abdominal fluid that develops during the resuscitation phase that is critical in DCS [13]. This is compounded by lateral retraction of the skin and fascial edges [37]. As seen in our study, the times to abdominal closure were longest in the cohort managed with BB.

Previous studies raise concern that negative pressure vacuum therapy may potentiate further bleeding and risk enteric injury [22, 38]. However, the results from our study oppose these findings. The outcome improvements in our population may potentially be related to development of systems like ABT, which allow for better distribution of negative pressure and more uniform drainage of effluent from the peritoneal cavity [39]. Decreased intra-abdominal fluid allows for decreased intra-abdominal pressure, while also maintaining continued fascial traction toward the midline, thus allowing for earlier abdominal closure. Earlier and improvised methods of negative pressure vacuum therapy rely on a centralized negative pressure source which is both uneven and may leave areas of the peritoneal cavity undrained.

Effective drainage of the peritoneal cavity during TAC may offer additional benefits outside of pressure-related

Table 4 Odds ratios (ORs) and associated 95% confidence intervals (CIs) for the association between initial abdominal closure technique and complications

	N (%)	Odds ratio	95% confidence interval	
			Lower	Upper
Fascial closure				
Skin only	133 (96.4)	3.38	1.08	10.55
ABThera	34 (94.4)	1.83	0.38	8.75
Bogotá bag	50 (83.3)	0.26	0.09	0.73
Barker's vacuum packing	4 (80.0)	0.35	0.03	3.69

*Multivariate logistic regression adjusted for Injury Severity Score, admission lactate, admission base deficit, and massive transfusion requirement (> 10 units RBC/24 h)

effects. Recent studies have highlighted the profound role that the peritoneal cavity may play as an inflammatory reservoir [20, 40]. New techniques incorporating peritoneal resuscitation with dialysate in conjunction with existing negative pressure vacuum TAC have been reported with significant decreases in mortality, time to closure, and rates of PFC [41, 42]. While other methods for TAC have sought to improve outcomes by preventing fascial retraction using various devices to physically keep the fascia at midline, increasing basic and translational research suggests that the benefits of direct peritoneal resuscitation stem from drainage of inflammatory mediators and modulation of organ damage, while also better providing resuscitative fluids [43–47]. Additional research efforts should be directed into the role of peritoneal resuscitation and drainage given these promising early results, which include a single-center, randomized, prospective trial [41].

Our study is not without limitations. Given its retrospective nature and the inherent limits of our medical record, we were unable to assess patients for abdominal compartment syndrome, as there is no regular recording of intra-abdominal pressure. Additionally, variation in practice patterns may have influenced outcomes. Though primarily validated in the treatment of hemorrhagic shock and traumatic coagulopathy, enthusiasm for DCS has encouraged use of the procedure for re-visualization or delayed repair of hollow viscus injury. Coupled with the potential of surgeons to use one personally preferred method of TAC, this may have introduced selection bias into the different cohorts. Finally, more patients are required to adequately evaluate the use of BVP and conclusions cannot be drawn regarding its use given our limited sample size. In spite of these limitations, we provide a large examination of multiple methods for TAC. To our knowledge, this is among the largest series reported on use of PSC or BB for DCS in the era of DCR.

Conclusions

Our findings suggest that PSC is a viable option in the initial management of the open abdomen. This recommendation must acknowledge that these patients demonstrated less injury burden in comparison to others within our study. Concern for overuse of DCS has previously been raised and fervor for the procedure should be tempered with the knowledge that the risk of complications for patients managed with TAC is greater for those who may undergo definitive closure at the initial operation [36, 48]. Use of vacuum-assisted dressings continues to be the preferred method for TAC in DCS for trauma.

Abbreviation
ABT: ABThera™ VAC system; BB: Bogota bag; BVP: Barker's vacuum-packing; DCR: Damage control resuscitation; DCS: Damage control surgery; LOD: Loss of abdominal domain; PFC: Primary fascial closure; PSC: Primary skin closure; TAC: Temporary abdominal closure

Authors' contributions
PH was responsible for the principle design and overview of the project. PH performed all statistical analysis. All authors were responsible for acquisition and interpretation of data as well as manuscript preparation. All authors read and approved the final manuscript.

Competing interests
The authors declare that they have no competing interests.

Author details
[1]Division of Acute Care Surgery, Department of Surgery, University of Alabama at Birmingham, Birmingham, AL, USA. [2]Division of Acute Care Surgery, Department of Surgery, University of Alabama at Birmingham, 701 19th Street South, 112 Lyons-Harrison Research Building, Birmingham, AL 35294, USA. [3]Department of Surgery, University of Alabama at Birmingham, Birmingham, AL, USA.

References
1. Evans JA, et al. Epidemiology of traumatic deaths: comprehensive population-based assessment. World J Surg. 2010;34(1):158–63.
2. Mitra B, et al. Acute coagulopathy and early deaths post major trauma. Injury. 2012;43(1):22–5.
3. Tieu BH, Holcomb JB, Schreiber MA. Coagulopathy: its pathophysiology and treatment in the injured patient. World J Surg. 2007;31(5):1055–64.
4. Kochanek K, et al. Deaths: final data for 2014. In: D.o.H.a.H. Services, editor. Centers for Disease Control and Prevention. Hyattsville: National Center for Health Statistics; 2016.
5. Rotondo MF, et al. 'Damage control': an approach for improved survival in exsanguinating penetrating abdominal injury. J Trauma. 1993;35(3):375–82. discussion 382–3
6. Tremblay LN, et al. Skin only or silo closure in the critically ill patient with an open abdomen. Am J Surg. 2001;182(6):670–5.
7. Stone HH, Strom PR, Mullins RJ. Management of the major coagulopathy with onset during laparotomy. Ann Surg. 1983;197(5):532–5.
8. Mattox KL. Introduction, background, and future projections of damage control surgery. Surg Clin North Am. 1997;77(4):753–9.
9. Raeburn CD, et al. The abdominal compartment syndrome is a morbid complication of postinjury damage control surgery. Am J Surg. 2001; 182(6):542–6.
10. Brock WB, Barker DE, Burns RP. Temporary closure of open abdominal wounds: the vacuum pack. Am Surg. 1995;61(1):30–5.
11. Barker DE, et al. Vacuum pack technique of temporary abdominal closure: a 7-year experience with 112 patients. J Trauma. 2000;48(2): 201–6. discussion 206–7
12. Cheatham ML, et al. Prospective study examining clinical outcomes associated with a negative pressure wound therapy system and Barker's vacuum packing technique. World J Surg. 2013;37(9):2018–30.
13. Rutherford EJ, Skeete DA, Brasel KJ. Management of the patient with an open abdomen: techniques in temporary and definitive closure. Curr Probl Surg. 2004;41(10):815–76.
14. Diaz JJ Jr, et al. The management of the open abdomen in trauma and emergency general surgery: part 1-damage control. J Trauma. 2010;68(6): 1425–38.
15. Chiara O, et al. International consensus conference on open abdomen in trauma. J Trauma Acute Care Surg. 2016;80(1):173–83.
16. Godat L, et al. Abdominal damage control surgery and reconstruction: world society of emergency surgery position paper. World J Emerg Surg. 2013;8(1):53.
17. Cheatham ML, Safcsak K. Is the evolving management of intra-abdominal hypertension and abdominal compartment syndrome improving survival? Crit Care Med. 2010;38(2):402–7.
18. Acosta S, et al. Multicentre prospective study of fascial closure rate after

open abdomen with vacuum and mesh-mediated fascial traction. Br J Surg. 2011;98(5):735–43.

19. Bjorck M, et al. Classification--important step to improve management of patients with an open abdomen. World J Surg. 2009;33(6):1154–7.

20. Cheatham ML, Safcsak K, Sugrue M. Long-term implications of intra-abdominal hypertension and abdominal compartment syndrome: physical, mental, and financial. Am Surg. 2011;77(Suppl 1):S78–82.

21. Miller PR, et al. Prospective evaluation of vacuum-assisted fascial closure after open abdomen: planned ventral hernia rate is substantially reduced. Ann Surg. 2004;239(5):608–14. discussion 614–6

22. Barker DE, et al. Experience with vacuum-pack temporary abdominal wound closure in 258 trauma and general and vascular surgical patients. J Am Coll Surg. 2007;204(5):784–92. discussion 792–3

23. Navsaria PH, et al. Temporary closure of open abdominal wounds by the modified sandwich-vacuum pack technique. Br J Surg. 2003;90(6):718–22.

24. Cothren CC, et al. One hundred percent fascial approximation with sequential abdominal closure of the open abdomen. Am J Surg. 2006;192(2):238–42.

25. Smith PC, Tweddell JS, Bessey PQ. Alternative approaches to abdominal wound closure in severely injured patients with massive visceral edema. J Trauma. 1992;32(1):16–20.

26. Kirshtein B, et al. Use of the "Bogota bag" for temporary abdominal closure in patients with secondary peritonitis. Am Surg. 2007;73(3):249–52.

27. Huang Q, Li J, Lau WY. Techniques for abdominal wall closure after damage control laparotomy: from temporary abdominal closure to early/delayed fascial closure-a review. Gastroenterol Res Pract. 2016;2016:2073260.

28. Doyon A, et al. A simple, inexpensive, life-saving way to perform iterative laparotomy in patients with severe intra-abdominal sepsis. Color Dis. 2001; 3(2):115–21.

29. Burch JM, et al. Abbreviated laparotomy and planned reoperation for critically injured patients. Ann Surg. 1992;215(5):476–83. discussion 483–4

30. Balogh Z, et al. Secondary abdominal compartment syndrome is an elusive early complication of traumatic shock resuscitation. Am J Surg. 2002;184(6): 538–43. discussion 543–4

31. Balogh Z, et al. Both primary and secondary abdominal compartment syndrome can be predicted early and are harbingers of multiple organ failure. J Trauma. 2003;54(5):848–59. discussion 859–61

32. Harvin JA, et al. Mortality after emergent trauma laparotomy: a multicenter, retrospective study. J Trauma Acute Care Surg. 2017;83(3):464–8.

33. Holcomb JB, et al. Damage control resuscitation: directly addressing the early coagulopathy of trauma. J Trauma. 2007;62(2):307–10.

34. Brandstrup B, et al. Effects of intravenous fluid restriction on postoperative complications: comparison of two perioperative fluid regimens: a randomized assessor-blinded multicenter trial. Ann Surg. 2003;238(5):641–8.

35. Cannon JW, et al. Damage control resuscitation in patients with severe traumatic hemorrhage: a practice management guideline from the Eastern Association for the Surgery of Trauma. J Trauma Acute Care Surg. 2017;82(3):605–17.

36. George MJ, et al. The effect of damage control laparotomy on major abdominal complications: A matched analysis. Am J Surg. 2018;216(1):56-59.

37. Regner JL, Kobayashi L, Coimbra R. Surgical strategies for management of the open abdomen. World J Surg. 2012;36(3):497–510.

38. Smith LA, et al. Vacuum pack technique of temporary abdominal closure: a four-year experience. Am Surg. 1997;63(12):1102–7. discussion 1107-8

39. Delgado A, Sammons A. In vitro pressure manifolding distribution evaluation of ABThera() active abdominal therapy system, V.A.C.((R)) abdominal dressing system, and Barker's vacuum packing technique conducted under dynamic conditions. SAGE Open Med. 2016;4: 2050312115624988.

40. Kubiak BD, et al. Peritoneal negative pressure therapy prevents multiple organ injury in a chronic porcine sepsis and ischemia/reperfusion model. Shock. 2010;34(5):525–34.

41. Smith JW, et al. Randomized controlled trial evaluating the efficacy of peritoneal resuscitation in the management of trauma patients undergoing damage control surgery. J Am Coll Surg. 2017;224(4):396–404.

42. Smith JW, et al. Direct peritoneal resuscitation accelerates primary abdominal wall closure after damage control surgery. J Am Coll Surg. 2010; 210(5):658–64. 664-7

43. Weaver JL, et al. Direct peritoneal resuscitation alters leukocyte infiltration in the lung after acute brain death. Shock. 2017; https://doi.org/10.1097/SHK. 0000000000001069.

44. Weaver JL, et al. Direct peritoneal resuscitation alters hepatic miRNA expression after hemorrhagic shock. J Am Coll Surg. 2016;223(1):68–75.

45. Zakaria el R, et al. Hemorrhagic shock and resuscitation-mediated tissue water distribution is normalized by adjunctive peritoneal resuscitation. J Am Coll Surg. 2008;206(5):970–80. discussion 980–3

46. Hurt RT, et al. Hemorrhage-induced hepatic injury and hypoperfusion can be prevented by direct peritoneal resuscitation. J Gastrointest Surg. 2009; 13(4):587–94.

47. Garrison RN, et al. Direct peritoneal resuscitation as adjunct to conventional resuscitation from hemorrhagic shock: a better outcome. Surgery. 2004; 136(4):900–8.

48. Hatch QM, et al. Impact of closure at the first take back: complication burden and potential overutilization of damage control laparotomy. J Trauma. 2011;71(6):1503–11.

24

Blunt cerebrovascular injury in elderly fall patients: are we screening enough?

Vincent P. Anto, Joshua B. Brown, Andrew B. Peitzman, Brian S. Zuckerbraun, Matthew D. Neal, Gregory Watson, Raquel Forsythe, Timothy R. Billiar and Jason L. Sperry[*]

Abstract

Background: Blunt cerebrovascular injuries (BCVI) are generally associated with high-energy injury mechanisms. Less is known regarding lower-energy injuries in elderly patients. We sought to determine the incidence of BCVI and characterize current BCVI screening practices and associated complications in elderly ground-level fall patients (EGLF, ≥ 65 years). We hypothesized that BCVI in EGLF patients would be clinically significant and screening would be less common.

Methods: A retrospective study was performed utilizing the National Trauma Data Bank (NTDB, 2007–2014) and single institutional data. BCVI risk factors and diagnosis were determined by ICD-9 codes. Presenting patient characteristics and clinical course were obtained by chart review. The NTDB dataset was used to determine the incidence of BCVI, risk factors for BCVI, and outcomes in the EGLF cohort. Local chart review focused on screening rates and complications.

Results: The incidence of BCVI in EGLF patients was 0.15% overall and 0.86% in those with at least one BCVI risk factor in the NTDB. Upper cervical spine fractures were the most common risk factor for BCVI in EGLF patients. In EGLF patients, the diagnosis of BCVI was an independent risk factor for mortality (OR1.8, 95% C.I. 1.5–2.1). The local institutional data (2007–2014) had a BCVI incidence of 0.37% ($n = 6487$) and 1.47% in those with at least one risk factor ($n = 1429$). EGLF patients with a risk factor for BCVI had a very low rate of screening (44%). Only 8% of EGLF patients not screened had documented contraindications. The incidence of renal injury was 9% irrespective of BCVI screening.

Conclusions: The incidence of BCVI is clinically significant in EGLF patients and an independent predictor of mortality. Screening is less common in EGLF patients despite few contraindications. This data suggests that using age and injury mechanism to omit BCVI screening in EGLF patients may exclude an at-risk population.

Trial registration: IRB approval number: PRO15020269. Retrospective trial not registered

Keywords: Blunt cerebrovascular injury, Elderly, Falls, Screening, Incidence, Intravenous contrast

Background

Blunt cerebrovascular injury (BCVI) is an injury to the carotid or vertebral arteries which can result in devastating consequences. BCVI is estimated to occur in 1–2% of blunt traumatic hospital admissions [1–3]. Appropriate screening is of paramount importance due to the morbidity and mortality of ischemic events attributable to BCVI if not diagnosed and properly managed [1, 4]. Detection of BCVI before the onset of symptoms allows

for appropriate treatment and greatly reduces the risk of neurological sequelae [5]. There have been considerable research efforts made to determine the appropriate risk factors for BCVI that warrant screening. Current screening guidelines for BCVI are based in part on anatomic risk factors such as cervical spine injuries and basilar skull fractures [6–8].

Despite the general research interest in BCVI, the injury has not been specifically investigated in elderly patients. Elderly trauma admissions have increased as the population of Americans over the age of 65 continues to grow [9]. Injuries in the elderly often involve low-energy

* Correspondence: sperryjl@upmc.edu
Division of General Surgery and Trauma, Department of Surgery, University of Pittsburgh Medical Center, 200 Lothrop Street, Pittsburgh, PA 15213, USA

mechanisms [10]. Fall injuries are particularly common in the elderly population [9]. Low-energy injuries in the elderly often involve risk factors for BCVI that would generally mandate screening. In clinical practice, BCVI screening is often associated with higher-energy injury mechanisms which may predispose practitioners not to screen as commonly in low-energy injuries [8]. The risk of BCVI in these low-energy injuries has not been adequately characterized. Due to limited knowledge regarding the incidence of BCVI in elderly trauma patients, screening may be less prevalent in the elderly.

We undertook a retrospective review of the National Trauma Data Bank (NTDB 2007–2014) as well as the local institutional registry data at the University of Pittsburgh (2007–2014) to characterize BCVI in elderly trauma patients, particularly those with low-energy fall injuries. The study aims to define the incidence of BCVI in this patient cohort and explore the frequency of risk factors for BCVI. Screening rates, complications of screening for BCVI in the elderly, and outcomes are also investigated to see if current practices need to be modified to provide better care to this subset of patients. We hypothesized that the incidence of BCVI in low-energy falls would be clinically significant in the elderly population and screening rates would be lower relative to younger patients and elderly patients with non-fall injury mechanisms.

Methods

We conducted a retrospective review of two large datasets from 2007 to 2014 using only blunt injured patients. Patients were divided by age with elderly patients being considered to be at least 65 years of age at the time of admission. The National Trauma Data Bank (NTDB) is a collection of data from over 900 US trauma centers [11]. Over 1 million elderly patients with blunt injuries were used to determine the incidence of BCVI in the elderly population, specifically those involved in low-energy mechanisms of injury. Prominent risk factors that could be obtained from the data set were analyzed to examine their relationship to the incidence of BCVI.

The incidence of BCVI in all blunt patients was obtained from the NTDB using ICD-9 codes for BCVI injuries (900.00, 900.01, 900.03, 900.82, 900.89, 900.90). Elderly ground-level fall (EGLF) patients were defined by those with low-energy falls using ICD-9 E-codes specific for such injury mechanisms (880.1, 884.2–884.6, 885.9, 888.1, 888.8, 888.9). Falls from a height and falls down stairs were not included in the EGLF group as they were considered high-energy injury mechanisms. Such high-energy falls and any other non-fall blunt trauma were defined as the elderly non-GLF group. Risk factors for BCVI that could be extracted from the NTDB included cervical spine injuries (fractures and subluxations), basilar skull fractures, Le Fort

II and III fractures, and mandible fracture [7]. These were selected using corresponding ICD-9 codes (801.0–801.9, 802.2–802.39, 805.0–805.18, 806.0–806.19, 839–839.18). Upper cervical spine fractures were defined as fractures in vertebrae 1–3 and lower spine were fractures in cervical vertebrae 4–7. This was done to reflect the difference in risk for BCVI depending on the location of the cervical spine fracture [7].

The incidence of BCVI was determined in young patients 18–64 years of age with or without a GLF mechanism, elderly non-GLF patients, and EGLF patients for all blunt injury patients and in those patients with at least one screening risk factor for BCVI. We then compared EGLF patients who suffered BCVI to those EGLF patients without BCVI to characterize differences between the two groups. Finally, we utilized logistic regression to determine if BCVI in EGLF patients was independently associated with mortality in this cohort after controlling for confounding factors.

Local data from the University of Pittsburgh Medical Center trauma registry, an urban level 1 trauma center with 5000 trauma patients per year, was used to determine incidence and characteristics of patients who suffered BCVI, associated outcomes, screening rates, and complications associated with screening. Our institution had a BCVI screening protocol during the time of the study (2007–2014) which followed the most up-to-date published guidelines [7].

BCVI incidence from the local institutional data was determined by selecting all patients ≥ 18 years of age with an ICD-9 code for BCVI. The incidence of BCVI in younger patients, elderly non-GLF patients, and EGLF patients with and without risk factors for BCVI was determined. Specific screening practices, complications from screening, and outcomes were then obtained via chart review. BCVI injury grade was defined by the BCVI grading scale [12]. Radiology reports that indicated that the injury was more likely due to a pre-existing process (atherosclerotic changes) were not included in the positive BCVI groups.

Patients with specific risk factors for BCVI were examined to determine screening rates at our institution. Upper cervical spine fractures were studied in depth as this injury complex was the most common risk factor for BCVI in the elderly. Additionally, local institutional screening protocol recommends screening for all upper cervical spine fractures. Screening rates were calculated by selecting all patients with an upper cervical spine fracture who survived for at least 24 h. Rates of BCVI screening with computed tomography angiography (CTA), magnetic resonance angiography (MRA), or digital subtraction angiography (DSA) within 72 h of admission were determined via chart review. Time until BCVI screening was defined as the amount of time between admission and BCVI radiologic screening exam. Patients with BCVI screening were compared to those that were not screened for all patients with upper cervical spine fractures. Demographics, injury characteristics, renal function (estimated glomerular filtration rate [eGFR]), and pre-injury anti-thrombotic (aspirin, $p2y_{12}$ inhibitors, heparin, warfarin, and novel oral anticoagulants) were compared between the two groups.

Lastly, we compared creatinine levels between patients screened for BCVI ($n = 442$) and a randomly selected elderly group ($n = 200$) that received no IV contrast during their hospital stay. Renal injury was defined as an increase in baseline creatinine by 25% or by 0.5 within 72 h of receiving contrast or an increase within 72 h from admission for those patients who did not receive intravenous contrast. The definition for renal injury is based upon previous studies of contrast-induced nephropathy [13, 14].

All data are presented as a mean (standard deviation [SD]), median (interquartile range [IQR]), or percentage. Univariate comparisons were made using Student's t test for normally distributed data, Mann-Whitney U test for non-parametric data, and chi-square test for proportions. An α of 0.05 was considered significant. Multivariate comparisons for mortality were performed by logistic regression and adjusted for baseline demographics, injury severity, pertinent associated injuries, and presenting vital signs. The C statistic was used to characterize model discrimination and calibration curves were used to characterize model fit.

Results

There were over 1.2 million blunt trauma patients aged 65 and older in the NTDB dataset during the time period of this study. BCVI injuries and associated injury mechanisms were selected using appropriate ICD-injury codes and E-codes respectively. Ground-level falls accounted for 67% of blunt traumatic injuries in the ≥ 65-year-old cohort. EGLF injuries were found to have an overall BCVI incidence of 0.15% in the elderly cohort (Table 1). This was significantly lower than the incidence in younger patients. Despite the overall lower incidence, EGLF injuries accounted for 33% of the cases of BCVI

in the elderly cohort due to the prevalence of this injury mechanism. Less than 5% of BCVI injuries in the younger population were a result of low-energy falls.

When selecting patients with at least one risk factor for BCVI using specific ICD-9 injury codes, the incidence of BCVI increased in all groups as expected. The incidence in patients with EGLF injuries was almost six times higher with at least one injury risk factor being present (Table 1).

EGLF patients with and without documented BCVI injuries were compared (Table 2). Patients with BCVI were more commonly male, had higher injury severity, and more commonly had injuries associated with BCVI. Upper cervical spine fractures were common in EGLF BCVI patients, occurring in 32% of patients. This is much higher than any other risk factor screened for in the NTDB. Cervical spine injuries in general (fractures or subluxations anywhere in the cervical spine) occurred in 45% of BCVI patients. While risk factors for BCVI are much more prevalent in patients with BCVI, they still are frequently present in EGLF patients who did not have BCVI injury codes. Mortality was significantly higher in patients with BCVI.

Multivariate logistic regression was used to determine if BCVI was an independent risk factor for mortality in the EGLF cohort after controlling for important confounders (Table 3). BCVI was significantly associated with over 77% higher odds of mortality after adjusting for demographics, injury severity, and other injuries which are risk factors for BCVI screening. Visual inspection of the model calibration plot demonstrated excellent calibration as the observed and predicted mortality correlated closely across predicted mortality risk deciles.

In the 6520 EGLF patients at our institution, the incidence of BCVI was 0.37%; this was significantly lower compared to that of younger patients and elderly patients with high-energy injury mechanisms (Table 4). There was no significant difference in BCVI incidence when comparing the 18–64 age group to the elderly non-GLF group. The trends of BCVI incidence based upon injury mechanism and risk factors were similar when comparing the local institutional data to the NTDB data. The incidence was roughly twice as high in

Table 1 Incidence of BCVI based upon ICD-9 code from the NTDB (2007–2014), stratified by age (18–64, 65+) and injury mechanism

	All blunt injuries	≥ 1 risk factor for BCVI	p
18–64 non-ground-level fall	0.70% (14497)	2.8% (10758)	< 0.001
18–64 ground-level fall	0.20% (715)	1.1% (388)	< 0.001
Elderly non-ground level fall	0.59% (2330)*	2.49% (1810)*	< 0.001
Elderly ground level fall	0.15% (1168)† ‡	0.86% (652)† ‡	< 0.001

All data are presented as incidence (number of patients with BCVI)
*Statistically significant difference relative to 18–64 non-ground-level fall group ($p < 0.05$)
†Statistically significant difference relative to elderly non-ground-level fall group ($p < 0.05$)
‡Statistically significant difference relative to 18–64 ground-level fall group ($p < 0.05$)

Table 2 Elderly ground-level fall (EGLF) patient comparison with and without documented BCVI

	BCVI injury		
	No	Yes	
	n = 796,021	n = 1168	p
Age (years)	81.0 (7.5)	80.2 (7.4)	< 0.001
Male sex	33.0%	45.8%	< 0.001
Admission GCS	15 (15-15)	15 (14-15)	< 0.001
Admission SBP (mmHg)	149 (29)	151 (33)	0.007
Upper cervical spine fracture	3.7%	31.9%	< 0.001
Lower cervical spine fracture	1.3%	9.0%	< 0.001
Any cervical spine injury	5.6%	44.5%	< 0.001
Basilar skull fracture	2.5%	11.2%	< 0.001
Le Fort fracture	1.9%	5.50%	< 0.001
Mandible fracture	0.4%	0.60%	0.371
At least 1 injury risk factor for BCVI	9.1%	56.0%	< 0.001
Greater than 1 risk factor for BCVI	1.2%	8.30%	< 0.001
Mortality	5.0%	19.0%	< 0.001

Data are presented as mean (SD), percentage, or median (IQR). p values are calculated by Mann Whitney U test or chi-square test

the local data compared to the BCVI data in all groups which may signify differences between the respective data sets. When selecting only patients with risk factors for BCVI, the incidence increased significantly in all groups. The incidence remained lower in the EGLF group compared to that of the other two patient groups (Table 4).

We characterized all elderly BCVI patients at our institution during the time period of the study (Table 5). EGLF injuries accounted for 31% of the BCVI in the institutional data. This was similar to findings in the NTDB data (33%). Upper cervical spine fractures were the most common risk factor for BCVI. Most EGLF patients had a least one risk factor for BCVI screening. The severity of BCVI included grade 1 thru grade 4 injuries. EGLF mechanism still resulted in serious BCVI

injuries with 25% of the low-energy injuries resulting in vessel occluding grade 4 injuries. The incidence of cerebral ischemic events in the EGLF patients was similar to patients aged 18–64 (4.2% compared to 5.3% p = 0.81).

The NTDB and local institutional data indicated that patients with cervical spine fractures were at a high risk for BCVI. All patients with ICD-9 codes (805.01–805.03) for upper cervical spine fractures were then selected from the local trauma registry. Appropriate BCVI screening (CTA, MRA, DSA) for these 1387 patients was then determined via chart review. BCVI screening rates differ significantly based on age and injury mechanism. In elderly non-GLF patients, screening was 65.9% with a decrease to 44.0% in EGLF patients (Fig. 1).

Elderly patients with upper cervical spine fractures who were screened for BCVI were compared to those who were not screened (Table 6). Patients not screened for BCVI were significantly older and more likely to have suffered a ground-level fall. Patients who did not undergo BCVI screening were more likely to have compromised renal function on initial laboratory assessment. An eGFR of < 30 mL/min/1.73 m^2 was used as a surrogate for renal insufficiency and is considered a relative contraindication for IV contrast at our institution. Rates of pre-injury anti-thrombotic medication were not different between those screened for BCVI and those not screened.

Patients who received IV contrast (n = 442) for BCVI screening were compared to a randomly selected group of elderly trauma patients who did not receive IV contrast (n = 200). Rates of renal injury did not differ between those who received IV contrast for BCVI screening compared to those patients who did not receive contrast from the random sample (8.7 vs 9.4% p = 0.84). The injury severity score was higher in the group that underwent BCVI screening (median 10 vs 9, p = 0.04). Of the 8.7% (n = 38) of patients who were screened and had renal injury, seven patients had persistent increases in their creatinine for over 1 week and a single patient required initiation of dialysis.

Table 3 Logistic regression model to determine independent risk factors of in-hospital mortality in elderly ground-level falls (n = 1168)

	Coefficient	S.E.	Wald	Odds ratio	95% C.I.	p
Age (years)	0.046	.001	2525	1.047	1.045–1.049	< 0.001
Male sex	0.483	.013	1442	1.621	1.581–1.662	< 0.001
ISS	0.091	.001	12,574	1.096	1.094–1.097	< 0.001
Admission SBP (mmHg)	− 0.005	.000	720	0.995	0.994–0.995	< 0.001
Admission GCS	− 0.280	.002	25,836	0.756	0.753–0.758	< 0.001
BCVI	0.571	.097	35	1.770	1.464–2.139	< 0.001
≥ 1 BCVI screening injury risk factor	0.379	.017	495	1.461	1.413–1.511	< 0.001
Constant	− 3.401	.082	1720			< 0.001

Logistic regression model for predictors of in-hospital mortality. p values are calculated by the Wald test. Area under the cross-validated receiver operating characteristic curve for the model is 0.8233

CI confidence interval, SE standard error

Table 4 Local institution BCVI incidence data 2007–2014

	All blunt injuries	≥ 1 risk factor for BCVI	p
18–64	1.17% (290)	5.68% (270)	< 0.001
Elderly non-ground-level fall	1.12% (53)	4.87% (52)	< 0.001
Elderly ground-level fall	0.37% (24)*	1.47% (21)*	< 0.001

All data are presented as incidence (number of patients with BCVI). Incidence of BCVI based upon ICD-9 code from registry data from 2007 to 2014, stratified by age (18–64, 65+) and injury mechanism
*Statistically significant difference relative to elderly non-GLF (p < 0.05)

Discussion

The diagnosis and incidence of BCVI have increased over time corresponding with documented increased screening rates [15, 16]. Despite this increased screening and the growing elderly population in the USA, little is known about risk of BCVI in elderly patients with low-energy injury mechanisms, particularly ground-level falls [8]. Such low-energy injuries are associated with higher rates of fractures and other complications compared to younger patients [10, 17, 18]. This is due to osteopenia and altered biomechanics in elderly patients [18, 19]. We speculated that these low-energy mechanisms would still result in injuries such as cervical spine and basilar skull fractures which would place patients at risk for BCVI.

The current analysis provides evidence for the decreased incidence of BCVI in elderly ground-level fall patients compared to patients with other injury mechanisms. However, those patients with risk factors for BCVI screening had an incidence of BCVI similar to the general trauma population approaching 1–2% [1–3]. Approximately 1 in 10 EGLF patients had at least one risk factor for BCVI in the current study. The diagnosis of BVCI was found to be an independent risk factor for mortality in the EGLF cohort after controlling for other

Table 5 Elderly ground-level fall patients with BCVI

	(n = 24)
Demographics	
Age (years)	81.6 (7.6)
Male sex	50%
ISS	9.5 (5.8–13)
Admission GCS	15 (14–15)
Pre-injury anti-thrombotic	75.0%
Upper cervical spine fracture	79.2%
Any risk factor for BCVI	87.5%
BCVI location	
Carotid	25%
Vertebral	75%
Grade	
1 (intimal irregularity with < 25% narrowing)	50%
2 (dissection, intramural hematoma, or intimal flap with > 25% narrowing)	12.5%
3 (pseudoaneurysm)	12.5%
4 (vessel occlusion)	25%
Treatment	
Aspirin	16
Aspirin + clopidogrel	1
Heparin	2
Stenting + aspirin	1
None	4
Outcome	
BCVI attributable stroke	4.2%
Mortality	8.3%

Data presented as a mean (SD), median (IQR), or percentage of the patient population

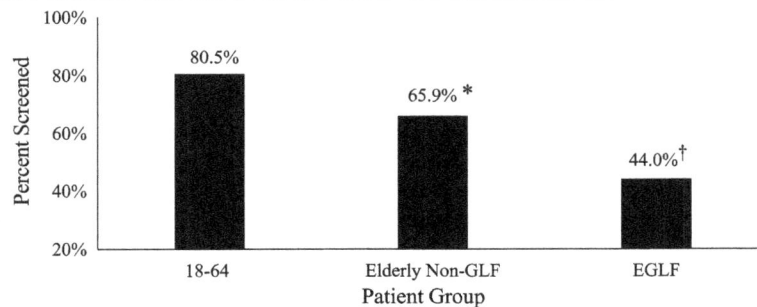

Fig. 1 Screening rates for BCVI with known upper cervical spine fracture. *p < 0.05 relative to 18–64-year-old group; †p < 0.05 relative to elderly non-GLF group

important variables which impact mortality. BCVI was associated with a 4.2% rate of cerebral ischemic events in the EGLF patients.

Despite having a well-defined BCVI screening protocol at our institution, screening rates were significantly lower in EGLF patients even when injuries known to be BCVI risk factors were present. Screening was significantly less common in elderly patients compared to that in younger patients regardless of injury mechanism. Providers may justify omitting BCVI screening for many reasons: if patients are already on BCVI treatment (anti-thrombotic therapy), fear of contrast-induced nephropathy, and lack of perceived benefit due to assumptions that elderly patients are at low risk for having BCVI. The current study suggests that many of the above reasons to omit screening elderly patients may not be evidence-based.

When examining BCVI screening, there was no difference in the proportion of patients already on pre-injury anti-thrombotic medication. Contrast-induced nephropathy does not appear to be a reason to avoid screening if risk factors for BCVI are present. There was no significant difference in renal injury between patients who received IV contrast for BCVI screening relative to those without IV contrast imaging. This is consistent with previous studies that demonstrate that the risk of contrast-induced renal injury is low and that rates of renal injury are not different from patients who do not receive contrast [13, 14]. The patients in the unscreened group were found to have significantly higher mortality. This is likely attributable to older age and increased comorbidities in this patient group. Lastly, this study indicates that elderly patients have a lower incidence of BCVI but are still at clinically significant risk. Even with a low-energy injury mechanism, EGLF patients have a BCVI incidence of 0.86–1.47% when a screening risk factor was present.

As seen in the local data, patients can have high-grade BCVI injuries and ischemic events regardless of injury mechanism. All cases of cerebral ischemia occurred in patients before proper treatment was initiated. This is consistent with other published data on BCVI [4, 5]. Early screening in patients with risk factors can allow for proper treatment and prevention of debilitating or deadly ischemic events.

Table 6 Comparison of elderly patients with upper cervical spine fractures with and without BCVI screening

	Screened		
	Yes	No	
	n = 442	n = 412	p
Age (years)	79.9 (8.0)	83.9 (8.2)	< 0.001
Male sex	39.0%	41.0%	0.44
ISS	9 (5–14)	9 (5–13)	0.32
Admission GCS	15 (15–15)	15 (14–15)	< 0.001
Admission SBP (mmHg)	151 (30)	149 (29)	0.67
Pre-injury anti-thrombotic	66.0%	64.0%	0.41
EGLF injury	54.7%	72.0%	< 0.001
Admission eGFR < 30 (mL/min/1.73 m^2)	2.70%	8.00%	< 0.001
Time to BCVI screening (hours)	9 (14.3)	N/a	N/a
Mortality	7.0%	12.6%	0.006

Data are presented as mean (SD), median (IQR), or percentage of the patient population. p values are calculated by Mann Whitney U test or chi-square test

This analysis has several limitations which should be considered when interpreting the results. One major limitation of this study is the retrospective nature of the analysis. It is impossible to know how many patients had BCVI injuries but were not screened or were not properly coded for a BCVI diagnosis. It is known that BCVI incidence has increased over time with increased screening [15, 16]. We can speculate that the true incidence of BCVI in the elderly is significantly higher than what was determined in this study and future estimates will need to account for low screening rates seen in the elderly population. Lower screening rates likely contribute to the lower incidence in EGLF patients compared to that in younger patients with GLF injuries.

There are inherent limitations of large national datasets like the NTDB. The NTDB includes a disproportionate number of large hospitals with younger and more severely injured patients which may skew the true incidence of BCVI in the elderly. Hospital variability in screening rates and data reporting could significantly impact the outcomes of this study. From the NTDB data, screening rates in EGLF patients could not be determined. Lower screening rates may contribute to the difference in BCVI incidence in the NTDB compared to local institutional data. Future multi-center trials would be needed to examine screening practices at other institutions. Due to the large sample size of the NTDB cohort, our group comparisons were highly statistically significant, even though some differences were not clinically different. We attempted to highlight those differences which were clinically relevant in our interpretation of the results. For our regression model, the covariates of interest were also highly significant due to the large sample size which limits the conclusions which can be formulated from the results.

We utilized our local trauma registry to overcome limitations attributable to large national datasets. This limits the applicability to other centers across the country. To compare screening rates, we focused on the most common and robust BCVI risk factor, upper cervical spine fracture, to select our cohort. This may bias our conclusions relative to other types of injuries associated with BCVI. Despite this limitation, we fully characterized the radiographic workup for over 1300 trauma patients and performed a thorough medical record review for over 850 elderly trauma patients. Radiographic diagnosis and grade of BCVI were complicated by presence of atherosclerotic disease in elderly patients. Local radiologists generally indicated which arterial abnormalities were more likely related to a pre-existing process. When comparing the effects of IV contrast on renal injury, some patients screened for BCVI had multiple scans with IV contrast which may affect the results.

Conclusions

The novel results of this retrospective study demonstrate that despite having lower energy injuries, elderly patients remain at risk for BCVI. Current BCVI screening of elderly ground-level fall patients is less common relative to younger patients and elderly patients with high-energy injury mechanisms. This lower screening rate exists in spite of similar risks of stroke with a BCVI diagnosis. The current data demonstrates that patients who present with risk factors for BCVI, even in those who suffer low-energy injury mechanisms, are at significant risk for BCVI. Patients should be screened for the injury when feasible and safe to allow for appropriate diagnosis and treatment. Screening decisions should not be biased by age or injury mechanism when patients meet criteria for BCVI screening.

Abbreviations
BCVI: Blunt cerebrovascular injury; CTA: Computed tomography angiography; DSA: Digital subtraction angiography; eGFR: Estimated glomerular filtration rate; EGLF: Elderly ground-level fall (age ≥ 65 years); GCS: Glasgow Coma Scale; GLF: Ground-level fall; ICD: International Classification of Diseases; IQR: Interquartile range; ISS: Injury severity score; MRA: Magnetic resonance angiography; NTDB: National Trauma Data Bank; SBP: Systolic blood pressure; SD: Standard deviation

Authors' contributions
VPA and JLS contributed to the study design, data collection, data analysis, data interpretation, writing, and critical revision. JBB, BSZ, and MDN contributed to study design, data collection, and data analysis. GW and RF contributed to the study design and data interpretation. ABP and TRB contributed to the critical revision. All authors read and approved the final manuscript.

Competing interests
The authors declare that they have no competing interests.

References
1. Bromberg WJ, Collier BC, Diebel LN, Dwyer KM, Holevar MR, Jacobs DG, Kurek SJ, Schreiber MA, Shapiro ML, Vogel TR. Blunt cerebrovascular injury practice management guidelines: the eastern association for the surgery of trauma. J Trauma. 2010;68(2):471-7.
2. Franz RW, Willette PA, Wood MJ, Wright ML, Hartman JF. A systematic review and meta-analysis of diagnostic screening criteria for blunt cerebrovascular injuries. J Am Coll Surg. 2012;214(3):313-27.
3. Harrigan MR, Falola MI, Shannon CN, Westrick AC, Walters BC. Incidence and trends in the diagnosis of traumatic extracranial cerebrovascular injury in the nationwide inpatient sample database, 2003-2010. J Neurotrauma. 2014;31(11):1056-62.
4. DiCocco JM, Fabian TC, Emmett KP, Magnotti LJ, Zarzaur BL, Bate BG, Muhlbauer MS, Khan N, Kelly JM, Williams JS, et al. Optimal outcomes for patients with blunt cerebrovascular injury (BCVI): tailoring treatment to the lesion. J Am Coll Surg. 2011;212:549-57. discussion 557-59
5. Edwards NM, Fabian TC, Claridge JA, Timmons SD, Fischer PE, Croce MA. Antithrombotic therapy and endovascular stents are effective treatment for blunt carotid injuries: results from long term follow up. J Am Coll Surg. 2007;204(5):1007-13. discussion 1014-15
6. Biffl WL, Moore EE, Offner PJ, Brega KE, Franciose RJ, Elliott JP, Burch JM. Optimizing screening for blunt cerebrovascular injuries. Am J Surg. 1999; 178:517-22.

7. Burlew CC, Biffl WL, Moore EE, Barnett CC, Johnson JL, Bensard DD. Blunt cerebrovascular injuries: redefining screening criteria in the era of noninvasive diagnosis. J Trauma Acute Care Surg. 2012;72:330–5.

8. Cothren CC, Moore EE, Biffl WL, Ciesla DJ, Ray CE Jr, Johnson JL, Moore JB, Burch JM. Anticoagulation is the gold standard therapy for blunt carotid injuries to reduce stroke rate. *Arch Surg*. 2004;139:540–5. discussion 545–546

9. Kozar RA, Arbabi S, Stein DM, Shackford SR, Barraco RD, Biffl WL, Brasel KJ, Cooper Z, Fakhry SM, Livingston D, et al. Injury in the aged: geriatric trauma care at the crossroads. J Trauma Acute Care Surg. 2015;78(6):1197–209.

10. Daffner RH, Goldberg AL, Evans TC, Hanlon DP, Levy DB. Cervical vertebral injuries in the elderly: a 10-year study. Emerg Radiol. 1998;5:38–42.

11. NTDB User Manual 2017. Available at: https://www.facs.org/~/media/files/quality%20programs/trauma/ntdb/ntdb_rds_archived_user_manuals.ashx. Accessed 5 Oct 2017.

12. Biffl WL, Moore EE, Offner PJ, Brega KE, Franciose RJ, Burch JM. Blunt carotid arterial injuries: implications of a new grading scale. J Trauma. 1999;47:845–53.

13. McGillicuddy EA, Schuster KM, Kaplan LJ, Maung AA, Lui FY, Maerz LL, Johnson DC, Davis KA. Contrast-induced nephropathy in elderly trauma patients. J Trauma. 2010;68(2):294–9.

14. Finigan R, Pham J, Mendoza R, Lekawa M, Dolich M, Kong A, Bernal N, Lush S, Barrios C. Risk for contrast-induced nephropathy in elderly trauma patients. Am Surg. 2012;78:1114–7.

15. Jacobson LE, Ziemba-Davis M, Herrera AJ. The limitations of using risk factors to screen for blunt cerebrovascular injuries: the harder you look, the more you find. World J Emerg Surg. 2015;10:46.

16. Shahan CP, Croce MA, Fabian TC, Magnotti TJ. Impact of continuous evaluation of technology and therapy: 30 years of research reduces stroke and mortality from blunt cerebrovascular injury. J Am Coll Surg. 2017;224(4):595–9.

17. Miriam T. Aschkenasy, Todd C. Rothenhaus. Trauma and falls in the elderly. Emerg Med Clin North Am 2006; 24 (2):413-432.

18. Schrag SP, Toedter LJ, McQuay N Jr. Cervical spine fractures in geriatric blunt trauma patients with low-energy mechanism: are clinical predictors adequate? Am J Surg. 2008;195:170–3.

19. Lockhart TE, Smith JL, Woldstad JC. Effects of aging on the biomechanics of slips and falls. Hum Factors. 2005;47(4):708–29.

25

Risk factors for mortality in the late amputation of necrotizing fasciitis

Chia-Peng Chang[1], Cheng-Ting Hsiao[1,2], Chun-Nan Lin[1] and Wen-Chih Fann[1,2*]

Abstract

Background: Necrotizing fasciitis (NF) is a rapidly progressive infectious disease that primarily involves the fascia and subcutaneous tissue. If not promptly treated, it can lead to morbidity as well as mortality. It can affect any part of the body, most commonly the extremities. Early and aggressive surgical treatment is the proper way of management. The purpose of this study was to identify the risk factors for mortality in late amputation among NF patients that may be used in routine clinical practice to prevent mortality.

Methods: A retrospective cohort study of hospitalized patients with NF was conducted in a tertiary teaching hospital in Taiwan between March 2015 and March 2018. All collected data were statistically analyzed.

Results: A total of 582 patients with NF were included; 35 of them had undergone amputation (7 primary and 28 late amputations), with a 6% amputation rate. Thirteen amputated patients still died eventually (all in the late amputation group). Significant risk factors for mortality identified in the late amputation group included hemorrhagic bullae ($p = 0.001$, OR 4.7, 95% confidence interval (CI) 2.68–8.69), peripheral vascular disease ($p < 0.001$, OR 3.2, 95% CI 1.12–10.58), bacteremia ($p = 0.021$, OR 2.87, 95% CI 2.07–5.96), and Laboratory Risk Indicator of Necrotizing Fasciitis (LRINEC) score > 8 ($p < 0.001$, OR 1.97, 95% CI 1.28–4.61). *Vibrio vulnificus* was the main causative organism based on our study, but the microbiology results showed no significant correlation.

Conclusion: NF patients with hemorrhagic bullae, comorbidity with peripheral vascular disease, presence of bacteremia, or LRINEC score > 8 should receive early and primary amputation in order to prevent mortality.

Keywords: Necrotizing fasciitis, Amputation, Soft tissue infection, Risk factor, LRINEC

Background

Necrotizing fasciitis (NF) is a serious form of infection involving rapidly spreading inflammation and extensive necrosis of the skin, subcutaneous tissue, and superficial fascia [1]. In order to successfully treat NF, two important factors must always be present: awareness of the disease, in spite of its rare occurrence, and consequently immediate therapy (surgical and antibiotic treatment). The treatment of choice for NF is rapid surgical debridement and broad-spectrum antibiotic therapy [2]. Delayed treatment may result in extensive loss of soft tissue associated with limb loss; moreover, the risk of mortality is also increased. Even with aggressive treatment, patients may suffer significant morbidity such as amputation and organ failure [3–5]. Various predictors of mortality based on predisposing factors have been reported by different investigators. Previous studies have identified advanced age (> 60 years), *Aeromonas* and *Vibrio* infection, liver cirrhosis, cancer, hypotension, band polymorphonuclear neutrophils > 10%, and serum creatinine level > 2 mg/dL to be independent predictors of mortality in NF cases [6, 7]. Khamnuan et al. identified that clinical predictors for amputation in patients with NF included diabetes mellitus, soft tissue swelling, skin necrosis, gangrene, and serum creatinine values > 1.6 mg/dL on admission [8]. Lee et al. reported that treatment delayed beyond 3 days was an independent factor indicating a poor prognosis in *Vibrio* NF [9]. However, limited data exist with regard to with

* Correspondence: dr5853@cgmh.org.tw
[1]Department of Emergency Medicine, Chang Gung Memorial Hospital, No.6, Sec. W., Jiapu Rd, Puzi City, Chiayi County 613, Taiwan
[2]Department of Medicine, Chang Gung University, Taoyuan, Taiwan

mortality and delayed amputation. This study investigated factors associated with mortality in late amputation among NF patients that could be used in clinical practice.

Methods

The institutional review board of our hospital approved this retrospective study. In all, 582 patients were enrolled based on two criteria: (1) surgically proven diagnosis of NF and (2) treatment received between March 2015 and March 2018. Thirty-five patients underwent amputation during hospitalization, of which 7 were amputated within 3 days of admission, defined as primary amputation, while the other 28 were amputated beyond 3 days, defined as late amputation. Thirteen amputated NF patients died during hospitalization. We defined the variables as follows: wound, the presence of any wound on the affected limb, toe, or finger; hemorrhagic bullae, confirmed as hemorrhagic bullae by the emergency physician in the medical records and clinical photos. Comorbidities and admission laboratory data were extracted through chart review. All patients were assessed by emergency physicians as soon as they were admitted. They received broad-spectrum antibiotic treatment for anaerobic and aerobic bacteria as well as early surgical debridement including fasciotomy or primary amputation post-diagnosis. Each patient's medical record was screened for documentation of NF to confirm the diagnosis. Those with NF involving the head, neck, or trunk were excluded. Amputation sites included the fingers, toes, hands, forearms, and below and above the knee. Baseline demographic characteristics, laboratory findings, and clinical presentation were compared between mortality in the late amputation and survival of the amputation groups.

Statistical analysis

All data were analyzed using SPSS Statistics version 20.0 (IBM Corp., Armonk, NY, USA). Continuous variables were analyzed using the t test, and categorical variables were analyzed using the chi-square test, except where 20% of cells had expected counts of < 5, in which case Fisher's exact test was used. Multivariate logistic regression analysis was performed to identify the predictors of mortality in the late amputation NF cohort along with the odds ratio (OR) and 95% confidence interval (CI). p values less than 0.05 were considered to be statistically significant.

Results

From a total number of 582 patients, 35 were amputated resulting in an amputation rate of 6%. Among 35 amputated patients, 7 were categorized as primary, while 28 were categorized as late amputations. Thirteen amputated patients died during hospitalization, who all belonged to the late amputation group, and the other 22 patients survived. As shown in Table 1, in the analysis of

clinical condition, comorbidity, and laboratory evaluations, there were statistically significant differences with hemorrhagic bullae (53.8% vs. 15.4%; $p = 0.001$), diabetes mellitus (76.9% vs. 41.4%; $p = 0.004$), peripheral artery disease (23.1% vs. 1.2%; $p < 0.001$), C-reactive protein level (191.9 mg/dL vs. 134.1 mg/dL), bacteremia (69.2% vs. 36.0%; $p = 0.001$), and Laboratory Risk Indicator for Necrotizing Fasciitis (LRINEC) score > 8 (61.5% vs. 36.7%; $p < 0.001$) between mortality in the late amputation and survival in the amputation groups. All significant variables (with $p < 0.05$) were included in the multivariable logistic regression analysis. The multivariate logistic regression analysis revealed that independent risk factors for mortality in late amputation included hemorrhagic bullae ($p = 0.001$, OR 4.75, 95% CI 2.68–8.69), peripheral vascular disease ($p < 0.001$, OR 3.2, 95% CI 1.12–10.58), LRINEC score > 8, ($p < 0.001$, OR 1.97, 95% CI 1.28–4.61), and the presence of bacteremia ($p = 0.021$, OR 2.87, 95% CI 2.07–5.96) (Table 2).

Microbiology data regarding blood culture are shown in Table 3. In all, 159 patients (27.4%) were found to have positive isolated organisms. *Vibrio vulnificus* was the most frequent causative organism (34.6%). *Streptococcus* species and polymicrobial infections both accounted for 13.2% of infections. However, no difference between the amputation and non-amputation groups was found according to the isolated organisms.

Discussion

A number of studies have investigated risk factors associated with NF patient mortality, but only a limited amount of literature is available on the association between mortality and late amputation. In the mortality group, all 13 patients received fasciotomy and debridement at the first day of admission, 10 of them received multiple debridement and amputated at last and 3 of them amputated at second times of operation beyond 3 days after admission. Inadequate initial debridement for infection control, unexpectedly deteriorated clinical condition, and delay recognition may be the source of delay amputation, which led to mortality. Besides, few patients refused to receive primary amputation which caused delay amputation, which was also documented in the medical chart. Therefore, early recognition of high-risk NF patients is an important issue. Our findings suggest that an NF case should be treated early and aggressively and that primary amputation will prevent high-risk factors in patients that lead to mortality. Khamnuan et al. reported that clinical predictors for amputation in patients with NF included soft tissue swelling, skin necrosis, and gangrene [8]. Krieg et al. also reported that the presence of visible skin necrosis as an independent predictor of mortality emphasizes the outstanding importance of early diagnosis and prompt

Table 1 Clinical characteristics between mortality in the late amputation and survival in the amputation group

Variable	Mortality in late amputation (n = 13)		Survival in amputation (n = 22)		p value
Mean age (years)	65.08	± 10.94	66.35	± 14.76	0.762
Clinical condition, no.(%)					
Wound	9	(69.2%)	9	(42.0%)	0.059
Hemorrhagic bullae	7	(53.8%)	13	(35.4%)	0.001[*]
Comorbidity, no. (%)					
Diabetes mellitus	10	(76.9%)	8	(36.4%)	0.014[*]
CKD	5	(38.5%)	10	(45.5%)	0.286
Liver cirrhosis	1	(7.7%)	5	(22.7%)	0.327
PAD	5	(38.5%)	2	(9.1%)	< 0.001[*]
Admission data					
WBC count ($\times 10^3$/μL)	13.9	(± 6.5)	14.8	(± 7.8)	0.693
CRP (mg/dL)	191.9	(± 103.3)	134.1	(± 111.7)	0.012[*]
Creatinine (mg/dL)	2.4	(± 1.5)	1.6	(± 0.8)	0.139
Albumin (g/dL)	3.1	(± 0.6)	3.3	(± 0.6)	0.266
Na (mmol/L)	133	(± 4.3)	134	(± 3.6)	0.125
Lactate, mg/dL	33.9	(± 30.4)	23.2	(± 18.6)	0.086
LRINEC score > 8, n (%)	8	(61.5%)	8	(36.7%)	< 0.001[*]
Bacteremia, n (%)	9	(69.2%)	8	(36.4%)	0.001[*]
Hospital stay (days)	41.2	(± 16.9)	33.7	(± 21.1)	

Values are presented as mean ± standard deviation or number (%)
PAD, peripheral artery disease, *CKD* chronic kidney disease, *WBC* white blood cell, *CRP* C-reactive protein, *LRINEC* Laboratory Risk Indicator for Necrotizing Fasciitis
*p < 0.05

treatment to improve the prognosis [10]. Our study demonstrated that hemorrhagic bullae were highly associated with mortality in late amputation in NF, which is more precise than skin necrosis, also a late clinical manifestation and indicates an unfavorable progression of NF. Su et al. studied the LRINEC cut-off value associated with poor outcomes in 209 NF patients and demonstrated higher mortality and amputation rates in patients based on LRINEC scores [10]. The rates of early diagnosis (64 vs 70%), early operation (71 vs 70%), and time for operation (30 ± 51 vs 27.5 ± 51 min) were comparable between the two LRINEC groups. The overall mortality and amputation rates were 16% and 26%, respectively,

Table 2 Independent risk factors for mortality in late amputation NF using a multivariate analysis

Risk factor	OR	95% CI	p value
Hemorrhagic bullae	4.75	2.68–8.69	0.001[*]
Diabetes mellitus	1.62	1.15–7.14	0.15
PAD	3.20	1.12–10.58	0.001[*]
CRP	1.06	0.99–1.87	0.204
LRINEC score > 8	1.97	1.28–4.61	0.001[*]
Bacteremia	2.87	2.07–5.96	0.021[*]

OR odds ratio, *CI* confidence interval, *PAD* peripheral artery disease, *CRP* C-reactive protein, *LRINEC* Laboratory Risk Indicator for Necrotizing Fasciitis
*p < 0.05

whereas the rates of mortality (21% vs. 11%) and amputation (36% vs. 17%) in patients with LRINEC score ≥ 6 were higher than those who had LRINEC < 6 [11]. Wong et al. described the LRINEC that categorizes patients as "high risk" if the score is ≥ 8 [12]. El-Menyar et al. published results suggesting the LRINEC score might be useful for risk stratification and prognosis, in which cut-off value for predicting hospital mortality was 8 points in their study [13]. In our study, LRINEC score > 8 showed a statistically significant difference between mortality of the primary and late amputation groups. Chen et al. identified vascular disease as a common comorbidity of necrotizing soft tissue infections [14]. On the basis of this study, we found that peripheral artery disease was an important independent factor associated with mortality in late amputation. Chen et al. reported that the presence of *Streptococcus* group A in blood cultures was associated with a high risk of mortality in NF [15]. In our study, all NF patients underwent blood culture; the positivity rate was 27.4%. NF patients with bacteremia were more susceptible to death in the late amputation group.

Some individuals might be more susceptible to *V. vulnificus* infection following the consumption of contaminated seafood or following exposure of an open wound to seawater or marine animals, especially in situations where there is underlying chronic liver disease [16]. Most of our

Table 3 Microorganisms identified in blood culture in amputation and non-amputation groups with NF

Pathogens	Amputation group (n = 35)	Non-amputation group (n = 124)	Total, n (%) (n = 159)
MSSA	0 (0)	2 (1.3)	2 (1.3)
MRSA	4 (2.5)	6 (3.8)	10 (6.3)
Streptococcus species	4 (2.5)	17 (10.7)	21 (13.2)
Escherichia coli	1 (0.6)	2 (1.3)	3 (1.9)
Pseudomonas aeruginosa	7 (4.4)	3 (1.6)	10 (6.3)
Vibrio vulnificus	4 (2.5)	51 (32.1)	55 (34.6)
Aeromonas species	3 (1.6)	8 (5.0)	11 (6.9)
Other gram-positive	3 (1.6)	9 (5.7)	11 (6.9)
Other gram-negative	2 (1.3)	12 (7.5)	14 (8.8)
Polymicrobial	7 (4.4)	14 (8.8)	21 (13.2)

Microorganisms identified in blood culture did not show statistically significant differences between the two groups ($p > 0.05$). Values are shown as n (%)
MSSA methicillin-sensitive *Staphylococcus aureus*, MRSA methicillin-resistant *Staphylococcus aureus*

patients lived near the ocean and worked in fisheries, which is in support of the abovementioned findings. Tsai et al. reported that among patients with *Vibrio* NF, a systolic blood pressure of 90 mmHg, low platelet count, and a combination of hepatic dysfunction were associated with a higher mortality rate [17]. Although *Vibrio* NF has high mortality, our study showed that this had no clinical correlation with mortality in late amputation. Jabbour et al. reported that among gram-positive bacteria in NF, *Streptococcus* and *Staphylococcus* were the most commonly identified organisms [18]. In our study, *V. vulnificus* accounted for 34.6%, while *Streptococcus* species and polymicrobial infection both accounted for 13.2% of cases.

Lee et al. previously reported that early diagnosis and prompt treatment within 3 days post-injury or symptom onset should be the goal for treating patients with NF caused by *V. vulnificus* [9]. Wong et al. identified that delay in surgery for more than 24 h was correlated with increased mortality [1]. Hong et al. reported that early initiation of simple incision and drainage under regional anesthesia followed by complete debridement 24 h later is more feasible and effective for patients with *Vibrio* NF complicated by septic shock, as compared with the aggressive surgical debridement strategy [19]. Based on our findings, NF patients with hemorrhagic bullae, comorbidity with peripheral vascular disease, LRINEC score > 8, or the presence of bacteremia should receive early and primary amputation in order to prevent mortality. More studies are necessary to determine the benefit from surgical time and intervention for NF patients.

Most of the limitations of our study are related to its relatively small sample size. This results in a wide range in the confidence interval of our factors and also limits the evaluation of more factors.

Conclusions

Emergency physicians are often the first to evaluate patients with NF and therefore should be aware of the risk and management of this disease. This study confirmed that peripheral artery disease, presence of hemorrhagic bullae, bacteremia, and LRINEC score > 8 are independent risk factors, which contribute to mortality in late amputation of NF. Patients with any of these predictors should be monitored closely and receive early aggressive treatment as primary amputation to prevent mortality. More studies are required to determine the significance of these findings and develop guidelines for management.

Abbreviations
CI: Confidence interval; CKD: Chronic kidney disease; CRP: C-reactive protein; LRINEC: Laboratory Risk Indicator of Necrotizing Fasciitis; MRSA: Methicillin-resistant *Staphylococcus aureu*; MSSA: Methicillin-sensitive *Staphylococcus aureus*; NF: Necrotizing fasciitis; OR: Odds ratio; PAD: Peripheral artery disease; WBC: White blood cell

Acknowledgements
The authors thank all the participants who participated in this study.

Authors' contributions
CPC conceived of the study, and participated in its design and coordination, and helped to draft the manuscript. CNL participated in drafting the manuscript and statistical analysis. CTH participated in the design of the study and statistical analysis. WCF participated in the design of study and drafted the manuscript. All authors read and approved the final manuscript.

Competing interests
The authors declare that they have no competing interests.

References

1. Wong C-H, Chang H-C, Pasupathy S, Khin L-W, Tan J-L, Low C-O. Necrotizing fasciitis: clinical presentation, microbiology, and determinants of mortality. J Bone Joint Surg Am. 2003;85-A:1454–60.
2. Headley AJ. Necrotizing soft tissue infections: a primary care review. Am Fam Physician. 2003;68:323–8.
3. Ozalay M, Ozkoc G, Akpinar S, Hersekli MA, Tandogan RN. Necrotizing soft-tissue infection of a limb: clinical presentation and factors related to mortality. Foot Ankle Int. 2006;27:598–605.
4. Roje Z, Roje Z, Matić D, Librenjak D, Dokuzović S, Varvodić J. Necrotizing fasciitis: literature review of contemporary strategies for diagnosing and management with three case reports: torso, abdominal wall, upper and lower limbs. World J Emerg Surg. 2011;6:46.
5. Hakkarainen TW, Kopari NM, Pham TN, Evans HL. Necrotizing soft tissue infections: review and current concepts in treatment, systems of care, and outcomes. Curr Probl Surg. 2014;51:344–62.
6. Huang K-F, Hung M-H, Lin Y-S, Lu C-L, Liu C, Chen C-C, et al. Independent predictors of mortality for necrotizing fasciitis: a retrospective analysis in a single institution. J Trauma. 2011;71:467–73 discussion473.
7. Hsiao C-T, Weng H-H, Yuan Y-D, Chen C-T, Chen I-C. Predictors of mortality in patients with necrotizing fasciitis. Am J Emerg Med. 2008;26:170–5.
8. Khamnuan P, Chongruksut W, Jearwattanakanok K, Patumanond J, Tantraworasin A. Necrotizing fasciitis: epidemiology and clinical predictors for amputation. Int J Gen Med. 2015;8:195–202.
9. Lee YC, Hor LI, Chiu HY, Lee JW, Shieh SJ. Prognostic factor of mortality and its clinical implications in patients with necrotizing fasciitis caused by *Vibrio vulnificus*. Eur J Clin Microbiol Infect Dis. 2014;33:1011–8.
10. Krieg A, Dizdar L, Verde PE, Knoefel WT. Predictors of mortality for necrotizing soft-tissue infections: a retrospective analysis of 64 cases. Langenbeck's Arch Surg. 2014;399:333–41.
11. Su YC, Chen HW, Hong YC, et al. Laboratory risk indicator for necrotizing fasciitis score and the outcomes. ANZ J Surg. 2008;78:968–72.
12. Wong CH, Khin LW, Heng KS, et al. The LRINEC (Laboratory Risk Indicator for Necrotizing Fasciitis) score: a tool for distinguishing necrotizing fasciitis from other soft tissue infections. Crit Care Med. 2004;32(7):1535–41.
13. El-Menyar A, Asim M, Mudali IN, et al. The laboratory risk indicator for necrotizing fasciitis (LRINEC) scoring: the diagnostic and potential prognostic value. Scand J Trauma Resus Emerg Med. 2017;25(1):28.
14. Chen KJ, Klingel M, McLeod S, Mindra S, Ng VK. Presentation and outcomes of necrotizing soft tissue infections. Int J Gen Med. 2017;10:215–20.
15. Chen IC, Li WC, Hong YC, Shie SS, Fann WC, Hsiao CT. The microbiological profile and presence of bloodstream infection influence mortality rates in necrotizing fasciitis. Crit Care. 2011;15:R152.
16. Bross MH, Soch K, Morales R, Mitchell RB. *Vibrio vulnificus* infection: diagnosis and treatment. Am Fam Physician. 2007;76:539–44.
17. Tsai Y-H, Hsu RW-W, Huang K-C, Huang T-J. Laboratory indicators for early detection and surgical treatment of vibrio necrotizing fasciitis. Clin Orthop Relat Res. 2010;468:2230–7.
18. Jabbour G, El-Menyar A, Peralta R, Shaikh N, Abdelrahman H, Mudali IN, et al. Pattern and predictors of mortality in necrotizing fasciitis patients in a single tertiary hospital. World J Emerg Surg. 2016;11:40.
19. Hong GL, Dai XQ, Lu CJ, Liu JM, Zhao GJ, Wu B, et al. Temporizing surgical management improves outcome in Vibrio necrotizing fasciitis complicated with septic shock on admission. Burns. 2014;40:446–54.

26

Pediatric falls from windows and balconies: incidents and risk factors as reported by newspapers in the United Arab Emirates

Michal Grivna[1*], Hanan M. Al-Marzouqi[2], Maryam R. Al-Ali[2], Nada N. Al-Saadi[2] and Fikri M. Abu-Zidan[3]

Abstract

Background: Falls of children from heights (balconies and windows) usually result in severe injuries and death. Details on child falls from heights in the United Arab Emirates (UAE) are not easily accessible. Our aim was to assess the incidents, personal, and environmental risk factors for pediatric falls from windows/balconies using newspaper clippings.

Methods: We used a retrospective study design to electronically assess all major UAE national Arabic and English newspapers for reports of unintentional child falls from windows and balconies during 2005–2016. A structured data collection form was developed to collect information. Data were entered into an Excel sheet and descriptive analysis was performed.

Results: Newspaper clippings documented 96 fall incidents. After cleaning the data and excluding duplicate cases and intentional injuries, 81 cases were included into the final analysis. Fifty-three percent (n = 42) were boys. The mean (range) age was 4.9 years (1–15). Thirty-eight (47%) children fell from windows and 36 (44%) from balconies. Twenty-two (27%) children climbed on the furniture placed on a balcony or close to a window. Twenty-five (31%) children were not alone in the apartment when they fell. Twenty-nine children fell from less than 5 floors (37%), 33 from 5 to 10 floors (42%) and 16 from more than 10 floors (21%). Fifteen children (19%) were hospitalized and survived the fall incident, while 66 died (81%).

Conclusions: Newspapers proved to be useful to study pediatric falls from heights. It is necessary to improve window safety by installing window guards and raising awareness.

Keywords: Falls from windows, Balconies, Children, UAE

Background

Unintentional falls are the second leading cause of injury-related hospitalization for all ages accounting for about 30% of injury admissions and 15% of all Emergency Department visits [1, 2]. Falls of children from heights (balconies and windows) often result in severe injuries and death [3]. These falls were described in a chapter called "Falling out of a window" in "The Book of Accidents" 1830. The authors stressed the importance of supervision and vigilance of parents and maids [4]. Community education and installation of window guards, starting in 1970s in several US cities, led

to successful decrease of these injuries [3]. The famous intervention "Children Cannot Fly" targeting parents with extensive educational campaign and distribution of free window guards in New York City in 1976 resulted in 96% reduction of unintentional window falls [5, 6].

United Arab Emirates is a Middle-East country with a fast economic development characterized by diversification from the oil industry to other sectors, as tourism, retail and manufacturing. The population of the UAE increased rapidly and recently reached over 9 million inhabitants, of whom less than 18% are UAE Nationals [7]. Children less than 15 years old constitute about 20% of the population [7]. The country is a federation of seven emirates (Abu Dhabi, Ajman, Dubai, Fujairah, Ras Al Khaimah, Sharjah, and Umm al-Quwain).

* Correspondence: m.grivna@uaeu.ac.ae
[1]Institute of Public Health, College of Medicine and Health Sciences, UAE University, Al-Ain, United Arab Emirates
Full list of author information is available at the end of the article

Despite improvements in the health care, injuries remain a leading cause of morbidity and mortality in the UAE, especially among children and youth [8]. The injury death rate for children under 15 years old was 13.6 per 100.000 person-years during 2000–2008 [8]. Various ethnic groups with diverse socio-cultural, religious and educational background pose a special challenge for safety promotion in the UAE [8].

Details on child falls from heights in the United Arab Emirates (UAE) are not easily accessible. Our aim was to assess the incidents, activities and risk factors for pediatric falls from windows/balconies in the UAE using newspaper clippings.

Methods

We used a retrospective survey to assess eight UAE national Arabic and English newspapers for reports on unintentional child falls from heights (windows, balconies) at residential buildings during 2005–2016. Children 0–15 years were included. Intentional injuries, as suicide, homicide, and from other buildings (school, hotel) were excluded. We searched newspapers electronically using key words including child/boy/girl/baby/toddler and fall/fell/died and window/balcony/height. A structured data collection form was designed.

Variables collected included demography, location of injury (Emirate), supervision of a child, equipment (furniture), environmental factors (balcony or window, number of floors) and outcome (died on spot, died in the hospital, survived). Nationality was divided into four categories (UAE national, Asian, other Arabs, and others). Four investigators did the search independently checking for completeness of reporting. Data of fall incidents were entered into an Excel sheet. Descriptive analysis was performed. Official letters were written to health authorities (Ministry of Health, Health Authority Abu Dhabi, Dubai Health Authority) in order to obtain mortality and morbidity reports on falls. The websites of health authorities were also checked. We searched also for information about safety policy and interventions.

Fisher's exact test was used to compare categorical data of two or more independent groups. A p value of less than 0.05 was accepted as significant. Data were analyzed using Statistical Package for the Social Sciences (IBM-SPSS version 23.0, Chicago, Il, USA).

Results

Data from health authorities lacked details on personal and environmental risk factors and could not be studied. Newspaper clippings documented 96 fall incidents of children 0–15 years during the study period. After cleaning the data and excluding duplicate cases (3 cases), non-residential cases (1 at hotel, 1 at the airport, 1 at school) and intentional injuries (5 suicides; 3 homicides; 1 child was thrown from window during a fire by a mother), 81 cases were included in the final analysis. Fifty-three percent ($n = 42$) were boys and 4% ($n = 3/75$) were UAE-nationals. Male to female ratio was 1:1.1. The mean (range) age was 4.9 years (1–15) (Fig. 1, Table 1). Forty-nine percent ($n = 39$) were from the Emirate of Sharjah. Thirty-eight (47%) children fell from windows, 36 (44%) from balconies, and 7 (9%) cases were unknown. Twenty-two (27%) children climbed on the furniture placed on a balcony or close to a window.

Information about supervision was available in 43 cases (53%). There was another person present in the apartment when the child fell in 25 cases (31%) mother, father, or both parents in 18/25 cases (72%), grandmother or aunt in 2 cases, maid in 2 cases and older

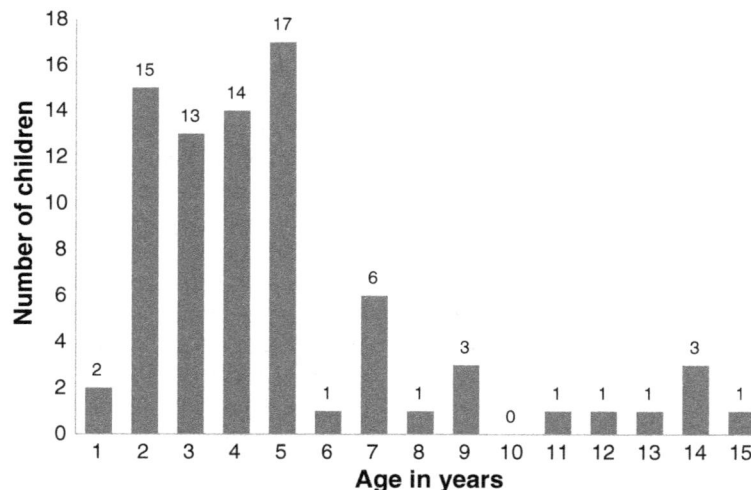

Fig. 1 Pediatric falls from windows/balconies by age ($n = 81$)

Table 1 Demographic variables

Variable		n	%
Gender			
	Male	42	52.5
	Female	38	47.5
Age group			
	0–5	61	77.2
	6–10	11	13.9
	11–15	7	8.9
Nationality			
	UAE	3	4
	Asian	24	32
	Other Arab	40	53.3
	Other	8	10.7
Emirate			
	Sharjah	39	48.7
	Abu Dhabi	16	20
	Dubai	10	12.5
	Ajman	9	11.3
	Fujeirah	4	5
	RAK	2	2.5
Supervision			
	Yes	25	54.3
	No	21	45.7

UAE United Arab Emirates, *RAK* Ras Al Khaimah

sibling in one case). Children were alone in 21 cases. One child was autistic.

Twenty-nine children fell from less than 5 floors (37%), 33 from 5 to 10 floors (42%), and 16 from more than 10 floors (21%) (Fig. 2). Falls were more frequent in May ($n = 12$; 15%) (Fig. 3), in the evening ($n = 19$; 38%), and on Tuesday ($n = 14$; 19%), (Fig. 4). Forty-nine children died on spot (60%), 11 children died in the hospital (13%), and 15 (19%) were hospitalized and survived the fall incident. The place of death was unknown in six children (7%). 6/8 (75%) children falling from 1 to 2 floors survived, 7 out of 26 (26.9%) falling from 3 to 5 floors survived and 2/38 (5.3%) falling from more than 5 floor survived ($p < 0.001$, Fisher's Exact test). We identified local governmental efforts to introduce new building regulations and increase public awareness. Changes in regulations were usually triggered by fatal fall incidents.

Discussion

Children under 5 years old and those living in Sharjah Emirate were at high risk of falling from windows or balconies. Majority of those who fell from higher levels died. Many children were not alone in the apartments when they fell.

The male preponderance has been described in many studies [3, 9–11]. In contrast, our study showed a gender male/female ratio of 1:1.1. UAE-nationals were only 4% of all victims. UAE nationals usually live in villas having less number of floors with better supervision by maids. Similar to others, majority of our cases were children under 5 years of age [3, 9, 12]. Small actively moving children who love to explore things without appreciation

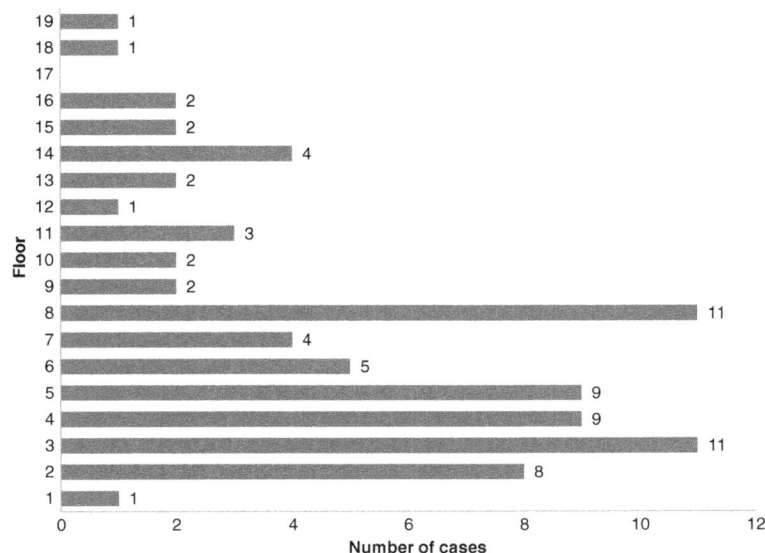

Fig. 2 Pediatric falls from windows/balconies by floor ($n = 78/81$)

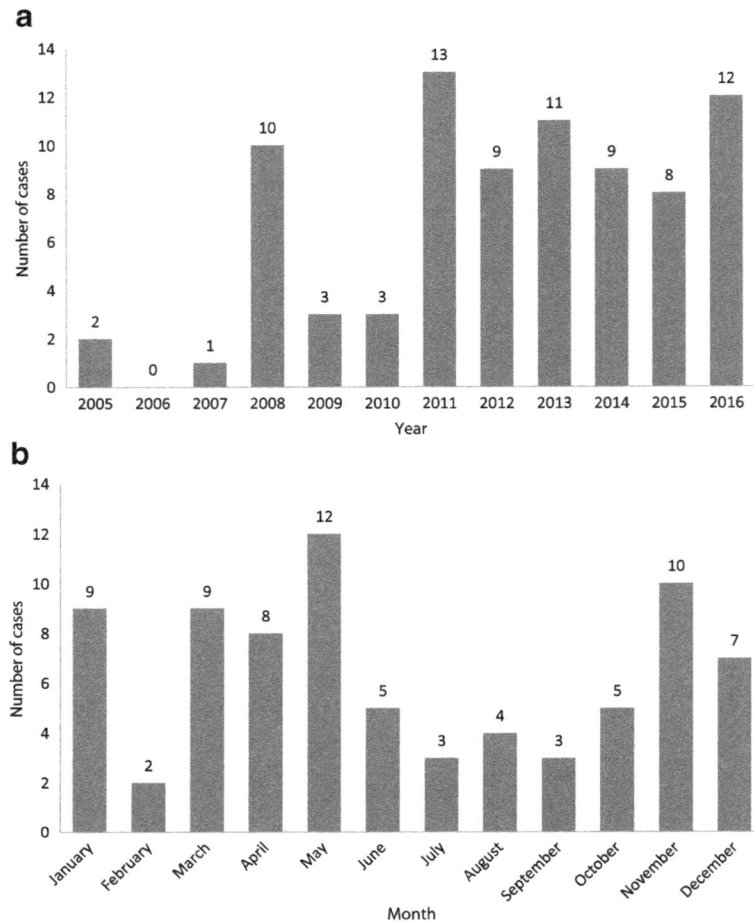

Fig. 3 Pediatric falls from windows/balconies by year (a) and month (b) (n = 77/81)

of risks are more vulnerable to injuries [13]. A small body of a child can easily squeeze through small window gaps or railings of balconies.

The high incidence of falls in Sharjah Emirate can be explained by the high proportion of high buildings, and residents having low socio-economic status. If both parents are working and cannot afford to appoint a maid or if the mother is busy working at home, then there is lack of supervision of children.

Falls are more serious if they are from higher levels [12, 14, 15]. Children who fell from less than two floors in our study had a better chance to survive. Furthermore, kinetic energy absorbing surfaces, such as grass or vegetation may reduce the fall impact [15].

Fall incidents occurred more often in cooler months when there was no need to use air conditioning because families tend to open windows and balconies at that time. In other countries, there were more fall cases during the hot summer, especially among families with low-income living in buildings without air-conditioning [3, 10, 16]. Less falls occurred during the summer in our study. The exceptionally hot weather in our setting discourages opening the windows because of the air-conditioned environment. Furthermore, many families travel overseas for summer holidays.

More incidents occurred during the working days of the week and decreased during the weekends, possibly due to increased supervision by parents and older siblings. The time of incidents differs in the literature. Some studies showed more falls in the afternoon [3, 5], while others in the evening [9].

The information about supervision in newspapers was limited. Nevertheless, many of the children were not alone during the incident similar to a US study, in which more than half the falls occurred when a parent was at home [3]. In another study from Switzerland, the supervising person did not see the fall of the child. The child was left alone at home or left unattended for a short period of time [11]. Parents, maids, or siblings may have difficulty to watch children all the time. They may be distracted by other activities. Many parents undermine the importance of limiting access of children to

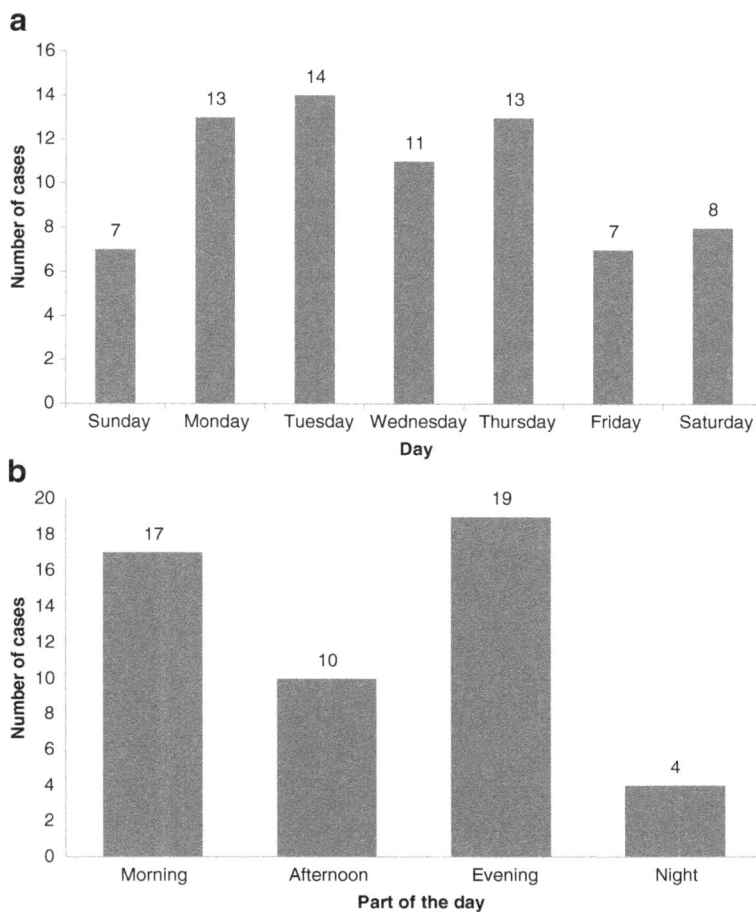

Fig. 4 Pediatric falls from windows/balconies by day of the week (a) and part of the day (b) (*n* = 77/81; 24/81)

balconies or windows. One alarming case study occurred when police saved a child sitting at the kitchen window by breaking into the apartment. The police warned the parents. Nevertheless, the same child fell to death from the balcony later on [17].

Our data suggest that furniture placed near a window or at a balcony is a contributing risk factor for falls, because the child has an easier access to the window. This was reported by others [3, 11, 16].

The government, municipalities, police, and building construction sectors in the UAE reacted to the fall incidents and have made active efforts to reduce the burden of falls over the last few years. This included introduction of new building and construction laws, enforcement of window guards, requiring minimum heights for railing at balconies, and educational campaigns. The challenge remains with the high turn-over of working expatriate families having different educational, cultural and socio-economic background, and various languages. The broad base public education should not focus only on parents, but also on maids, building owners, and managers [15].

Limitations of the study

We have to acknowledge that there are certain limitations of our study. There is debate about the value of using newspaper clippings for injury prevention [18–20]. Despite that debate, we can observe the high precision of information on the floor level from which children fell and their associated mortality. We could not previously reach that level of accuracy in our prospectively collected data of a trauma registry [21]. We have previously studied charts of pediatric injured patients who fell from height and found that detailed information on risk factors was missing [22]. Furthermore, 60% of our cases in the present study died on scene having no hospital charts.

Available data reports on mortality and morbidity is usually lacking details on personal and environmental risk factors which can affect appropriate local prevention strategies. There is no unified health information system in the United Arab Emirates. Every health authority has its own injury data collection.

Although newspaper clippings contained rich information, some cases could have been missed, including less serious cases which may be treated in emergency rooms or hospitals. There is a possibility for selection bias by newspapers as they capture more serious conditions, while milder cases may have survived. Our study population represents only the tip of an iceberg. The exact time of incidents is lacking in our study. We could not also verify the reported information with official death reports. Although death reports in our setting improved by introducing an electronic reporting system, the access to data is limited. Some of our unintentional falls could be cases of child abuse or may include suicide attempts, especially among older children.

Conclusions

Newspaper clippings proved to be useful to study national pediatric falls from heights. It is necessary to improve window safety by installing window guards and raising awareness among parents, maids, and building owners and managers.

Acknowledgements
Not applicable.

Authors' contributions
MG did the newsletter search, analyzed data, drafted the manuscript, and approved the final version for submission. HMA, MRA, and NNA were working together on the newsletter search did partial data analysis, critically reviewed, and approved final version of manuscript for submissions. FMA helped in data analysis, drafted with MG the manuscript, and approved the final version for submission.

Competing interests
All authors declare that they have no competing interests.

Author details
[1]Institute of Public Health, College of Medicine and Health Sciences, UAE University, Al-Ain, United Arab Emirates. [2]Medical Student, College of Medicine and Health Sciences, UAE University, Al-Ain, United Arab Emirates. [3]Department of Surgery, College of Medicine and Health Sciences, UAE University, Al-Ain, United Arab Emirates.

References
1. Scuffham P, Chaplin S, Legood R. Incidence and costs of unintentional falls in older people in the United Kingdom. J Epidemiol Community Health. 2003;57:740–4.
2. World Health Organization. WHO global report on falls prevention in older age. Geneva: World Health Organization; 2007.
3. Vish NL, Powell EC, Wiltsek D, Sheehan KM. Pediatric window falls: not just a problem for children in high rises. Inj Prev. 2005;11:300–3.
4. Author unknown. The book of accidents. New Haven: Designed for Young Children; 1830.
5. Spiegel CN, Lindaman FC. Children Can't fly: a program to prevent childhood morbidity and mortality from window falls. Am J Public Health. 1977;12:1143–7.
6. Barlow B, Niemirska M, Gandhi RP, Leblanc W. Ten years of experience with falls from height in children. J Pediatr Surg. 1983;18:509–11.
7. Central Intelligence Agency. The world Factbook 2017. https://www.cia.gov/library/publications/the-world-factbook/geos/ae.html Accessed 6 June 2017.
8. Grivna M, Aw TC, El-Sadeg M, Loney T, Sharif A, Thomsen J, et al. The legal framework and initiatives for promoting safety in the United Arab Emirates. Int J Inj Control Saf Promot. 2012;19:278–89.
9. Istre GR, McCoy MA, Stowe M, Davies K, Zane D, Anderson RJ, et al. Childhood injuries due to falls from apartment balconies. Inj Prev. 2003;9:349–52.
10. Pressley JC, Barlow B. Child and adolescent injury as a result of falls from buildings and structures. Inj Prev. 2005;11:267–73.
11. Mayer L, Meuli M, Lis U, Frey B. The silent epidemic of falls from buildings: analysis of risk factors. Pediatr Surg Int. 2006;22:743–8.
12. Freyne B, Doyle J, McNAmara R, Nicholson AJ. Epidemiology of high falls from windows in children. Ir Med J. 2014;2:57–9.
13. Melo JRT, Di Rocco F, Lemos-Junior LP, Roujeau T, Thelot B, Sainte-Rose C, et al. Defenestration in children younger than 6 years old: mortality predictors in severe head trauma. Childs Nerv Syst. 2009;25:1077–83.
14. Khambalia A, Joshi P, Brussoni M, Raina P, Morrngiello B, McArthur C. Risk factors for unintentional injuries due to falls in children aged 0-6 years: a systematic review. Inj Prev. 2006;12:378–81.
15. American Academy of Pediatrics, Committee on Injury and Poison Prevention. Falls from heights: windows, roofs and balconies. Pediatrics. 2001;107:1188–91.
16. Hussain N, Mewasingh L, Gosalakkal J. Is the heat wave increasing the number of falls from open windows among children? Arch Dis Child. 2007;92:90.
17. Gulf News. Parents of toddler who fell from building face jail. 2012. http://gulfnews.com/news/uae/emergencies/parents-of-toddler-who-fell-from-building-face-jail-1.976534. Accessed 6 June 2017.
18. Barss P, Subait OM, Ali MHA, Grivna M. Drowning in a high-income developing country in the Middle East: newspapers as an essential resource for injury surveillance. J Sci Med Sport. 2009;12:164-170.
19. Baullinger J, Quan L, Bennett E, Cummings P, Williams K. Use of Washington state newspapers for submersion injury surveillance. Inj Prev. 2001;7:339–42.
20. Rainey DY, Runyan CW. Newspapers: a source for injury surveillance. Am J Public Health. 1992;82:745–6.
21. Grivna M, Hani OE, Abu-Zidan FM. Epidemiology, morbidity and mortality from fall-related injuries in the United Arab Emirates. Scand J Trauma Resusc Emerg Med. 2014;22:51.
22. Grivna M, Barss P, Stanculescu C, Hani OE, Abu-Zidan FM. Home and other nontraffic injuries among children and youth in a high-income middle eastern country: a trauma registry study. Asia Pac J Public Health. 2015;27:NP1707–18.

27

CD4$^+$CD25$^+$CD127 high cells as a negative predictor of multiple organ failure in acute pancreatitis

Wei Wang[1], He-Ping Xiang[1], Hui-Ping Wang[2], Li-Xin Zhu[3] and Xiao-Ping Geng[4*]

Abstract

Background: It has been suggested that severity of the immune response induced by immune cells is associated with morbidity and mortality from acute pancreatitis. The authors investigated and evaluated the relationship between distinct peripheral lymphocyte subsets at admission and clinical outcome prior to hospital discharge so as to find a predictor to the prognosis of acute pancreatitis in lymphocyte profile.

Methods: Lymphocyte subsets in admission peripheral venous blood were tested through flow cytometry on 48 patients with acute pancreatitis. Clinical data was recorded as well. The primary observational outcomes were multiple organ failure (MOF) and infection.

Results: There was a significant difference in natural killer cells between two subgroups sorted by the presence or absence of infection (25.5 ± 4.47 [95% CI 14.4, 36.6] vs 14.8 ± 7.62 [95% CI 12.5,1 7.1] p = 0.021). Patients who developed MOF had lower CD4 + CD25 + CD127^{high} (4.49 ± 1.5 (MOF) [95% CI 3.83, 5.16] vs 6.57 ± 2.65 (non-MOF) [95% CI 5.5, 7.64] p = 0.002) and higher CD127low/high cell counts (1.35 ± 0.66 [95% CI 1.06, 1.65] vs 0.97 ± 0.44 [95% CI 0.79, 1.15] p = 0.02). MOF patients were significantly older (55 ± 14.58 [95% CI 48.49,61.42] vs 46 ± 15.59 [95% CI 39.39,51.99] p = 0.04), and had higher Acute Physiology and Chronic Health Evaluation IIscores (7 ± 3.66 [95% CI 5.5,7.64] vs 4 ± 2.89 [95% CI 2.45,4.78] p = 0.001) and C reactive protein (100.53 ± 94.38 [95% CI 58.69,142.48] vs 50.8 ± 59.2 [95% CI 26.88,74.71] p = 0.04). In a multivariate regression model, only CD4 + CD25 + CD127^{high} cell was a significant predictor of non-MOF. For the detection of non-MOF, CD4 + CD25 + CD127^{high} cell generated a receiver operating characteristic (ROC) curve with an area under the curve of 0.74.

Conclusion: CD4 + CD25 + CD127^{high} cell at early phase of acute pancreatitis yields good specificity in detecting non-MOF at a suggested cutoff value 6.41%. Patients with fewer natural killer cells may be at risk in developing secondary infection.

Keywords: Acute pancreatitis, Prognosis, Multiple organ failure, CD4 + CD25 + CD127^{high} cell, Regulatory T cell, Natural killer cells

Background

Acute pancreatitis (AP) is an inflammatory disorder associated with high morbidity and mortality rate. The annual incidence of acute pancreatitis ranges from 13 to 45 per 100 000 people [1]. AP is the leading discharge diagnosis in patients admitted with gastrointestinal or liver problems in countries such as the United States [2].

Prognosis of the disease varies widely, from self-limiting to severe or critical, and mortality reaches 30% in severe cases [3].

Irrespective of the etiology of pancreatitis, early pathophysiology events include activation of digestive enzymes by lysosomal hydrolases, autodigestive processes, intraparenchymal inflammatory response and the systemic inflammatory response syndrome (SIRS). The initial protease cascade doesn't necessarily determine the severity of AP [4]. In contrast, evidence is accumulating of a crucial relationship between innate immune components

* Correspondence: xp_geng@163.net
[4]Department of General Surgery, The Second Affiliated Hospital of Anhui Medical University, Hefei 230601, Anhui Province, People's Republic of China
Full list of author information is available at the end of the article

involved in AP pathogenesis and disease severity [5–7]. Neutrophils and macrophages are the first line of the immune system's defense. T-lymphocytes, which are mainly involved in the cell-mediated immune response, also play a vital role in AP [5]. CD4 + T cells increase the severity of AP due to macrophage activation via antigen presentation and pro-inflammatory cytokine release as well as through direct cytotoxicity effects [5]. Immunological suppression mediated by regulatory T cells (Tregs) expressing transcription factor forkhead box P3 (FOXP3) has been reported to be the critical mechanism controlling the inflammatory response for which the immune system is primed after serious injury such as severe AP (SAP) [8]. However, these studies focused on a single lymphocyte subgroup rather than the broad subgroups of lymphocyte in patients with AP.

In present study, we evaluated the relationship between multiple peripheral lymphocyte subsets (i.e., T lymphocyte cells, T Helper cells, cytotoxic T cells, Tregs, activated effector T cells, natural killer (NK) cells and B cells) through flow cytometry done early during hospitalization vs. patient outcome. We then compared the accuracy of activated effector T cells estimation to predict non-MOF with Acute Physiology and Chronic Health Evaluation (APACHE) IIscores and C reactive protein (CRP) estimation of MOF.

Methods

This prospective clinical observational study was performed between June 2015 and August 2015 in the second affiliated hospital of Anhui Medicine University. The study was approved by the hospital's Ethics Committee. Written informed consent was obtained from patient surrogates before study inclusion.

Eligible criteria and treatment

Patients who achieved two of the following three features were diagnosed as having AP and screened for participation in the study: acute epigastric pain with or without radiation through to the back; serum amylase or lipase activity greater than three times the upper limit of normal; and characteristic features on cross-sectional abdominal computer tomography (CT) imaging consistent with the diagnosis of acute pancreatitis [9].Exclusion criteria were: age <18 or >80 years, previous or chronic treatment with immunological suppressants such as cortisone or its analogues, immunodeficiency diseases such as acquired immune deficiency syndrome (AIDS), malignant tumor, ongoing radiotherapy or chemotherapy, pregnancy, or patients without written permission or complete data. Of the 60 cases identified, 48 patients were eligible for inclusion in the study. Among 12 patients who were excluded from the study, 8 patients exceeded the study age limit, 2 patients were pregnant, 1 patient persisted in taking glucocorticoid due to rheumatoid arthritis, and the last one was undergoing chemotherapy after radical gastrectomy.

Eligible patients were included as soon as possible at time of hospital admission. All patients were treated according to standard guidelines including fluid resuscitation, enteral nutrition, endoscopic retrograde cholangiopancreatography (ERCP), catheter drainage (Fig. 1) and necrosectomy when indicated [10].

Sample collection and preparation

Each patient's peripheral venous blood (2 ml) was collected in an anticoagulation tube containing heparin within two hours of admission. Heparin (100ul) was added to each blood sample in 2 tubes separately. Next, 10ul of mixed antibodies was added to one of the tubes. A second control tube was mixed with 10ul Isotype Control Antibodies. The tubes were mixed gently and incubated for 15 min in the dark. A hemolytic agent (0.83% NH_4Cl) was put in 2 tubes and incubated for 10 mins in a 37 °C water bath.

Flow cytometry analysis

Lymphocyte subsets in blood were phenotyped by flow cytometry (Beckman-Coulter, Brea, CA) according to the manufacturer's instructions. We first gated on lymphocytes based on forward scatter and side scatter; >10,000 cells within gate were obtained for every sample. Each antibody was matched with a respective isotype IgG1 as a control, and the gating threshold was set accordingly. Cells were labeled with specific mono-antibodies in different combinations. Lymphocyte subsets were selected for detailed phenotypic analysis as follows: T lymphocyte cells were CD3+ T cells; T Helper cells were CD3 + CD4+ T cells; cytotoxic T cells were CD3 + CD8+ T cells; NK cells were CD3-CD16 + CD56+ T cells; B cells were CD19 + CD20 + CD45+ T cells; Tregs were CD4 + CD25 + CD127^{low} T cells; and activated effector T cells were CD4 + CD25 + CD127^{high} T cells. Representative gating figures are shown in Fig. 2.

Endpoints and outcome assessment

The primary observational endpoints of the study were MOF and infection. Severity of AP was divided into three categories: mild, moderate severity (MSAP), and severe (SAP) according to the new revised Atlanta consensus. Organ failure was defined as a Sepsis-related Organ Failure Assessment (SOFA) score ≥2. MOF was defined as failure of two or more organs [11]. Infection was diagnosed based on ongoing signs of sepsis and/or the combination of clinical signs and CT imaging when extra-luminal gas was present within areas of necrosis in the pancreatic and/or peri-pancreatic tissues (Fig. 1). Balthazar scores were used to assess the extent of local inflammatory changes [1]. Second study endpoints were

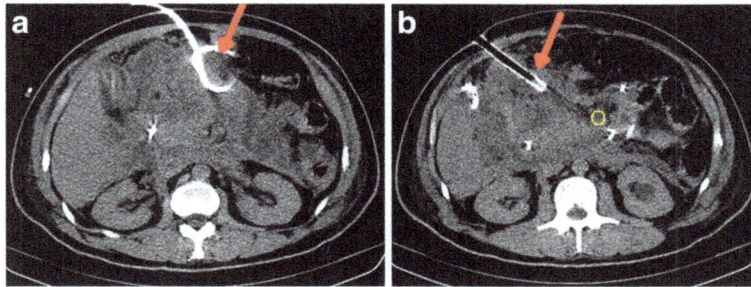

Fig. 1 A 28-year-old man with acute necrotizing pancreatitis complicated by infected pancreatic necrosis requiring multiple percutaneous catheter drainage (red arrow in A and B). There is a large heterogeneous area of necrosis in the pancreatic and peri-pancreatic area with impacted gas bubbles (yellow ring in B)

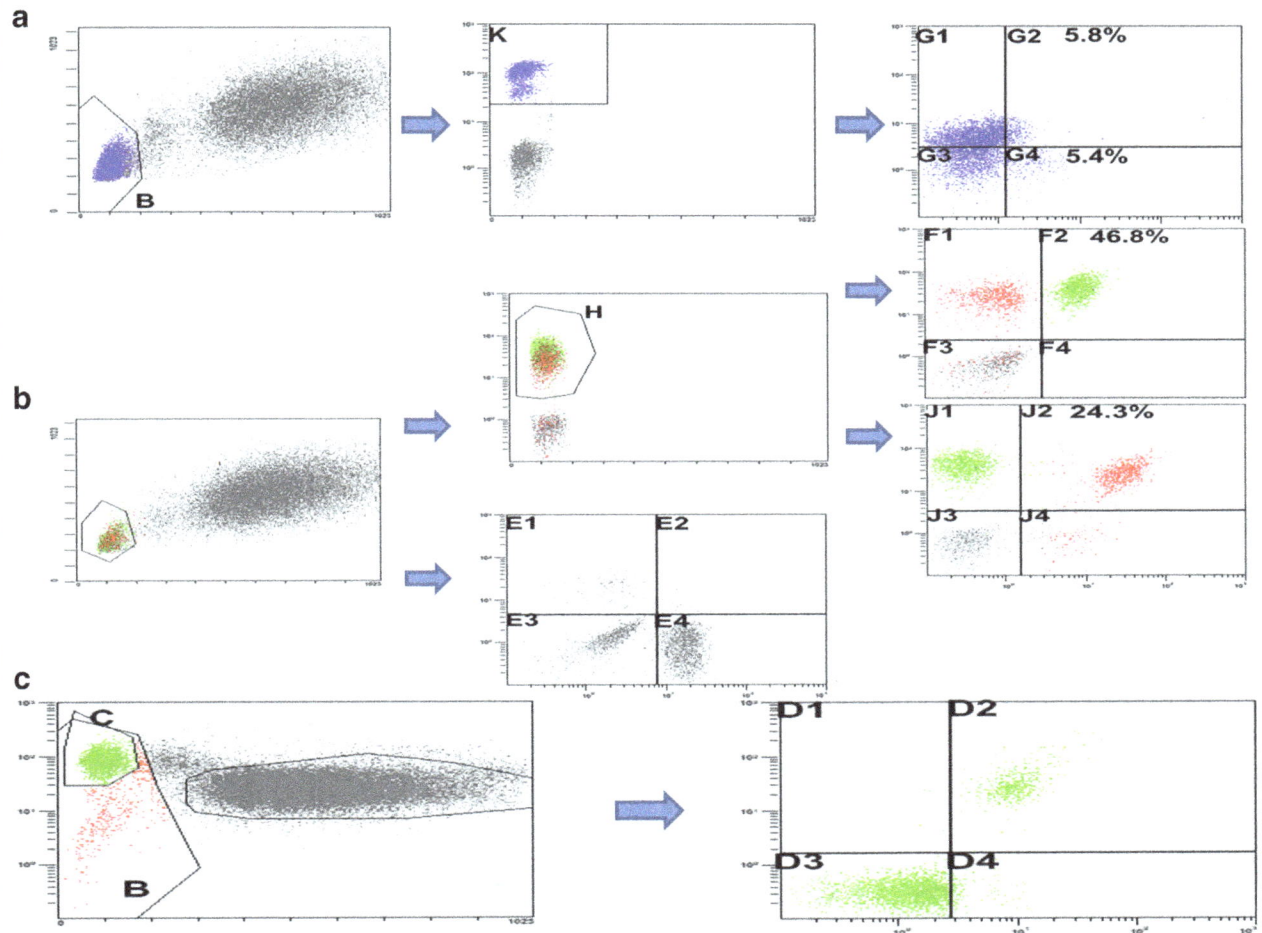

Fig. 2 Gating strategy of peripheral lymphocyte population (**a**) Gating strategy for CD4+ T cell subdivided into CD4 + CD25 + CD127^{low} and CD4 + CD25 + CD127^{high} subpopulation. B indicate lymphocyte divided from leukocyte based on forward scatter and side scatter, K indicate CD4+ T cells, G2 indicate CD4 + CD25 + CD127^{high} cells and G4 CD4 + CD25 + CD127^{low} cells. **b** Gating strategy for lymphocyte subdivided into T Helper cells, cytotoxic T cells and NK cells subpopulation. H indicate CD3+ T cells, F2 indicate CD3 + CD4+ T cells and J2 CD3 + CD8+ T cells, E1 indicate CD3-CD16 + CD56+ cells which were divided from CD3- T cells. **c** Gating strategy for B cells. C indicate lymphocyte divided from leukocyte according to CD45 and side scatter. D2 indicate CD19 + CD20 + CD45+ cells

mortality before discharge and intensive care unit (ICU) length of stay (LOS).

We recorded demographic data, comorbid, clinical laboratory values, treatment procedure and outcome and calculated the APACHE II score, SOFA score and Balthazar score in the first 24 h after admission. All data were entered into a secure and pre-established case report form by trained research assistants.

Statistical analysis

The study population was characterized using descriptive statistics. Categorical variables are provided as counts with frequencies and continuous variables as means with standard deviations (SD) or medians with quartiles depending on the normality of the data. Kolmgorov-Smirnov test was used to test the normal distribution of the data.

Group comparisons used the Student t-test for continuous variables, Chi-square for categorical data, and the ANOVA test and Mann–Whitney test for ordinal data. Spearman correlation analysis was used to determine the degree of relationship between lymphocytes substrate and other laboratory values and scores. Binary logistic regression was used for multivariate analysis. Only variables which were significantly associated with primary outcomes (including MOF and infection in univariate analysis) were introduced into the multivariate logistic model. Receiving operator characteristic (ROC) curves were generated with corresponding area under curve (AUC) analysis and computation of 95% confidence intervals (CI). The AUC was calculated as a measure of the ability for each marker to distinguish between groups. The optimum predictor cut-off was calculated as a trade-off between sensitivity and specificity. All hypothesis tests were two-sided, with a significance level of $p < 0.05$. Statistical analyses were performed using SPSS version 19.0 (IBM, Chicago, IL).

Results

Patient characteristics

The study included 48 patients. No patients were lost to follow up and no included patients had incomplete clinical data. The mean age for the complete study population was 50 (SD: 16) years and 26 (54%) were male. Gallstones were the major cause of AP with an incidence of 39.6%. Baseline patient characteristics including laboratory tests at admission are presented in Table 1. Three (6.25%) patients developed infection and presented with sepsis and pancreatic abscess (Fig. 1). All recovered fully after receiving appropriate antibiotics and multiple percutaneous, CT-guided external drainages (Fig. 1). All abscess pathogens were confirmed Gram-negative bacteria including Escherichia coli and Enterococcus faecium. Twenty-two patients (45.8%) developed subsequent MOF. One of these patients (2%) died before hospital discharge. Median hospital LOS was 10 days.

Table 1 Selected baseline characters of the study patients[abc]

Age(years)	50 ± 16
Male sex	26(54.17%)
Etiology	
gallstone	19(39.6%)
hypertriglyceride	15(31.2%)
alcohol	4(8.3%)
idiopathic	10(20.9%)
Category	
MAP	21(43.8%)
MSAP	19(39.6%)
SAP	8(16.6%)
Amylase(IU) at admission	720(349.5–1581.25)
CRP(mg/L) at admission	73.59 ± 80.44
Comorbidities	17(35.42%)
APACHEIIscores at enrollment	5.19 ± 3.66
SOFA scores at enrollment	2(1–3)
Balthazar scores at enrollment	2(2–3.75)
Lymphocyte (%)	16.24 ± 9.60
Lymphocyte subsets	
B cell (%)	7.84 ± 5.89
T cell (%)	68.92 ± 9.69
Helper T cell (%)	42.65 ± 11.31
Cytotoxic T cell (%)	23.38 ± 7.46
NK cell (%)	15.49 ± 7.88
Tregs (%)	5.55 ± 1.69
Activated effector T cell (%)	5.62 ± 2.42
CD4+/CD8+	2.13 ± 1.18
CD127low/high	1.15 ± 0.58

[a]Categorical variables are presented as count (frequency) and continues variables as mean (standard deviation) or median (quartiles) depending on the normality of the data
[b]CRP: C-reactive protein, APACHE: Acute Physiology and Chronic Health Evaluation, Tregs: T regular cell
[c]the value of the lymphocyte subsets including B cell, T cell, Helper T cell, Cytotoxic T cell, NK cell is the percentage to total lymphocytes. Whereas the value of two subsets including Treg cell and activated effector T cell is the percentage to helper T cell

Univariate analysis

Patients were stratified to two subgroups based on the presence or absence of MOF and infection, and the clinical variables were compared between subgroups. Figure 3 shows that NK cells increased significantly in the infection subgroup ($p = 0.021$). Activated effector T cells were significantly decreased in the MOF subgroup ($p = 0.002$) while the ratio of CD4 + CD25 + CD127^{low} and CD4 + CD25 + CD127^{high} subsets (CD127low/CD127high) was significantly increased in the MOF subgroup ($p = 0.02$). There was no difference in other lymphocytes subsets between subgroups. Patients in the MOF subgroup were older ($p = 0.04$) and had higher APACHEIIscores

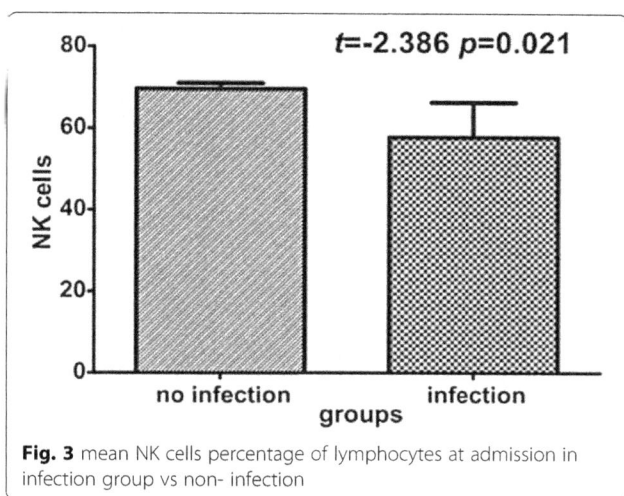

Fig. 3 mean NK cells percentage of lymphocytes at admission in infection group vs non- infection

(p = 0.001) and CRP (p = 0.04) (Table 2). There were no associations between LOS and either MOF (rho = 0.084 p = 0.573) or infection (rho = 0.213 p = 0.147).

Multivariate analysis for MOF

Multivariate logistic regression was performed adjusting for the effects of potentially confounding variables to predict MOF as a function of activated effector T cells, CD127low/high, and age. These variables were selected by investigating the association of all variables in Table 2 with MOF and selecting variables with significant associations as potential confounders. Using this multivariate regression model, only the variable, activated effector T cells (OR = 0.564 p = 0.042 95% CI [0.324, 0.98]), was a significant negative predictor of MOF (Table 3).

ROC Curve of activated effector T cells in Predicting non-MOF and APACHEIIscores and CRP in predicting MOF

Figure 4 illustrates the superiority of activated effector T cells (area under the curve 0.74) in predicting non-MOF. Activated effector T cells at 6.41% could be used as a cut-off point to predict non-MOF with a sensitivity of 53.8%, specificity of 90.9%. In contrast, both

Table 2 Univariate analysis of selected variables between subgroups sorting with MOF

	MOF (n = 22)	Non-MOF (n = 26)	P value
Age(years)	55 ± 14.58	46 ± 15.59	0.04
APACHEIIscores	7 ± 3.66	4 ± 2.89	0.001
CRP(mg/L)	100.53 ± 94.38	50.8 ± 59.2	0.04
Tregs (%)	5.51 ± 1.87	5.59 ± 1.56	0.879
Activated effector T cell (%)	4.49 ± 1.5	6.57 ± 2.65	0.002
CD4+/CD8+	2.2 ± 1.34	2.07 ± 1.04	0.71
CD127low/high	1.35 ± 0.66	0.97 ± 0.44	0.02

CRP C-reactive protein, *APACHE* Acute Physiology and Chronic Health Evaluation, *Tregs* T regular cell, *MOF* multiple organ failure

Table 3 Multiple logistic regression model for MOF

predictor	Frequency of MOF		
	OR	95%CI	P value
age	1.044	0.996–1.094	0.073
Activated effector T cell (%)	0.564	0.324–0.98	0.042
CD127low/high	0.881	0.156–4.977	0.886

MOF multiple organ failure

APACHEIIand CRP exhibited powerful ability to predict MOF with areas under the curves of 0.802 and 0.701, respectively, indicating that the former was superior than the latter based on the ROC curves (Fig. 5).

Discussion

The principle findings of our study are: (1) among peripheral lymphocyte subsets, only activated effector T cells phenotyped by CD4 + CD25 + CD127^{high} have a significant negative correlation with MOF and can be used as a predictor of non-MOF estimation in AP; and (2) there is a statistically significant association between NK cells at admission and secondary infection.

AP can present as a severe acute abdominal disease with a high mortality. Patients with AP can develop an early-onset phase of SIRS within 2 weeks, and/or an infection phase due to pancreatic necrosis. MOF and/or infection signal the presence of severe disease, and there is a high risk of death if both are present [11]. Thus, both MOF and infection are unfavorable prognostic signs in AP patients.

In the present study, we did not find correlations between activated effector T cells and both SOFA scores and Balthazar scores (r = –0.276 p = 0.058 and r = –0.140 p = 0.342 respectively). In contrast, there were correlations between activated effector T cells and both APACHE IIscores and CRP. Furthermore, there were significant differences in the level of activated effector T cells among three subgroups stratified by Revision of Atlanta criteria (F = 5.26 p = 0.009), and the severe AP patients had the lowest level of activated effector T cells (5.36% ± 1.31%). From the result, it was demonstrated that activated effector T cells enrollment was in accordance with Ranking criteria, APACHE IIscores and CRP rather than Balthazar scores and SOFA scores. Balthazar scores based on the CT findings focus on local complications of AP and it is hard to reflect the systematic immunology condition. In terms of SOFA scores, it is not a normal clinical predictor in assessing severity of AP. considering the potential confounding bias caused by accumulative SOFA scores, it was just utilized for judging whether it was MOF individually in the present study.

An accurate predictor to prognosis would be helpful for clinicians by allowing patients with a predicted

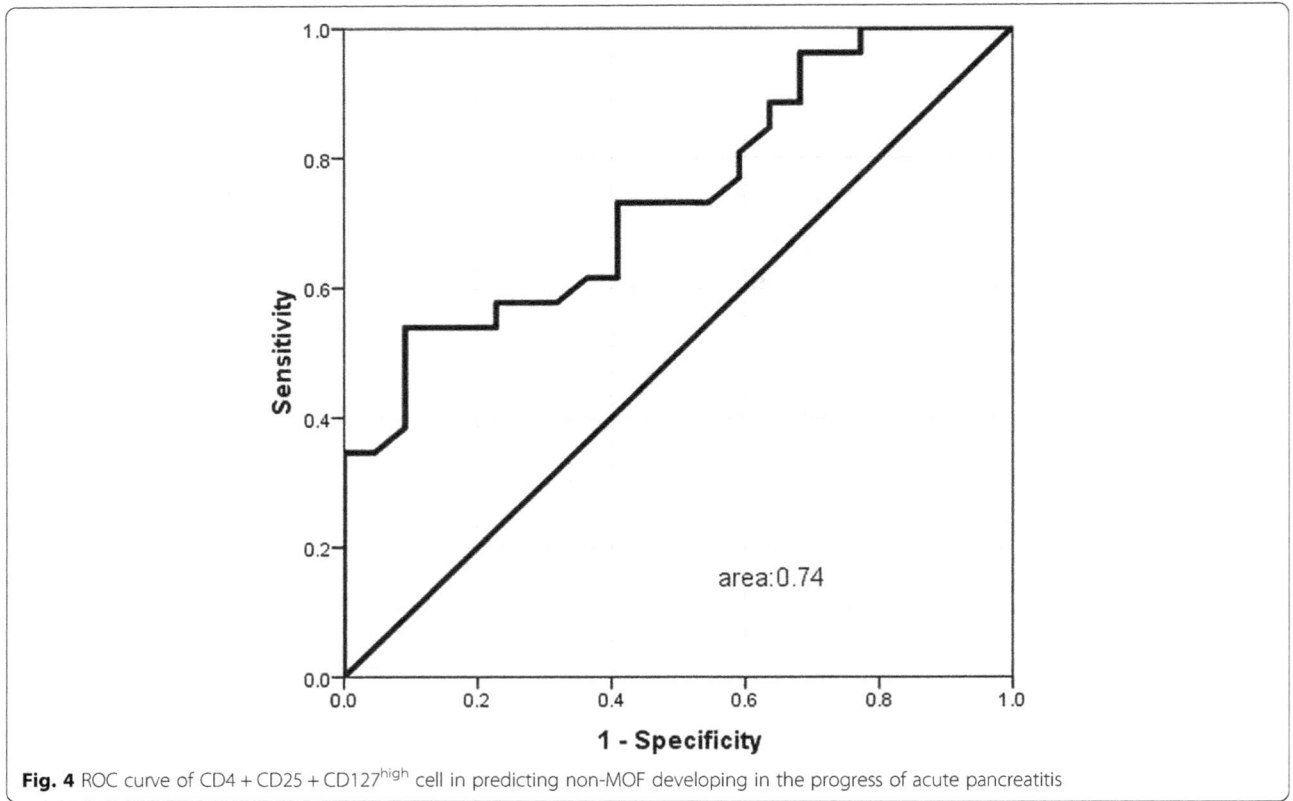

Fig. 4 ROC curve of CD4 + CD25 + CD127^high cell in predicting non-MOF developing in the progress of acute pancreatitis

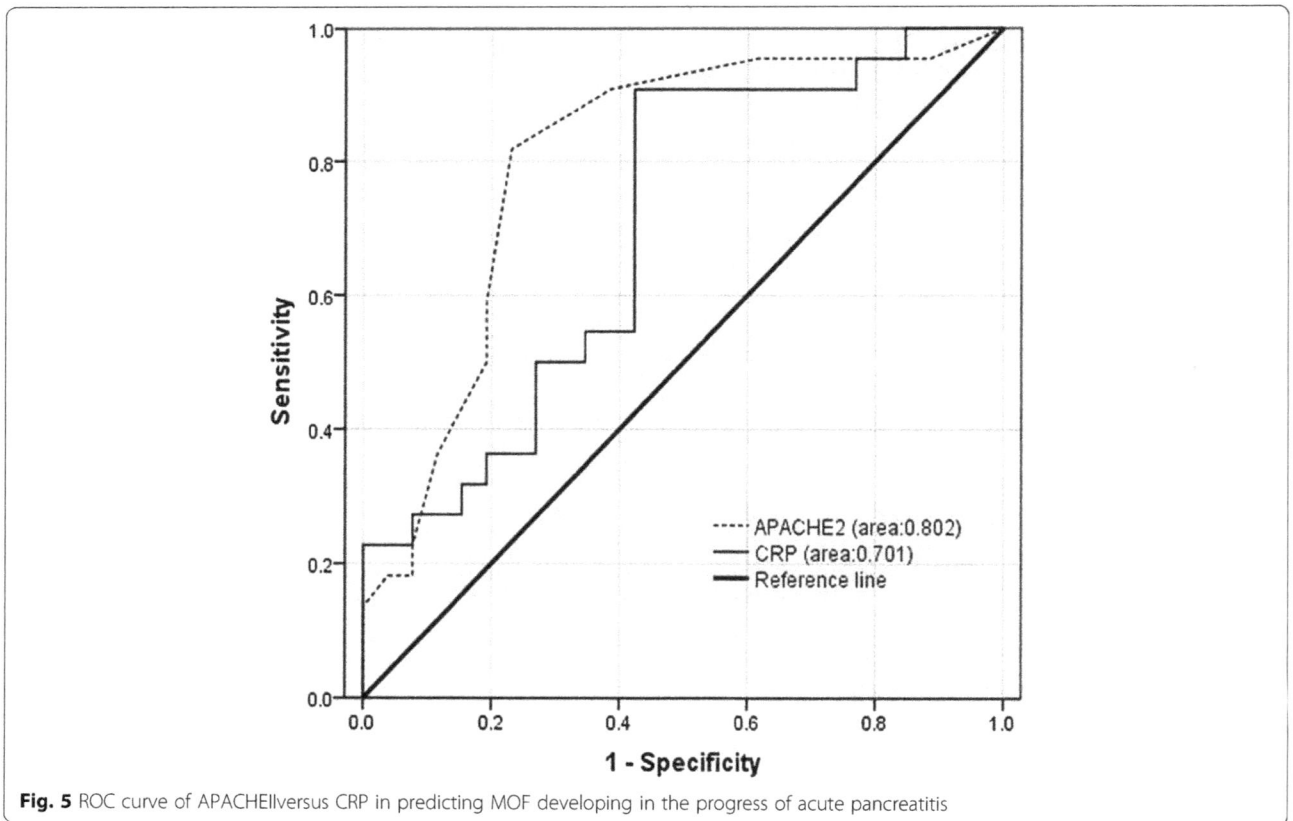

Fig. 5 ROC curve of APACHEIIversus CRP in predicting MOF developing in the progress of acute pancreatitis

severe course to be transferred to an intensive care unit while patients with a predicted mild course may be treated in an outpatient setting. Severity scoring systems such as APACHEIIand laboratory testing such as CRP have been used to accurately predict an unfavorable outcome, which we have confirmed in the present study [12, 13]. However, there has not been a validated, published strategy to predict a favorable outcome, which is important to avoid overtreatment. In the present study, only a special T cell subset called CD4 + CD25 + CD127^{high} cells using the cutoff value >6.41% at admission was a statistically significant negative predictor of AP severity upon patient presentation to the hospital. Even though this predictor had a low sensitivity of 53.8%, we believe that the specificity of such a value is of more clinical importance than its sensitivity because conservative and supportive management is the initial care for patients with AP and it seems unnecessary to apply drastic remedies for those with higher CD4 + CD25 + CD127^{high} cells. This test's potential as a superior predictor of a favorable prognosis will require confirmation in a larger population.

Lymphocytes play important roles in both adaptive and innate immune responses. The main function of the lymphocytic immune response is to mediate and resolve the nonspecific inflammatory process in AP. CD4+ T cells may act as co-stimulators for macrophage activation via antigen presentation and pro-inflammatory cytokine release as well as through direct cytotoxic effects (on acini) through Fas ligand expression on CD4+ T cells [14]. In addition, a distinct set of CD4 + CD25 + FOXP3 + Tregs presenting immunological tolerance and homeostasis have been identified with anti-inflammatory functions in AP [15]. These cells could bind to multiple effector immune cells and prevent their secretion of cytokines. They also secrete anti-inflammatory cytokines such as interleukin (IL)-10 and transforming growth factor (TGF)-β. Tregs have also been reported to restrain SIRS [16]. It was impossible to purify living Tregs in vivo previously because of the exclusive intracellular expression of FOXP3 as a critical factor for Tregs function. Recently, CD127 (IL-7 receptor a chain), whose expression was reverse to FOXP3, was recommended as an marker of Treg and has confirmed superiority compared to other cell surface markers [17, 18]. As indicated in previous study, serum sCD163, a biomarker released from macrophages, was increased in AP, but not associate with disease severity [19]. In present study, we used the sorting strategy of combining CD4+, CD25+, and CD127low to obtain viable, expandable Treg cells. There was no significant difference in Tregs between the two groups statistically, and we also found the mean number of Tregs as a percentage of CD4+ T cells was 5.55 ± 1.69%, which was a little lower than the 6.25 ± 0.26% in healthy people reported in previous research [18].

Prior studies have come to different conclusions regarding variation of Tregs in SIRS or the early phase of AP. Xue H et al. [20] reported that CD4 + CD25 + Tregs increased in SIRS and suppressed the excessive inflammatory response. In contrast, other investigators have reported that positive CD4 + CD25+ T cells significantly declined in a mouse SAP model [8]. Data on Tregs in humans with AP is limited and our data may be of value as a reference for future study.

Interestingly, the novel subgroup CD4 + CD25 + CD127^{high} cells had predictive value for the development of non-MOF in this investigation. This subset was previously thought to be a contaminant interfering with the suppressive function of Tregs and was neglected previously.[18] However, research by Michel L indicates that this specific population in multiple sclerosis (MS) appears more proliferative and secretes more interferon-γ (IFN-γ) and interleukin-2 (IL-2), both pro-inflammatory cytokines, than healthy individuals [21]. Similar observation has been made in CD4 + CD25 + CD127^{high} cells infiltrating rejected human allografts, in which allo-specific CD4 + CD25 + CD127^{high} cells were able to secrete effector cytokines such as tumor necrosis factor-α (TNF-α) and IFN-γ [22]. The ratio of CD127low/high also was statistically different in subgroups with and without MOF, but had no correlation with MOF in our multivariate regression model. Thus, CD4 + CD25 + CD127^{high} cells counts may be the sole factor which are associated with MOF estimation, and it is postulated that increment of CD4 + CD25 + CD127^{high} cells have a protective function to reflect the progress of AP independent of Tregs. The exact mechanism of CD4 + CD25 + CD127^{high} cell function in the setting of AP needs further study.

NK cells with phenotype marker CD3-CD16 + CD56+ are the type of cytotoxic lymphocytes critical to the innate immune system and secrete TNF-α and IFN-γ to control viral infection [23]. Dabrowski A et al. [24] found a dramatic depletion of peripheral NK cells in SAP compared to MAP and control, which indicates that there may be a correlation between NK cells and severity of AP. Our research further found that a lower number of NK cells at admission were associated with the development of secondary infection in AP patients. Since most pathogens causing secondary pancreatic infection are Gram-negative bacteria such as Escherichia coli originating from gut [25], we hypothesize that once circulating NK cells run into Gram-negative bacteria in a primary infection, they acquire memory function features which are a hallmark of T and B cells belonging to the adaptive immune system [26]. The memory-like, circulating NK cells then migrate into the pancreas at the early onset of AP and trigger a rapid immune response to the same antigen encountered again. In any case, patients with lower NK cells at admission may have a high risk of developing secondary infection in AP.

Limitations

Specific limitations need to be considered when interpreting results of our study. First, the number of study patients included ($n = 48$) and infection group ($n = 3$) was low. Furthermore, sepsis in the secondary progression of AP also triggers MOF which is more likely to happen due to SIRS in the first phase. The selection bias without intent may affect extrapolation of our outcomes, especially regarding the predictor role of activated effector T cells to non-MOF. Nonetheless, statistical significance was achieved for several analyses suggesting that these relationships could be clinically relevant. Second, the observational nature of this study indicated that relationships between dependent and independent variables are associations, and not cause and effect. Third, a separate test might be needed in different phases of the disease because of the essential dynamic progress of immune function during the development of AP. The present study did not dynamically investigate the immune function. Therefore, it can't reflect comprehensive immunological fluctuation.

Conclusion

Increased peripheral CD4 + CD25 + CD127^{high} cells, whose physiological role in the early phase of AP is unclear in the early phase of AP, appear to be associated with a good (non-MOF) prognosis. In addition, patients with lower NK cells at admission may have a higher risk of developing secondary infection in AP. Further study is needed to confirm these observations.

Abbreviations

AIDS: Acquired immune deficiency syndrome; AP: Acute pancreatitis; APACHE: Acute Physiology and Chronic Health Evaluation; CD: Cluster of differentiation; CRP: C reactive protein; CT: Computer tomography; FOXP3: Forkhead box P3; ICU: Intensive care unit; IFN-γ: Interferon-γ; IL: Interleukin; LOS: Length of stay; MOF: Multiple organ failure; NK: Natural killer; ROC: Receiver operating characteristic; SIRS: Systemic inflammatory response syndrome; SOFA: Sepsis-related Organ Failure Assessment; TGF: Transforming growth factor; TNF: Tumor necrosis factor.; Tregs: Regulatory T cells

Acknowledgements

Not applicable.

Funding

The study was funded by Natural Science Foundation of Anhui Province (1508085SMH225).

Author contributions

Wang W, Zhu LX and Geng XP conceived and designed the study. Wang W, Xiang HP collected and assembled data. Wang HP performed flow cytometry analysis. Wang W performed data analysis and interpretation. Wang W contributed to manuscript writing. All authors read and approved the final version of the manuscript.

Competing interests

The authors declare that they have no competing interests.

Author details

[1]Department of Emergency Surgery, The Second Affiliated Hospital of Anhui Medical University, 678 Furong Road, Hefei 230601, Anhui Province, People's Republic of China. [2]Hematology department, The Second Affiliated Hospital of Anhui Medical University, Hefei 230601, Anhui Province, People's Republic of China. [3]Central lab of the First Affiliated Hospital of Anhui Medical University, Hefei 230022, Anhui Province, People's Republic of China. [4]Department of General Surgery, The Second Affiliated Hospital of Anhui Medical University, Hefei 230601, Anhui Province, People's Republic of China.

References

1. Lankisch PG, Apte M, Banks PA. Acute pancreatitis. Lancet. 2015;386:85–96.
2. Peery AF, Dellon ES, Lund J, Crockett SD, McGowan CE, Bulsiewicz WJ, et al. Burden of gastrointestinal disease in the United States: 2012 update. Gastroenterology. 2012;143:1179–87. e1-3.
3. Gravante G, Garcea G, Ong SL, Metcalfe MS, Berry DP, Lloyd DM, et al. Prediction of mortality in acute pancreatitis: a systematic review of the published evidence. Pancreatology. 2009;9:601–14.
4. Dawra R, Sah RP, Dudeja V, Rishi L, Talukdar R, Garg P, et al. Intra-acinar trypsinogen activation mediates early stages of pancreatic injury but not inflammation in mice with acute pancreatitis. Gastroenterology. 2011;141:2210–7. e2.
5. Zheng L, Xue J, Jaffee EM, Habtezion A. Role of immune cells and immune-based therapies in pancreatitis and pancreatic ductal adenocarcinoma. Gastroenterology. 2013;144:1230–40.
6. Kylanpaa ML, Repo H, Puolakkainen PA. Inflammation and immunosuppression in severe acute pancreatitis. World J Gastroenterol. 2010;16:2867–72.
7. Sun J, Bhatia M. Blockade of neurokinin-1 receptor attenuates CC and CXC chemokine production in experimental acute pancreatitis and associated lung injury. Am J Physiol Gastrointest Liver Physiol. 2007;292:G143–53.
8. Zheng YS WZ, Zhang LY, Ke L, Li WQ, Li N, Li JS. Nicotine ameliorates experimental severe acute pancreatitis via enhancing immunoregulation of CD4+ CD25+regulatory T cells. Pancreas. 2015;44:500–6.
9. Sarr MG, Banks PA, Bollen TL, Dervenis C, Gooszen HG, Johnson CD, et al. The new revised classification of acute pancreatitis 2012. Surg Clin North Am. 2013;93:549–62.
10. Working Group IAPAPAAPG. IAP/APA evidence-based guidelines for the management of acute pancreatitis. Pancreatology. 2013. doi:10.1016/j.pan.2013.07.063.
11. Petrov MS, Shanbhag S, Chakraborty M, Phillips ARJ, Windsor JA. Organ Failure and Infection of Pancreatic Necrosis as Determinants of Mortality in Patients With Acute Pancreatitis. Gastroenterology. 2010;139:813–20.
12. Liu Y, Wang L, Cai Z, Zhao P, Peng C, Zhao L, et al. The Decrease of Peripheral Blood CD4+ T Cells Indicates Abdominal Compartment Syndrome in Severe Acute Pancreatitis. PloS one. 2015. doi:10.1371/journal.pone.0135768.
13. Freeman ML, Werner J, van Santvoort HC, Baron TH, Besselink MG, Windsor JA, et al. Interventions for necrotizing pancreatitis: summary of a multidisciplinary consensus conference. Pancreas. 2012;41:1176–94.
14. Pezzilli R, Billi P, Gullo L, Beltrandi E, Maldini M, Mancini R, et al. Behavior of serum soluble interleukin-2 receptor, soluble CD8 and soluble CD4 in the early phases of acute pancreatitis. Digestion. 1994;55:268–73.
15. Chinen T, Volchkov PY, Chervonsky AV, Rudensky AY. A critical role for regulatory T cell-mediated control of inflammation in the absence of commensal microbiota. J Exp Med. 2010;207:2323–30.
16. Jia W, Cao L, Yang S, Dong H, Zhang Y, Wei H, et al. Regulatory T cells are protective in systemic inflammation response syndrome induced by zymosan in mice. PloS one. 2013. doi:10.1371/journal.pone.0064936.
17. Liu W, Putnam AL, Xu-Yu Z, Szot GL, Lee MR, Zhu S, et al. CD127 expression inversely correlates with FoxP3 and suppressive function of human CD4+ T reg cells. J Exp Med. 2006;203:1701–11.
18. Seddiki N, Santner-Nanan B, Martinson J, Zaunders J, Sasson S, Landay A, et al. Expression of interleukin (IL)-2 and IL-7 receptors discriminates between human regulatory and activated T cells. J Exp Med. 2006;203:1693–700.

19. Xue H, Wang W, Li Y, Shan Z, Li Y, Teng X, et al. Selenium upregulates CD4(+)CD25(+) regulatory T cells in iodine-induced autoimmune thyroiditis model of NOD. H-2(h4) mice. Endocr J. 2010;57:595–601.

20. Karrasch T, Brünnler T, Hamer OW, Schmid K, Voelk M, Herfarth H, et al. Soluble CD163 is increased in patients with acute pancreatitis independent of disease severity. Exp Mol Pathol. 2015;99:236–9.

21. Michel L, Berthelot L, Pettre S, Wiertlewski S, Lefrere F, Braudeau C, et al. Patients with relapsing-remitting multiple sclerosis have normal Treg function when cells expressing IL-7 receptor alpha-chain are excluded from the analysis. J Clin Invest. 2008;118:3411–9.

22. Codarri L, Vallotton L, Ciuffreda D, Venetz JP, Garcia M, Hadaya K, et al. Expansion and tissue infiltration of an allospecific CD4 + CD25 + CD45RO + IL-7Ralphahigh cell population in solid organ transplant recipients. J Exp Med. 2007;204:1533–41.

23. Rehermann B. Natural Killer Cells in Viral Hepatitis. Cell Mol Gastroenterol Hepatol. 2015;1:578–88.

24. Dabrowski A, Osada J, Dabrowska MI. Wereszczynska-Siemiatkowska U. Monocyte Subsets and Natural Killer Cells in Acute Pancreatitis. Pancreatology. 2008;8:126–34.

25. Frossard JL, Steer ML, Pastor CM. Acute pancreatitis. Lancet. 2008;371:143–52.

26. Rolle A, Pollmann J, Cerwenka A. Memory of infections: an emerging role for natural killer cells. PLoS Pathog. 2013. doi:10.1371/journal.ppat.1003548.

28

Effect of resuscitative endovascular balloon occlusion of the aorta in hemodynamically unstable patients with multiple severe torso trauma

Hiroyuki Otsuka*, Toshiki Sato, Keiji Sakurai, Hiromichi Aoki, Takeshi Yamagiwa, Shinichi Iizuka and Sadaki Inokuchi

Abstract

Background: Although resuscitative endovascular balloon occlusion of the aorta (REBOA) may be effective in trauma management, its effect in patients with severe multiple torso trauma remains unclear.

Methods: We performed a retrospective study to evaluate trauma management with REBOA in hemodynamically unstable patients with severe multiple trauma. Of 5899 severe trauma patients admitted to our hospital between January 2011 and January 2018, we selected 107 patients with severe torso trauma (Injury Severity Score > 16) who displayed persistent hypotension [≥ 2 systolic blood pressure (SBP) values ≤ 90 mmHg] regardless of primary resuscitation. Patients were divided into two groups: trauma management with REBOA ($n = 15$) and without REBOA ($n = 92$). The primary endpoint was the effectiveness of trauma management with REBOA with respect to in-hospital mortality. Secondary endpoints included time from arrival to the start of hemostasis. Multivariable logistic regression analysis, adjusted for clinically important variables, was performed to evaluate clinical outcomes.

Results: Trauma management with REBOA was significantly associated with decreased mortality (adjusted odds ratio of survival, 7.430; 95% confidence interval, 1.081–51.062; $p = 0.041$). The median time (interquartile range) from admission to initiation of hemostasis was not significantly different between the two groups [with REBOA 53.0 (40.0–80.3) min vs. without REBOA 57.0 (35.0–100.0) min]. The time from arrival to the start of balloon occlusion was 55.7 ± 34.2 min. SBP before insertion of REBOA was 48.2 ± 10.5 mmHg. Total balloon occlusion time was 32.5 ± 18.2 min.

Conclusions: The use of REBOA without a delay in initiating resuscitative hemostasis may improve the outcomes in patients with multiple severe torso trauma. However, optimal use may be essential for success.

Keywords: Resuscitative endovascular balloon occlusion of the aorta, Multiple lethal trauma, Resuscitation, Trauma management

Background

Recently, new concepts and technologies such as damage-control strategies, whole-body computed tomography (CT), endovascular treatment, and hybrid operating rooms have been developed for the treatment of trauma patients [1–7]. Similarly, resuscitative endovascular balloon occlusion of the aorta (REBOA) has been widely used in the management of hemorrhagic shock [8]. Its effectiveness for trauma patients has been evaluated in many large-scale studies [9–13]; however, the evidence base is weak and clear indications are lacking. Furthermore, although the time and place of balloon insertion, zone of balloon inflation, and inflation cutoff time are very important, they are heterogeneous factors [11, 14–18]. In addition, while it has been conceivable that REBOA may be effective in patients with severe trauma when integrated with surgery or interventional radiology (IVR) without delay [9], it remains

* Correspondence: hirootsu@is.icc.u-tokai.ac.jp
Department of Emergency and Critical Care Medicine, Tokai University
School of Medicine, 143 Shimokasuya, Isehara city, Kanagawa Prefecture
259-1193, Japan

challenging to successfully perform REBOA in patients with severe multiple torso traumas.

The aim of this study was to evaluate our trauma management with REBOA in hemodynamically unstable patients with multiple severe trauma.

Methods

Study design and selection criteria

A total of 5899 severe trauma patients were admitted to our hospital between January 2011 and January 2018. Among them, we selected 107 patients with severe torso trauma [Injury Severity Score (ISS) > 16] who displayed persistent hypotension [≥ 2 systolic blood pressure (SBP) values ≤ 90 mmHg] regardless of primary resuscitation (airway management, massive transfusion, and/or reversal of obstructive shock) without cardiopulmonary arrest on admission. The patients were divided into two groups: trauma management with REBOA or without REBOA (Fig. 1). The with REBOA group indicated REBOA used primarily, and not secondarily, after open aortic cross-clamping via resuscitative thoracotomy as part of the cardiopulmonary resuscitation procedure. We retrospectively evaluated the characteristics of the patients, hematological tests at the time of admission, severity of trauma, treatment-related characteristics, and outcomes. We defined the primary endpoint as the effectiveness of REBOA for in-hospital mortality. In addition, we set the following secondary endpoints to evaluate the effectiveness of REBOA: pre-hemostasis CT scan performance ratio, REBOA performance ratio before CT, ratio of patients who underwent hemostasis, total amount of red blood cells (RBCs) and fresh frozen plasma (FFP) transfused, ratio of patients who underwent surgery as primary hemostasis among those who underwent hemostasis, time course from arrival to the start of surgery/IVR, pre-hemostasis-administrated RBCs and FFP, and REBOA-related characteristics.

REBOA procedure

The use of REBOA at our institution was started between 20 and 25 years ago. The decision to use REBOA and performing the procedure was at the discretion of the emergency physicians (EPs) or trauma surgeons. All EPs in our hospital have completed a 3-month course of radiology training (mainly vascular IVR). We have used REBOA in patients with severe multiple trauma as follows: the use of REBOA should never result in any delay in the initiation of resuscitative surgery/IVR; REBOA is used to prevent cardiac arrest and not to improve the shock state in patients with severe hemorrhagic shock. However, we do not make any guidelines for the use of REBOA. REBOA has been used under simply primary doctor judgment. In our center, most trauma patients who deteriorated into a state of severe shock have received an insertion of 4-French sheath into the common femoral artery, for the continuous measurement of arterial pressure or performing IVR irrespective of whether REBOA was used or not. Femoral access was obtained through anatomic landmarks using sonography without a surgical incision. REBOA was performed by inserting a 12-French or 7-French sheath set in the common femoral artery. Through the sheath, a balloon catheter was blindly inserted and initially inflated in the aortic zone I [19], located between the left subclavian artery and the celiac artery.

Trauma management

Our institution is a tertiary referral hospital that includes a specialized department in trauma management and intensive care. Moreover, the CT scan, angiography suite (AS), and operating room (OR) are part of the emergency department (ED) in our hospital and available for use at all hours. All trauma surgeons in our hospital have been trained in emergency medicine and general

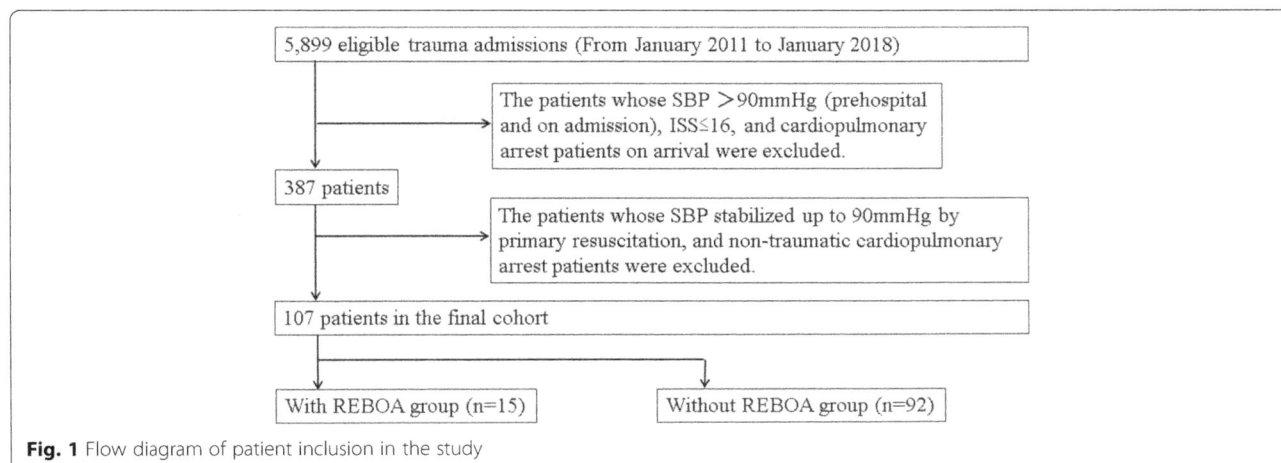

Fig. 1 Flow diagram of patient inclusion in the study

surgery and are also trained in cardiovascular surgery and IVR. The decision to perform surgery or IVR was made at the discretion of EPs or the trauma surgeons in the ED.

Data collection
The ED variables [Glasgow Coma Scale (GCS), respiratory rate (RR), SBP, body temperature (BT), pulse rate, pH, base excess, lactate value, D-dimer, and prothrombin time-international normalized ratio] were recorded as the initial set of vital signs and laboratory tests. Revised Trauma Score (RTS), ISS, and probability of survival calculated using the Trauma and Injury Severity Score (TRISS-Ps) were used for analyzing patient characteristics and severity.

Statistical analysis
Statistical analyses were performed using SPSS software (Windows version 22.0; SPSS Inc., Chicago, IL, USA). For the primary endpoint, multivariable logistic regression analysis was performed to evaluate the effectiveness of REBOA before cardiopulmonary arrest after adjusting for age, RTS, ISS, pre-hemostasis-administered RBCs, and the logarithm of time from admission to the start of hemostasis. For patients' baseline characteristics and secondary endpoints, categorical variables were compared using the χ^2 test or Fisher's exact test, and continuous variables were analyzed using the Student's t test or the Mann–Whitney U test. The values are presented as either the mean ± standard deviation or the median (interquartile range [IQR] 25–75). Statistical significance was defined as a p value of less than 0.05 or was assessed using 95% confidence intervals (CI).

This study was approved by the institutional review board for clinical research, Tokai University (approval no.: 17R-344).

Results
Fifteen patients were included in the with REBOA group, and 92 patients were included in the without REBOA group. Table 1 summarizes the patients' baseline characteristics. There were no significant differences between the two groups.

The primary endpoint is presented in Table 2. Although the 24-h and in-hospital mortality were not significantly different between the two groups when compared using the χ^2 test, REBOA was associated with a significant decrease in the in-hospital mortality when adjusted for age, RTS, ISS, pre-hemostasis-administered RBCs, and the logarithm of time from admission to initiating surgery/IVR, using the multivariable logistic regression analysis. Adjusted odds ratio (OR) of survival was 7.430, and 95% CI was 1.081–51.062 (p = 0.041).

The secondary endpoints are presented in Tables 3 and 4. The amount of pre-hemostasis-administered RBCs in the with REBOA group was higher than that in the without REBOA group when compared using the Mann–Whitney U test. However, there were no significant differences in any of the other parameters between both groups. Patients who were bleeding due to multiple injuries such as multiple facial bone fractures, skull base fractures with intracranial hemorrhage, mediastinal hematoma, chest wall hematoma, retroperitoneal hematoma, abdominal wall hematoma, or multiple extremities bone fractures, all of which were difficult to diagnose without CT, were not eligible for the hemostasis. These patients went into cardiac arrest before the hemostasis could be performed.

The REBOA-related characteristics analyzed in this study are shown in Table 5. The time from admission to the start of balloon occlusion was 55.7 ± 34.2 min. From the REBOA group, 12 (80%) patients underwent CT before hemostasis. Among them, 6 (50%) patients underwent REBOA prior to CT. Hemostasis was initiated in 5 patients before they could receive REBOA. SBP just before the inflation of REBOA was 48.2 ± 10.5 mmHg. Total time for balloon occlusion was 32.5 ± 18.2 min. Two patients received both the intermittent and partial methods. A rest of 1–2 min was allowed after every 10 min of occlusion. Prior to removal, the volume of the inflated balloon was gradually reduced. The total occlusion time of the 2 patients were 50 and 60 min, respectively.

REBOA-related complications occurred in two patients without severe atherosclerotic changes. One middle-aged male patient, for whom the duration of balloon occlusion was 61 min, accompanied with arterial dissection of the right common iliac artery, left limb ischemia that required below-knee amputation, and acute kidney injury (AKI) that required hemodialysis. The time from admission to the initiation of laparotomy was 40 min without CT scan, and the time from admission to the inflation of the balloon (12-Fr REBOA set) was 50 min. The systolic blood pressure just before the balloon occlusion was 48 mmHg, the RTS was 6.085, and the ISS was 50. To prevent cardiac arrest, the balloon should not be deflated until the final stage of hemostasis. Another patient only required the dissection of the common iliac artery using a 12-French set. The dissections in both patients were conservatively treated, and their condition improved. AKI also improved with time. Eventually, both patients were able to resume a normal life.

Discussion
The main finding of this study was that the use of REBOA was associated with reduced in-hospital mortality in patients with multiple severe torso trauma. Despite the use of REBOA in these patients, we were able to

Table 1 Characteristics and severity

	With REBOA (n = 15)	Without REBOA (n = 92)	p
Age, years	52.7 ± 19.8	52.1 ± 21.0	0.67
Male gender (%)	11 (73.3)	59 (64.1)	0.487
Mechanism of injury			
Motor vehicle accident	9	41	0.977
Fall from a height	5	34	
Stabbing	0	11	
Compression	1	4	
Gunshot	0	1	
Violence	0	1	
Vital signs on admission			
GCS total score	11.0 (3.0–14.0)	9.0 (4.25–14.0)	0.83
GCS < 9 (%)	6 (40.0)	45 (48.9)	0.522
RR, per min	24.0 (24.0–30.0)	24.0 (18.0–30.0)	0.643
SBP, mmHg	60.0 (52.0–90.0)	71.0 (56.5–84.5)	0.474
BT, Celsius	36.0 (35.0–36.8)	36.0 (35.4–36.7)	0.804
Pulse rate, beats per min	107.2 ± 24.4	108.7 ± 28.8	0.33
Laboratory evaluation			
pH	7.27 (7.13–7.44)	7.26 (7.08–7.35)	0.237
Base excess, mmol/L	− 9.7 (− 14.4 to − 3.2)	− 9.7 (− 18.3 to − 5.7)	0.353
Lactate, mg/dL	73.0 (36.0–91.0)	56.5 (36.0–100.0)	0.711
D-dimer, μg/mL	82.0 (27.6–117.7)	43.5 (15.9–99.9)	0.338
PT-INR	1.2 (1.0–1.4)	1.2 (1.0–1.4)	0.859
Trauma Score			
RTS	5.6 (2.6–6.6)	5.5 (3.5–6.6)	0.993
ISS	50.0 (41.0–66.0)	41.0 (29.0–50.0)	0.097
TRISS-Ps, %	43.3 (1.4–84.7)	36.9 (7.0–73.8)	0.76
Treatment outcome			
24-h mortality (%)	3 (20.0)	33 (35.9)	0.228
In-hospital mortality (%)	6 (40.0)	52 (56.5)	0.234

REBOA resuscitative endovascular balloon occlusion of the aorta, *GCS* Glasgow Coma Scale, *RR* respiratory rate, *SBP* systolic blood pressure, *BT* body temperature, *PT-INR* prothrombin time-international normalized ratio, *RTS* Revised Trauma Score, *ISS* Injury Severity Score, *TRISS-Ps* Probability of survival calculated by the Trauma and Injury Severity Score

initiate surgery/IVR early in the with REBOA group than in the without REBOA group.

In this study, we used age, RTS, ISS, pre-hemostasis-administrated RBCs, and time from admission to the start of hemostasis as confounding variables. Age, RTS, and ISS were selected to exclude the influence of aging as well as physiological and anatomical differences [20, 21]. Furthermore, we added pre-hemostasis-administrated RBCs and time from

Table 2 Primary endpoint

Variable	Adjusted odds ratio of survival (95% CI)	p-value
REBOA	7.430 (1.081 - 51.062)	0.041

REBOA resuscitative endovascular balloon occlusion of the aorta, *CI* confidence interval

admission to the start of hemostasis, which are the essentials for hemorrhage control in severely injured patients [22]. In addition, the results of time from admission to the start of hemostasis were skewed; therefore, we used the values for which logarithmic transformation was conducted. TRISS-Ps, lactate, base excess, and D-dimer values were used to evaluate the level of trauma severity between the two groups [23–25].

Inoue et al. [9] conducted a subgroup analysis of door-to-primary surgery time of < 60 min vs. ≥ 60 min and observed significant interactions, which may indicate that surgery time of ≥ 60 min could worsen in-hospital mortality. A delay in definitive hemostasis after REBOA may be one of the drawbacks that resulted in high mortality. Our analysis demonstrated that the

Table 3 Pre-hemostasis CT scan and hemostasis performance ratio and total amount of blood transfusions

	With REBOA (n = 15)	Without REBOA (n = 92)	p
Pre-hemostasis CT scan performance ratio (%)	12 (80.0)	60 (65.2)	0.258
The ratio of patients who underwent hemostasis (%)	14 (93.3)	81 (88.0)	0.643
Total amount of blood transfusions, units			
Red blood cells	16.0 (14.0–20.0)	16.0 (6.0–25.0)	0.175
Fresh frozen plasma	14.0 (6.0–20.0)	8.0 (4.0–18.0)	0.323

CT computed tomography, *REBOA* resuscitative endovascular balloon occlusion of the aorta

time from admission to the start of surgery/IVR with REBOA was approximately 60 min, while the time from admission to deflating the balloon was approximately < 90 min. These results suggested that hemorrhage could be controlled within 90 min with surgery/IVR/REBOA in patients with multiple lethal torso trauma. Taken together, the most important factor required to successfully perform REBOA in patients with multiple severe trauma may be the rapid achievement of complete hemostasis. In other words, the use of REBOA should not be a cause of delay in hemostasis.

Our usage of REBOA had the following unique features: shorter occlusion time despite longer time from arrival to the start of balloon occlusion and lower SBP just before REBOA insertion compared with other instances in current literature [11, 13, 14]; the ratio of the patients who underwent REBOA was, low and resuscitative hemostasis had been initiated in five patients before the insertion of REBOA. We had used REBOA based on permissive hypotension [1–4]. Although cardiac arrest should be avoided, we considered the possible harmful effects of not just the long aortic occlusion time but also the unnecessary rising of central SBP due to early use of REBOA, especially in patients with multiple injuries. Hence, unnecessary use of REBOA should be avoided. REBOA might be used to increase afterload with redistribution of blood flow and prevent cardiac arrest, rather than perform hemorrhage control of the distal arteries. The result showed that REBOA might exert effects that can help preserve brain and coronary blood flow while improving outcomes. However, the optimal patient selection is difficult, and the other effects of REBOA remain unclear. Further investigations are needed regarding selection guidelines.

Another notable drawback is REBOA-related complications. Despite technological advancements, REBOA is associated with significant risks due to complications of vascular access and reperfusion ischemia [26, 27]. The serious complication of lower limb ischemia, which may lead to amputation, occurred with high frequency (3/24 patients) in a previous study [28]. In our study, lower limb ischemia, which also required amputation, occurred in 1 of 15 patients. Moreover, there were some REBOA-related complications. Although the exact reasons for the occurrence of the severe complications observed in this study were unclear, we believe that the large size and rigidity of the 12-Fr REBOA and the long occlusion time in patients whose arteries might be in a state of vasospasm could explain such complications. To save the patient's life, some REBOA-related complications may even be inevitable, although all attempts should be made to avoid any adverse sequelae caused by REBOA-related complications. Some studies reported that small introducer sheaths for REBOA may be associated with fewer complications [27, 29] and that ultrasound should be optimized for REBOA [30]. Moreover, partial or intermittent REBOA should be considered in some cases [31, 32]. However, their effect remains unclear. Thus, prevention of REBOA-related morbidity is also important for successful trauma management with REBOA; however, we could not evaluate any possible harmful effects on mortality.

Statistically, this study may have some type 2 errors owing to a low-power analysis with the small sample size. However, our results suggest that there was non-inferiority at least with the REBOA group compared with the without-REBOA group. Therefore, we believe

Table 4 Surgery/IVR-related characteristics and total amount of preoperative blood transfusions in the patients with surgery/IVR

	With REBOA (n = 14)	Without REBOA (n = 81)	p
Patients who underwent surgery for PH (%)	8 (57.1)	38 (46.9)	0.643
Time to initiation PH, min	53.0 (40.0–80.3)	57.0 (35.0–100.0)	0.908
Preoperative blood transfusions, mL			
Red blood cells	840.0 (560.0–1120.0)	560.0 (280.0–1120.0)	0.037
Fresh frozen plasma	120.0 (0.0–300.0)	0 (0–240.0)	0.104

IVR interventional radiology, *REBOA* resuscitative endovascular balloon occlusion of the aorta, *PH* primary hemostasis

Table 5 REBOA related-characteristics

	With REBOA (n = 15)
Time from admission to start balloon occlusion, min	55.7 ± 34.2
The number of patients who underwent REBOA prior to CT (%)	6 (40.0)
The number of patients who started hemostasis before REBOA (%)	5 (33.3)
SBP just before inflation of the REBOA, mmHg	48.2 ± 10.5
Total length of balloon occlusion time, min	32.5 ± 18.2
The number of patients who received both intermittent and partial methods (%)	2 (13.3)
The morbidity of REBOA (%)	2 (13.3)
Arterial dissection (%)	2 (13.3)
Limb ischemia required below-the-knee amputation (%)	1 (6.7)
Acute kidney injury required HD (%)	1 (6.7)

REBOA resuscitative endovascular balloon occlusion of the aorta, *CT* computed tomography, *SBP* systolic blood pressure, *HD* hemodialysis

that these results may be of value in performing further prospective and multicenter studies.

There were several limitations to this study. Our study was conducted at a single center with a small sample size and retrospective study design. Our results were obtained using careful patient selection; however, the potential number of patients could have been higher. Therefore, there may be an obvious selection bias. Moreover, cases of severe trauma referred to our center were highly specific, complex, and had low interdisciplinarity. Medical equipment and techniques have progressed substantially. More cases should be assessed for investigation in future studies.

Conclusions

The use of REBOA without a delay in initiating resuscitative hemostasis may improve the outcomes in patients with multiple injuries associated with severe trauma. Optimal usage of REBOA may be beneficial in preventing cardiac arrest and preserving brain and coronary blood flow without harmful effects. Further studies to assess optimal usage criteria are needed.

Abbreviations

AKI: Acute kidney injury; AS: Angiography suite; CI: Confidence interval; CT: Computed tomography; ED: Emergency department; EPs: Emergency physicians; FFP: Fresh frozen plasma; ISS: Injury Severity Score; IVR: Interventional radiology; OR: Odds ratio; OR: Operating room; RBCs: Red blood cells; REBOA: Resuscitative endovascular balloon occlusion of the aorta; RTS: Revised trauma score; SBP: Systolic blood pressure

Acknowledgments

None.

Funding

This study did not receive any funding.

Authors' contributions

HO and SIn had full access to all the data in the study and take responsibility for the integrity and accuracy of the data. HO, TS, SK, HA, TY, and SIi

contributed to the creation of the strategy for resuscitation using REBOA in practice. The final version was read and approved by all authors.

Competing interests

The authors declare that they have no competing interests.

References

1. Rotondo MF, Schwab CW, McGonigal MD, Phillips GR 3rd, Fruchterman TM, Kauder DR, et al. 'Damage control': an approach for improved survival in exsanguinating penetrating abdominal injury. J Trauma. 1993;35:375–82 discussion 382-3.
2. Moore EE, Burch JM, Franciose RJ, Offner PJ, Biffl WL. Staged physiologic restoration and damage control surgery. World J Surg. 1998;22:1184–90 discussion 1190-1.
3. Shapiro MB, Jenkins DH, Schwab CW, Rotondo MF. Damage control: collective review. J Trauma. 2000;49:969–78.
4. Stahel PF, Smith WR, Moore EE. Current trends in resuscitation strategy for the multiply injured patient. Injury. 2009;40:S27–35.
5. Leidner B, Beckman MO. Standardized whole-body computed tomography as a screening tool in blunt multitrauma patients. Emerg Radiol. 2001;8:20–8.
6. Ball CG, Kirkpatrick AW, D'Amours SK. The RAPTOR: resuscitation with angiography, percutaneous techniques and operative repair: transforming discipline of trauma surgery. Can J Surg. 2011;54:E3–4.
7. Kinoshita T, Yamakawa K, Matsuda H, Yoshikawa Y, Wada D, Hamasaki T, et al. The survival benefit of a novel trauma workflow that includes immediate whole-body computed tomography, surgery, and interventional radiology, all in one trauma resuscitation room: a retrospective historical control study. Ann Surg. 2017. https://doi.org/10.1097/SLA. 0000000000002527.
8. Morrison JJ, Galgon RE, Jansen JO, Cannon JW, Rasmussen TE, Eliason JL. A systematic review of the use of resuscitative endovascular balloon occlusion of the aorta in the management of hemorrhagic shock. J Trauma Acute Care Surg. 2016;80:324–34.
9. Inoue J, Shiraishi A, Yoshiyuki A, Haruta K, Matsui H, Otomo Y. Resuscitative endovascular balloon occlusion of the aorta might be dangerous in patients with severe torso trauma: a propensity score analysis. J Trauma Acute Care Surg. 2016;80:559–66 discussion 566-7.
10. Moore LJ, Martin CD, Harvin JA, Wade CE, Holcomb JB. Resuscitative endovascular balloon occlusion of the aorta for control of noncompressible truncal hemorrhage in the abdomen and pelvis. Am J Surg. 2016;212:1222–30.
11. Gamberini E, Coccolini F, Tamagnini B, Martino C, Albarello V, Benni M, et al. Resuscitative endovascular balloon occlusion of the aorta in trauma: a systematic review of the literature. World J Emerg Surg. 2017;12:42.
12. Norii T, Crandall C, Terasaka Y. Survival of severe blunt trauma patients treated with resuscitative endovascular balloon occlusion of the aorta compared with propensity score-adjusted untreated patients. J Trauma Acute Care Surg. 2015;78:721–8.

13. Brenner M, Teeter W, Hoehn M, Pasley J, Hu P, Yang S, et al. Use of resuscitative endovascular balloon occlusion of the aorta for proximal aortic control in patients with severe hemorrhage and arrest. JAMA Surg. 2018;153:130–5.

14. Pieper A, Thony F, Brun J, Rodière M, Boussat B, Arvieux C, et al. Resuscitative endovascular balloon occlusion of the aorta for pelvic blunt trauma and life-threatening hemorrhage: a 20-year experience in a level I trauma center. J Trauma Acute Care Surg. 2018;84:449–53.

15. DuBose JJ. How I do it: partial resuscitative endovascular balloon occlusion of the aorta (P-REBOA). J Trauma Acute Care Surg. 2017;83:197–9.

16. Biffl WL, Fox CJ, Moore EE. The role of REBOA in the control of exsanguinating torso hemorrhage. J Trauma Acute Care Surg. 2015;78:1054–8.

17. Johnson MA, Davidson AJ, Russo RM, Ferencz SE, Gotlib O, Rasmussen TE, et al. Small changes, big effects: the hemodynamics of partial and complete aortic occlusion to inform next generation resuscitation techniques and technologies. J Trauma Acute Care Surg. 2017;82:1106–11.

18. Romagnoli A, Teeter W, Pasley J, Hu P, Hoehn M, Stein D, et al. Time to aortic occlusion: it's all about access. J Trauma Acute Care Surg. 2017;83: 1161–4.

19. Martinelli T, Thony F, Decléty P, Sengel C, Broux C, Tonetti J, et al. Intra-aortic balloon occlusion to salvage patients with life-threatening hemorrhagic shocks from pelvic fractures. J Trauma. 2010;68:942–8.

20. Champion HR, Sacco WJ, Copes WS, Gann DS, Gennarelli TA, Flanagan ME. A revision of the Trauma Score. J Trauma. 1989;29:623–9.

21. Baker SP, O'Neill B, Haddon W Jr, Long WB. The injury severity score: a method for describing patients with multiple injuries and evaluating emergency care. J Trauma. 1974;14:187–96.

22. Gruen RL, Brohi K, Schreiber M, Balogh ZJ, Pitt V, Narayan M, et al. Haemorrhage control in severely injured patients. Lancet. 2012;380:1099–108.

23. de Munter L, Polinder S, Lansink KW, Cnossen MC, Steyerberg EW. Mortality prediction models in the general trauma population: a systematic review. Injury. 2017;48:221–9.

24. Ibrahim I, Chor WP, Chue KM, Tan CS, Tan HL, Siddiqui FJ, et al. Is arterial base deficit still a useful prognostic marker in trauma? A systematic review. Am J Emerg Med. 2016;34:626–35.

25. Umebachi R, Taira T, Wakai S, Aoki H, Otsuka H, Nakagawa Y, et al. Measurement of blood lactate, D-dimer, and activated prothrombin time improves prediction of in-hospital mortality in adults blunt trauma. Am J Emerg Med. 2018;36:370–5.

26. Davidson AJ, Russo RM, Reva VA, Brenner ML, Moore LJ, Ball C, et al. The pitfalls of resuscitative endovascular balloon occlusion of the aorta: risk factors and mitigation strategies. J Trauma Acute Care Surg. 2018; 84:192–202.

27. Taylor JR 3rd, Harvin JA, Martin C, Holcomb JB, Moore LJ. Vascular complications from resuscitative endovascular balloon occlusion of the aorta: life over limb? J Trauma Acute Care Surg. 2017;83:S120–3.

28. Saito N, Matsumoto H, Yagi T, Hara Y, Hayashida K, Motomura T, et al. Evaluation of the safety and feasibility of resuscitative endovascular balloon occlusion of the aorta. J Trauma Acute Care Surg. 2015;78:897–903 discussion 904.

29. Teeter WA, Matsumoto J, Idoguchi K, Kon Y, Orita T, Funabiki T, et al. Smaller introducer sheaths for REBOA may be associated with fewer complications. J Trauma Acute Care Surg. 2016;81:1039–45.

30. Bogert JN, Patel BM, Johnson DJ. Ultrasound optimization for resuscitative endovascular balloon occlusion of the aorta. J Trauma Acute Care Surg. 2017;82(1):204–7.

31. Kuckelman J, Barron M, Moe D, Derickson M, Phillips C, Kononchik J, et al. Extending the golden hour for zone 1 REBOA: improved survival and reperfusion injury with intermittent versus continuous REBOA in a porcine severe truncal hemorrhage model. J Trauma Acute Care Surg. 2018. https://doi.org/10.1097/TA.0000000000001964.

32. Russo RM, Williams TK, Grayson JK, Lamb CM, Cannon JW, Clement NF. Extending the golden hour: partial resuscitative endovascular balloon occlusion of the aorta in a highly lethal swine liver injury model. J Trauma Acute Care Surg. 2016;80:372–8 discussion 378-80.

29

Developing and validating of Ramathibodi Appendicitis Score (RAMA-AS) for diagnosis of appendicitis in suspected appendicitis patients

Chumpon Wilasrusmee[1,2], Boonying Siribumrungwong[3], Samart Phuwapraisirisan[4], Napaphat Poprom[1,2], Patarawan Woratanarat[2,5], Panuwat Lertsithichai[1], John Attia[6] and Ammarin Thakkinstian[2*]

Abstract

Background: Diagnosis of appendicitis is still clinically challenging where resources are limited. The purpose of this study was to develop and externally validate Ramathibodi Appendicitis Score (RAMA-AS) in aiding diagnosis of appendicitis.

Methods: A two-phase cross-sectional study (i.e., derivation and validation) was conducted at Ramathibodi Hospital (for derivation) and at Thammasat University Hospital and Chaiyaphum Hospital (for validation). Patients with abdominal pain and suspected of having appendicitis were enrolled. Multiple logistic regression was applied to develop a parsimonious model. Calibration and discrimination performances were assessed. In addition, our RAMA-AS was compared with Alvarado's score performances using ROC curve analysis.

Results: The RAMA-AS consisted of three domains with seven predictors including symptoms (i.e., progression of pain, aggravation of pain, and migration of pain), signs (i.e., fever and rebound tenderness), and laboratory tests (i.e., white blood cell count (WBC) and neutrophil). The model fitted well with data, and it performed better discrimination than the Alvarado score with C-statistics of 0.842 (95% CI 0.804, 0.881) versus 0.760 (0. 710, 0.810). Internal validation by bootstrap yielded Sommer's D of 0.686 (0.608, 0.763) and C-statistics of 0.848 (0.846, 0.849). The C-statistics of two external validations were 0.853 (0.791, 0.915) and 0.813 (0.736, 0.892) with fair calibrations.

Conclusion: RAMA-AS should be a useful tool for aiding diagnosis of appendicitis with good calibration and discrimination performances.

Keywords: Appendicitis score, Derive phase, Validation phase, Calibration, Discrimination

Background

Appendicitis is one of the most common causes of acute abdominal pain, with an incidence of 110/100,000 [1]. Although, many attempts have been made to improve the diagnostic accuracy, false negative rates remain common with rates of negative appendectomy of 15 to 26% [2, 3] and perforated appendectomy of 10 to 30% [4].

The critical evaluation of appendicitis should balance between early operation to minimize complicated appendicitis (i.e., perforation, gangrene, and abscess) and a conservative approach reducing unnecessary operation. Several scores had been developed for screening of appendicitis, e.g., Alvarado [5], modified-Alvarado Fenyo [6], Eskelinen [7], etcetera. A systematic review of previous appendicitis scores was conducted to explore their methods used for developments, validations, and performances [8]. Surprisingly, about two-thirds of those studies developed scores based on univariate analysis, and none had evaluated their impacts on health outcome

* Correspondence: ammarin.tha@mahidol.ac.th
[2]Section for Clinical Epidemiology and Biostatistics, Faculty of Medicine Ramathibodi Hospital, Mahidol University, Bangkok, Thailand
Full list of author information is available at the end of the article

in clinical practice [9]. With poor methodology in previous score developments, we therefore conducted our study, which aimed to develop and externally validate Ramathibodi Appendicitis Score (RAMA-AS).

Methods
Study design
The design was a cross-sectional study consisting of derivation and validation phases. Derived data were collected at Ramathibodi Hospital (RH), whereas validated data were collected at Thammasat University Hospital (TH) and Chaiyaphum Hospital (CH) from January 2013 to May 2015. The RH and TH are the Schools of Medicine, whereas CH is a provincial hospital.

The study was conducted and reported according to Transparent Reporting of a Multivariable Prediction Model for Individual Prognosis Or Diagnosis (TRIPOD) [10] and STrengthening the Reporting of OBservational studies in Epidemiology (STROBE) [11]. Consecutive suspected appendicitis patients presenting with abdominal pain were included with following criteria: aged 15–60 years, right side abdominal pain within 7 days, had at least one of the following symptoms (i.e., right lower abdominal pain, migration of abdominal pain, anorexia, nausea, vomiting) and signs (i.e., raised body temperature, right lower quadrant tenderness, guarding, rebound tenderness, and decreased bowel sound), and willing to participate and gave consent. Exclusion criteria were patients who could not give the history of illness, had myocardial infarction or terminal illness, abdominal mass, tumor or malignancy of appendix.

Outcome and predictors
The interested outcome was acute appendicitis by histopathological diagnosis for operative patients. For those patients with conservative management, telephone was made to confirm the final diagnosis 6 weeks after visiting.

Sample size
As for our literature review, a total of 8–10 variables were potentially included in the final risk prediction score. A simulation study indicated that a number of events per variable of at least 10 to 30 yielded less bias in coefficient estimation of logistic regression [12], which was known as a rule of thumb as per recommendation [13].Using a rule of thumb of at least 20 appendicitis patients per variable required 200 appendicitis patients for 10 variables. The prevalence of appendicitis in our setting was 62% from our pilot study. As a result, 355 patients were needed. Taking into account for missing data of 20%, at least 388 patients were finally required. In addition, an additional 100 subjects (i.e., about 30% of derived subjects) were enrolled from each of the external sites for external validation.

Statistical analysis
Imputation
Multiple imputation was applied to predict missing variables using a simulation-based approach which assumed data were missing at random [14, 15]. A linear truncated regression was applied by regressing missing data on complete data with a number of 20 imputations as per recommendation [16]. Performance of imputation can be assessed using relative variance increase (RVI) and fraction of missing information (FMI). The RVI refers to average relative increase in variances of estimates because of missing variables (i.e., mean of variance of all coefficients from missing data); and as this value closes to 0, missing data reflect less on estimates. The FMI refers to the largest fraction of missing information of coefficient estimates due to missing data. The number of imputations should be roughly estimated based on a rule of thumb, i.e., FMI×100. For instance, if FMI = 0.15, the number of imputations = 0.15 × 100, i.e., at least 15 imputations are required.

Derivation
A simple logistic regression analysis was used to screen variables that might associate with appendicitis. Individual variables of 4 domains (i.e., demographic data, clinical symptoms, clinical signs, and laboratory tests) were fitted in a logit model, and a likelihood ratio (LR) test was used to select variables. Variables with p values < 0.20 were simultaneously considered in a multivariate logit model. Only significant variables were kept in a parsimonious-model. Goodness of fit was assessed whether the expected (E) or predicted and observed (O) values were close using chi-square Hosmer-Lemeshow test [17]. In addition, a calibration coefficient (O/E) and its 95% confidence interval (CI) were also estimated. The coefficients of the final parsimonious- model were used to create the RAMA-AS. The receiver operating characteristic (ROC) curve, which plotted sensitivity versus 1- specificity, was used to calibrate the score cutoff. Diagnostic parameters (i.e., sensitivity, specificity, likelihood ratio positive (LR+) and negative) were estimated for each distinct value of the scores. The area under ROC, called C-statistic, was estimated, and value close to one reflected higher discrimination of appendicitis from non-appendicitis [18].

Validation
Internal validation A bootstrap technique with 450 replications was applied for internal validation of the RAMA-AS [19]. For each bootstrap sample, the RAMA-AS score was calculated and fitted in the logit model. For calibration, the correlation between the observed and expected values of appendicitis was assessed using the Somer'D coefficient for all bootstrap data (called

D_{boot}) and derived data (called D_{org}). Calibration of the model was then assessed by subtracting the D_{org} from the mean D_{boot}, and lower value reflected less bias and thus better calibration. Likewise, the original C-statistic was compared to an average C-statistic from the bootstraps for discrimination performance.

External validation Data from the two external hospitals were used to validate the performances of RAMA-AS. Calibration performance was explored as mentioned above. In addition, model re-calibrations were performed by recalibrating intercept (called M1) and overall coefficient (called M2) [20, 21] as follows (see Additional file 1: Table S1: The M1 was constructed by fitting RAMA-AS on appendicitis. The estimated intercept was then used to re-calibrate by adding it up with the original intercept. The estimated coefficient from the M1 was then used to calibrate coefficient by multiplying it with overall coefficients (M2). Four model revisions were additionally performed from the M2 [10, 21–23], (see Additional file 1: Table S1). The M3 was constructed by fitting M2 plus significant predictors by LR test. The M4 was similar to M3 but added significant predictors by stepwise selections. The M5 re-estimated all coefficients of predictors. Finally, the M6 re-selected only significant predictors among all predictors.

Finally, the Alvarado score [5] was compared with the RAMA-AS using ROC curve analysis.

All analyses were performed using STATA version 14 (Stata Corp, College Station, Texas, USA) under mi estimate commands. A p value of less than 0.05 was taken as a threshold for statistical significance.

Results

A total of 396 suspected acute appendicitis patients were enrolled from RH. Among them, 132 patients (33.3%) were male, and mean age and BMI were 36.3 ± 14.6 and 22.8 ± 4.5, respectively. A total of 245/396 (61.8%; 95% CI 56.9%, 66.7%) patients were appendicitis, with a negative appendectomy rate of 4%.

Imputation

Two variables (i.e., WBC > 10,000 cell/mm³ and neutrophil > 75%) contained missing data of 43 (10.9%) and 40 (10.1%), respectively and imputed data were filled in for both variables. Performances of imputation were assessed, and the FMI was < 0.0001 for both variables, indicating 20 imputations were sufficient to fill in missing data, see Additional file 2: Table S2. The diagnostic plot was constructed by comparing missing versus observed values, suggesting no difference between the two values, see Additional file 2: Figure S1.

Model development
Derivation

A total of 16 out of 20 predictive variables were suggested from a univariate analysis that they might associate with appendicitis, see Table 1. These included eight symptoms (i.e., first location of pain, migration of pain, onset, progression of pain, right lower quadrant pain at presentation, nausea or vomiting, aggravation of pain by cough or movement, and fever), five signs (i.e., bowel sound, body temperature, tenderness at right lower quadrant of abdomen, rebound tenderness, and guarding), and two laboratory tests (i.e., WBC > 10,000 cell/mm³ and neutrophil > 75%).

These variables were simultaneously included in the logit model, in which only seven variables were remained in the final model. These were three symptoms (i.e., migration of pain, progression of pain, and aggravation of pain by cough or movement), two signs (i.e., body temperature ≥ 37.8 °C and rebound tenderness), two laboratory tests (i.e., WBC > 10,000 cell/mm³ and neutrophil > 75%), and odd ratios (OR) and 95% CI were reported, see Table 2. The predictive equation was

$$\ln[P/(1-P] = -3.37 + (0.80)\text{migration of pain}$$
$$+ (1.04)\text{progression of pain}$$
$$+ (0.78)\text{aggravation of pain by cough or movement}$$
$$+ (1.64)\text{Body temperature}$$
$$+ (1.53)\text{rebound tenderness}$$
$$+ (0.91)\text{white blood cell} + (0.69)\text{neutrophil}$$

Model performance

The estimated C-statistic was 0.842 (95% CI 0.804, 0.881), see (Additional file 3: Figure S2), indicating the model well discriminated appendicitis from non-appendicitis. Hosmer-Lemeshow goodness of fit test indicated the model fitted well with the data (chi-square test = 5.64, df = 8, p value = 0.687) with the O/E ratio of 0.95 (95% CI 0.83, 1.08).

The scoring scheme was constructed using the estimated 7 coefficients, which ranged from − 3.37 to 3.99 with a median of 0.86, see Table 2. The score cutoff was calibrated and stratified into four categories, i.e., very low (score < − 0.64), low (score − 0.64 to 0.84), moderate (score 0.85 to 1.74), and high risk (score > 1.74) groups, see Table 3. The estimated LR+ for these latter three groups were 1.98 (95% CI 1.65, 2.37), 5.25 (95% CI 3.39, 8.13), and 8.36 (95% CI 3.96 to 18.00) when compared to the lowest risk group. The post-test probabilities were 76.0, 89.0, and 93.0% for low, moderate, and high risk groups, respectively (see Fagan plot in Fig. 1).

Validation
Internal validation

The 450 bootstraps yielded estimated D_{org} and D_{boot}-coefficients of 0.686 and 0.695 (95% CI 0.692, 0.698) for

Table 1 Description of patients' characteristics in appendicitis and non-appendicitis groups

Characteristics	Non-appendicitis n = 155	Appendicitis n = 241	OR (95% CI)	p value
Demographic				
Age (year), mean (SD)	33.8 (11.9)	37.9 (15.9)		< 0.001
Age group				
< 40	99 (63.9)	140 (58.1)	1	0.251
≥ 40	56 (36.1)	101 (41.9)	1.3(0.8–1.9)	
Sex, number, (%)				
Male	39 (25.2)	93 (38.6)	1.9(1.2–2.9)	< 0.001
Female	116 (74.8)	148 (61.4)	1	
BMI, mean (SD)	22.4 (3.9)	22.95 (4.7)		0.230
Symptoms				
First location of pain				
Epigastrium	40 (25.8)	102 (42.3)	2.2(1.4–3.4)	< 0.001
Periumbilical	24 (15.5)	31 (12.9)	1.1(0.6–1.9)	
Other	91 (58.7)	108 (44.8)	1	
Type of pain				
Dull aching, constant	49 (31.6)	82 (34.0)	1.1(0.7–1.7)	0.620
Colicky	106 (68.4)	159 (65.9)	1	
Migration of pain				
Absence	108 (69.7)	111 (46.1)	1	< 0.001
Presence	47 (30.3)	130 (53.9)	2.7(1.8–4.1)	
Onset				
Insidious	120 (77.4)	146 (60.6)	1	< 0.001
Sudden	35 (22.6)	95 (39.4)	2.2(1.4–3.5)	
Progression of pain				
Yes	113 (72.9)	223 (92.5)	4.6(2.5–8.4)	
No	42 (27.1)	18 (7.5)	1	< 0.001
Right lower quadrant pain at presentation				
Yes	140 (90.3)	239 (99.2)	12.8(2.9–56.8)	
No	15 (9.7)	2 (0.8)	1	< 0.001
Time of pain before presentation (hours)				
≤ 48	126 (81.3)	204 (84.7)	1.3(0.7–2.2)	0.382
> 48	29 (18.7)	37 (15.4)	1	
Time of right lower quadrant pain before presentation (hours)				
≤ 12	67 (43.2)	107 (44.4)	1.1(0.7–1.6)	0.820
> 12	88 (56.8)	134 (55.6)	1	
Nausea or vomiting				
Yes	64 (41.3)	141 (58.5)	2.0(1.3–3.0)	
No	91 (58.7)	100 (41.5)	1	< 0.001
Aggravation of pain by cough or movement				

Table 1 Description of patients' characteristics in appendicitis and non-appendicitis groups *(Continued)*

Characteristics	Non-appendicitis n = 155	Appendicitis n = 241	OR (95% CI)	p value
Yes	88 (56.8)	199 (82.6)	3.6(2.3–5.7)	
No	67 (43.2)	42 (17.4)	1	< 0.001
Anorexia				
Yes	118 (76.1)	164 (68.1)	0.7(0.4–1.1)	0.083
No	37 (23.9)	77 (31.9)	1	
Fever				
Yes	135 (87.1)	154 (63.9)	0.3(0.2–0.5)	< 0.001
No	20 (12.9)	87 (36.1)		
Bowel sound				
Increase	20 (12.9)	37 (15.4)	1.4(0.8–2.5)	0.044
Decrease	16 (10.3)	45 (18.7)	2.1(1 .1–3.9)	
Normal	119 (76.8)	159 (65.9)	1	
Body temperature (°C)				
< 37.8	146 (94.2)	176 (73.0)	1	< 0.001
≥ 37.8	9 (5.8)	65 (26.9)	5.9 (2.8–12.4)	
Tenderness at right lower quadrant				
Yes	137 (88.4)	240 (99.6)	31.5 (4.2–238.8)	< 0.001
No	18 (11.6)	1 (0.4)	1	
Rebound tenderness				
Yes	37 (23.9)	155 (64.3)	5.8(3.7–9.1)	< 0.001
No	118 (76.1)	86 (35.7)	1	
Guarding				
Yes	26 (16.8)	82 (34.0)	2.6(1.6–4.2)	< 0.001
No	129 (83.2)	159 (65.9)	1	
Laboratory results				
WBC (cell/mm^3)				
≤ 10,000	55 (35.5)	26 (10.8)	1	< 0.001
> 10,000 cell/mm^3	100 (64.5)	215 (89.2)	4.6(2.7–7.7)	
Neutrophil (%)				
≤ 75%	80 (51.6)	54 (22.4)	1	< 0.001
> 75%	75 (48.4)	187 (77.6)	3.7(2.4–5.8)	

the derivative and bootstrap models, respectively. The bias was only − 0.009 (95% CI − 0.011, − 0.007), suggesting good calibration. The bootstrap C-statistics was 0.848 (95% CI 0.846, 0.849), with a bias of − 0.005 (95% CI − 0.006, − 0.004).

External validation

A total of 330 patients with suspected acute appendicitis (152 and 178 from TH and CH, respectively) were used to externally validate the RAMA-AS. Their characteristics were described in Table 4.

Thammasat University Hospital Comparing with RH, prevalence of appendicitis was much lower in TH,

i.e., 48.7 vs 61.8, %, but the mean age was quite similar (35.6 vs 36.3 years), although the male percentage was much lower (26.4 vs 35.8%), see Table 4. Among seven predictors, distributions of rebound tenderness (42.8 vs 48.5%), progression of pain (64.5 vs 84.8%), and aggravation of pain (51.4 vs 72.5%) were little to much lower, but migration of pain (48.0 vs 44.7%), body temperature (19.7 vs 18.7%) and WBC > 10,000 cell/mm^3 (82.2 vs 79.6%) and neutrophil > 75% (75.7 vs 66 .2%) were little to much higher differences. These variables were also described by appendicitis groups, indicating higher prevalence for all symptoms and signs, but not for laboratory tests, see Additional file 1: Table S3.

Table 2 Factor associated with appendicitis: multiple logistic regression analysis

Domain	Parameters	Coefficient	SE	p value	OR(95%CI)	Scoring
Symptoms	Progression of pain	1.04	0.4	0.007	2.8 (1.3–5.9)	1.04
	Aggravation of pain by cough or movement	0.78	0.3	0.009	2.2 (1.2–3.8)	0.78
	Migration of pain	0.80	0.3	0.004	2.6 (1.3–3.7)	0.77
Signs	Body temperature ≥ 37.8 °C	1.64	0.5	< 0.001	5.1 (2.1–12.1)	1.64
	Rebound tenderness	1.53	0.3	< 0.001	4.6 (2.7–7.7)	1.53
Lab results	WBC > 10,000 cell/mm^3	0.91	0.3	0.005	2.6 (1.3–5.0)	0.91
	Neutrophil > 75%	0.69	0.3	0.010	2.3 (1.2–4.1)	0.69
Constant						− 3.37
Total						3.99

WBC white blood cell count

The estimated RAMA-AS, which ranged from − 3.4 to 4.0, seemed to work well in TH with the estimated O/E ratio of 1.005 (95% CI 0.784, 1.225; Hosmer-Lemeshow = 8.219, (df = 4), p = 0.084). However, the calibration plot showed the predicted risk deviated from the reference line (see Additional file 4: Figure S3-A), i.e., under-estimated risk for lower score and over-estimated risk for higher scores. The intercept and overall coefficients were then calibrated (see Additional file 1: Table S4), and calibration plots were constructed (see Additional file 4: Figure S3-B-C) which suggested no improvement of calibrations.

Revision M3 models by LR test indicated that migration of pain, progression of pain, body temperature, WBC, and neutrophil were significant predictors, see Additional file 1: Table S4. Comparing coefficients of M3 versus coefficients of the original RH model in Table 2, coefficients of body temperature, WBC, and neutrophil were changed from positive to negative coefficients, whereas coefficients of

the rest of the predictors increased. Only migration of pain, progression of pain, and rebound tenderness were significant by stepwise selection for M4. Of these, progression of pain and rebound tenderness were much lower but migration of pain was higher than in RH, see Table 2 and Additional file 1: Table S4.

Calibration coefficients of these models were estimated, which resulted in the O/E ratio for revision M3 model and M4 of 0.940 (95% CI 0.729, 1.150; Hosmer-Lemeshow = 2.683, df = 4, p = 0.612) and 1.006 (95% CI 0.743, 1.269; Hosmer-Lemeshow = 5.00, df = 4, p = 0.287), respectively, which were much improved when compared to the M0. Calibration plots also showed better fits with the reference lines when compared to the M0, see Additional file 4: Figure S3 A, D-E. The M5 which entered all seven predictors or stepwise selection in M6 yielded similar results as M4, in which only three predictors (i.e., migration of pain, progression of pain, and rebound tenderness) were significant. The

Table 3 Risk stratification and predictive values of a RAMA-AS prediction score

Score	Risk groups	Score development for derivative phase						
		Outcome		% sensitivity (95% CI)	% specificity (95% CI)	LR+ (95% CI)	LR- (95% CI)	Post-positive test odds (%)
		AP	Non-AP					
<− 0.64	Very low	25	85	100.00	0	1.00	0	61.80
− 0.64 to 0.84	Low risk	61	51	89.75 (85.25–93.26)	54.97 (46.67–63.06)	1.98 (1.65–2.37)	0.19 (0.13–0.28)	76.00 (73.00–79.00)
0.85 to 1.74	Moderate	64	12	64.08 (57.73–70.09)	88.08 (81.82–92.78)	5.25 (3.39–8.13)	0.41 (0.34–0.49)	89.00 (85.00–93.00)
> 1.74	High	91	7	37.96 (31.86–44.36)	95.36 (90.68–98.12)	8.36 (3.96–18.00)	0.65 (0.59–0.72)	93.00 (86.00–97.00)

AP appendicitis, *LR* likelihood ratio

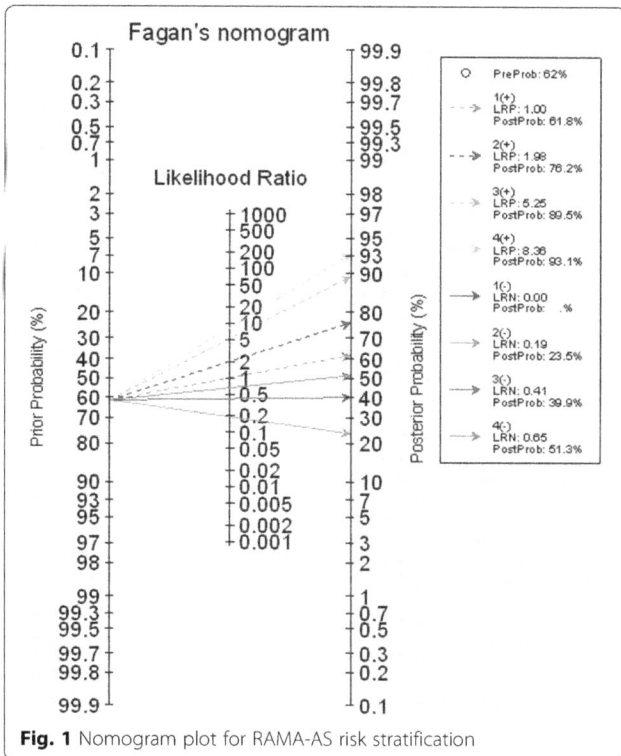

Fig. 1 Nomogram plot for RAMA-AS risk stratification

O/E ratios were 0.870 (0.578, 1.612) and 0.947 (95% CI 0.684, 1.209) and calibration plots showed better fit than M0, see Additional file 4: Figure S3 F-G.

C-statistics were estimated for all models, see Additional file 1: Table S5. These suggested that the M0 could well discriminate appendicitis from non-appendicitis with the C-statistics of 0.853 (95% CI 0.790,

0.915), and they were little improved for M3, M4, and M6, but not for M5, see Additional file 1: Table S5.

Chaiyaphum Hospital Comparing with RH (see Table 4), prevalence of appendicitis in CH was much higher (76.9 vs 61.8%), and mean age (42.9 vs 36.3 years) and male percentage were higher (39.9 vs 35.8%). Migration of pain (70.2 vs 44.7%), body temperature (37.6% vs 18.7%), and rebound tenderness (71.3 vs 48.5%) were more present, but aggravation of pain was much lower (58.4 vs 72.5%), whereas progression of pain (82.6 vs 84.8%), WBC > 10,000 cell/mm^3 (76.9 vs 79.6%) and neutrophil (63.5 vs 66.2%) were little lower than RH. Distribution of these predictors between appendicitis groups were described, and all except neutrophil were more prevalent in appendicitis than non-appendicitis groups, in Additional file 1: Table S3.

A median RAMA-AS was 1.6 (– 3.4, 4.0) with O/E ratio of 0.996 (95% CI 0.695, 1.333; Hosmer-Lemeshow = 6.640 (df = 4), p = 0.156), see Additional file 1: Table S5. Calibration models were constructed (see Additional file 1: Table S4) and plotted (see Additional file 5: Figure S4 A-G). These suggested that the M0 still deviated from the reference line particularly for low and high scores. M1 and M2 did not improve calibrations when compared to the original M0. Among revision models, M3-M6, M3-M4, and M6 were improved in calibrations, particularly the M6 was the best with O/E ratios of 1.021 (95% CI 0.905, 1.186), whereas the calibration plot of M5 showed quite poor performance.

The M0's discrimination performance was good, although it was lower than the original model (C-statistic = 0.813; 0.736, 0.892). The C-statistics for M3 to M6 were a bit higher than M0, see Additional file 1: Table S5.

Table 4 Describe characteristics of patients from derivation and external validation data

Characteristics	RA (n = 396)	TS (n = 152)	CP (n = 178)
Mean age (SD), years	36.3(14.6)	35.6(16 .9)	42.9(16.8)
Men	132 (35.8%)	40 (26.4%)	71 (39.9%)
Symptoms			
Progression of pain	336 (84.8%)	98 (64.5%)	147 (82.6%)
Aggravation of pain	287 (72.5%)	78 (51.4%)	104 (58.4%)
Migration of pain	177 (44.7%)	73 (48.0%)	125 (70.2%)
Signs			
Body temperature ≥ 37.8 °C	74 (18.7%)	30 (19.7%)	67 (37.6%)
Rebound tenderness	192 (48.5%)	65 (42.8%)	127 (71.3%)
Laboratory			
WBC	315 (79.6%)	125 (82.2%)	141 (79.2%)
Neutrophil	262 (66.2%)	115 (75.7%)	124 (69.7%)
Prevalence of appendicitis	245/396 (61.8%)	74/152 (48.7%)	137/178 (76.9%)

CP Chaiyaphum Hospital, *RA* Ramathibodi Hospital, *TS* Thammasat University Hospital

Comparison of RAMA-AS and previous score

Alvarado scores was calculated which ranged of 2 to 10 (mean = 7.04). The C-statistics was 0.752 (95% CI 0.710, 0.800) which was statistically lower than RAMA-AS (p value of < 0.001, see Fig. 2).

Discussion

We developed and internally and externally validated a RAMA-AS, for classifying very low, low, moderate, and high risk of having appendicitis. Predictive domains including three symptoms, two signs, and two laboratory tests were included. Internal validation showed the RAMA-AS performed well for both calibration and discrimination. The external validation showed fair calibrations and good discrimination with the O/E ratios of 1.01 (0.78, 1.23) and 0.996 (0.659, 1.333), with the C-statistics of 0.853 (95% CI 0.791, 0.915) and 0.817 (95% CI 0.736, 0.892), respectively.

Although most predictors of clinical signs, symptoms, and laboratory tests used in the RAMA-AS were similar to the Alvarado score, which was the most commonly used in prospective studies [6, 24–29], our performances were better. This might be due to difference in weighting or scoring for each predictor, distribution of predictors, and also prevalence of appendicitis itself. Our score was derived based on proper model construction, following the recommendation by TRIPOD [10], and let the data suggest proper weighting. Our finding was consistent to the appendicitis inflammatory response (AIR) [30], developed in 2008, which externally performed better than the Alvarado score. This score did not consider WBC and neutrophil, but instead included leukocyte and CRP in the model [30, 31], in which the CRP may be not a routine laboratory test in some developing countries. Thus, it is not easily applied in the setting where resources are limited. Our RAMA-AS and also these

scores could rule out well, but not rule in as per WSES Jarusalem guidelines [30], so high risk score may need confirmation by CT scan [31].

Calibration performance of RAMA-AS was fair in both external data sets. This could be explained as follows: first, prevalence of appendicitis in the derived RH and validated TH and CH's were reasonably different, i.e., 61.8 vs 48.7 vs 76.9%, respectively. Therefore, the original model over-estimated risk of appendicitis in TH, but under estimated risk in CH. We then re-calibrated the intercept in M1 models by minus and plus the original intercept (i.e., baseline risk) with estimated intercepts for TH and CH, respectively. These models were still not well calibrated, we thus moved further to recalibrate overall coefficient (M2), but this did not much improve. Differences in distributions of predictors between appendicitis groups across data sources may also play a role. For instance, all symptoms and signs were more present in appendicitis than in non-appendicitis groups for both external hospitals, but not for WBC and neutrophil. The revisions of models showed much improvement, which could be M4 or M6 for both TH and CH. Only two symptoms and one sign contributed in predictions for both hospitals, therefore, the predictive score containing only three symptoms (migration of pain, progression of pain, aggravation of pain) and one sign (rebound tenderness) without laboratory test is proposed. Its performances in calibration and discrimination was very much similar to M6 (data were not shown). Although the RAMA-AS did not perform well in the external data when compared to the derived data, it could still well discriminate appendicitis from non-appendicitis in provincial setting (CH) and School of Medicine setting (TH).

Using the RAMA-AS in practice

Our RAMA-AS should be applied in general hospitals where resources are limited. Data of seven variables can be collected from physical examination, interview, and CBC test. Applying the RAMA-AS is easy by inputting data in the equation. Probability of appendicitis is then estimated for each risk stratification using Fagan nomogram. In addition, the score can be straight forwardly classified as very low (score < − 0.64), low (score − 0.64 to 0.84), moderate (score 0.85 to 1.74), and high risk (score > 1.74) of having appendicitis. As for the ROC analysis, these cut-off thresholds were objectively selected based on LR+ (i.e., sensitivity/(1- specificity)), which had less bias than subjective selection [32]. Although our score could well discriminate appendicitis from non-appendicitis as for the C-statistics, clinical findings should also be incorporated for further decision making. Imaging investigation may be needed for moderate to high scores [31].

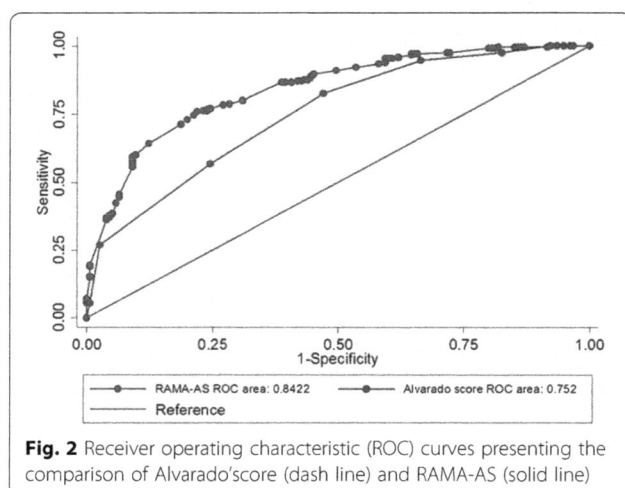

Fig. 2 Receiver operating characteristic (ROC) curves presenting the comparison of Alvarado'score (dash line) and RAMA-AS (solid line)

Counting number of positive of signs, symptoms, and laboratory results can be also applied. For instance, low risk appendicitis if having only positive for all items of signs, symptom, or laboratory tests; 1 positive item for each of 3 domains; 2 positive items among 3 domains (i.e., 1 symptom and sign, 1 symptom and laboratory test, 1 sign and 1 laboratory test); 3 symptoms with 1 laboratory test without sign; 3 symptoms plus one sign without laboratory test. The post-test probability would be 76.0%, so out-patient observation is recommended. The moderate risk requires three symptoms plus one sign of body temperature ≥ 37.8 °C, or three symptoms plus two laboratory tests without any sign. The post-test probability is from 85.0 to 93.0% for moderate risks, so other investigations such as ultrasound or CT scan may be needed for these patients.

The high risk group requires all symptoms and signs, or all symptoms plus one sign and laboratory test, all symptoms plus two signs plus any of laboratory test, or three symptoms plus two laboratory tests plus any of the signs. The post-test probability is about 93.0% and thus surgical treatment should be performed for high risk patients.

Our study has some strengths. We followed the recommendations for developing risk prediction score by Altman et al. [33] and TRIPOD [10]. We developed and both internally and externally validated the scores using prospective data collections. Imputation of missing data was applied, even though it occurred only on a few variables, which should yield better performances of risk prediction model than analysis of complete case only [34]. The RAMA-AS showed good performances for both calibration and discrimination in the derived setting, although one external setting had lower discrimination performance.

However, some limitations could not be avoided. The study was conducted at tertiary hospitals where the appendicitis prevalence was high. The RAMA-AS should be further validated in different populations and settings. In order to improve generalizability, big electronic health data or individual patient meta-analysis should be conducted [35]. Clinical impact of the RAMA-AS should be also further assessed. For instance, applying the score in a routine clinical practice, which will let us know whether our score, can still well rule out and rule in suspected patients with and without appendicitis. These suspected patients may be only observed or treated with operation or even non-operative treatment such as antibiotics. Previous cohort study showed long-term success and safety of antibiotics in suspected appendicitis [36]. However, this evidence was from observational study, which was prone to selection bias. Individual randomized controlled trial with appropriate methods should be conducted to test if non-operative treatment is non-inferior to operation [37].

Conclusions

Appendicitis is one of the most important clinical causes among acute abdominal pain. Several scoring systems had been developed for screening of appendicitis. Surprisingly, about two-thirds of studies developed prediction scores based on univariate analysis without applying statistical modeling. We have developed and internally/externally validated a clinical prediction score, called RAMA-AS, to classify risk of having appendicitis. The RAMA-AS showed good internal but fair external calibration, and it well discriminated for both internal and external validations. The RAMA-AS performed better than the Alvarado system (i.e., C-statistics 0.840 VS 0.710), which can suggest whether patients can be observed as out-patients, need further investigation or admit for appendectomy.

Additional files

Additional file 1: Table S1. Re-calibration and revision of models for external validations. **Table S2.** Report number of missing data. **Table S3.** Distributions of predictors by appendicitis groups and developed/validated data. **Table S4.** Estimation of intercept and coefficients for external validations using different update models. **Table S5.** Estimations of calibration coefficients and C-statistics for external validations using different re-calibration and revision methods. (DOCX 57 kb)

Additional file 2: Figure S1. Diagnosis plot between missing and observed values: A) WBC, B) Neutrophil. (PDF 157 kb)

Additional file 3: Figure S2. Receiver operating characteristic (ROC) curves of RAMA-AS for diagnosis of appendicitis. (PDF 153 kb)

Additional file 4: Figure S3. Calibration plots for external validations at Thammasat University Hospital using different update methods. (ZIP 298 kb)

Additional file 5: Figure S4. Calibration plots for external validations at Chaiyapum Hospital using different update methods. (ZIP 298 kb)

Abbreviations

CH: Chaiyaphum Hospital; CI: Confidence interval; E: Expected relative variance increase; FMI: Fraction of missing information; LR: Likelihood ratio; O: Observed; RAMA-AS: Ramathibodi Appendicitis Score; RH: Ramathibodi Hospital; ROC: receiver operating characteristic; RVI: Relative variance increase; STOBE: STrengthening the Reporting of OBservational studies in Epidemiology; TH: Thammasat University Hospital; TRIPOD: Transparent Reporting of a Multivariable Prediction Model for Individual Prognosis Or Diagnosis

Acknowledgements

Not applicable.

Funding

Not applicable.

Authors' contributions

CW initiated the idea, study conception and design, conducted the study and data analysis, interpreted the results, drafting of the manuscript, and critically revised the paper. BS is responsible for the acquisition of data of Thammasat University Hospital setting. SP helped in the acquisition of data of Phukhieo Hospital setting. NP helped in the acquisition of data of Ramathibodi Hospital setting and analysis. PW and PL helped in the study conception and design and critical revision. JA helped in the critical revision. AT helped in the study conception and design, data analysis, wrote the manuscript, interpretation of the results, and critical revision. All authors read and approved the final manuscript.

Competing interests
All authors declared that they had no competing interests.

Author details
[1]Department of Surgery, Faculty of Medicine Ramathibodi Hospital, Mahidol University, Bangkok, Thailand. [2]Section for Clinical Epidemiology and Biostatistics, Faculty of Medicine Ramathibodi Hospital, Mahidol University, Bangkok, Thailand. [3]Department of Surgery, Faculty of Medicine Thammasat University Hospital, Thammasat University, Pathumthani, Thailand. [4]Department of Surgery, Phukhieo Hospital, Chaiyaphum, Thailand. [5]Department of Orthopedics, Faculty of Medicine Ramathibodi Hospital, Mahidol University, Bangkok, Thailand. [6]School of Medicine and Public Health, The University of Newcastle, Newcastle, NSW, Australia.

References
1. Tepel J, Sommerfeld A, Klomp HJ, Kapischke M, Eggert A, Kremer B. Prospective evaluation of diagnostic modalities in suspected acute appendicitis. Langenbeck's Arch Surg. 2004;389(3):219–24.
2. Addiss DG, Shaffer N, Fowler BS, Tauxe RV. The epidemiology of appendicitis and appendectomy in the United States. Am J Epidemiol. 1990;132(5):910–25.
3. Horntrich J, Schneider W. Appendicitis from an epidemiological viewpoint. Zentralbl Chir. 1990;115(23):1521–9.
4. Temple CL, Huchcroft SA, Temple WJ. The natural history of appendicitis in adults. A prospective study. Ann Surg. 1995;221(3):278–81.
5. Alvarado A. A practical score for the early diagnosis of acute appendicitis. Ann Emerg Med. 1986;15(5):557–64.
6. Fenyo G, Lindberg G, Blind P, Enochsson L, Oberg A. Diagnostic decision support in suspected acute appendicitis: validation of a simplified scoring system. Eur J Surg. 1997;163(11):831–8.
7. Eskelinen M, Ikonen J, Lipponen P. The value of history-taking, physical examination, and computer assistance in the diagnosis of acute appendicitis in patients more than 50 years old. Scand J Gastroenterol. 1995;30(4):349–55.
8. Wilasrusmee C, Anothaisintawee T, Poprom N, McEvoy M, Attia J, Thakkinstian A. Diagnostic scores for appendicitis: a systematic review of scores' performance. Br J Med Med Res. 2014;4(2):11–20.
9. Steyerberg EW, Moons KG, van der Windt DA, Hayden JA, Perel P, Schroter S, Riley RD, Hemingway H, Altman DG: Prognosis research strategy (PROGRESS) 3: prognostic model research. PLoS Med 2013, 10(2):e1001381.
10. Moons KG, Altman DG, Reitsma JB, Collins GS. New guideline for the reporting of studies developing, validating, or updating a multivariable clinical prediction model: the TRIPOD statement. Adv Anat Pathol. 2015;22(5):303–5.
11. Vandenbroucke JP, von Elm E, Altman DG, Gotzsche PC, Mulrow CD, Pocock SJ, Poole C, Schlesselman JJ, Egger M, Initiative S. Strengthening the reporting of observational studies in epidemiology (STROBE): explanation and elaboration. Int J Surg. 2014;12(12):1500–24.
12. Peduzzi P, Concato J, Kemper E, Holford TR, Feinstein AR. A simulation study of the number of events per variable in logistic regression analysis. J Clin Epidemiol. 1996;49(12):1373–9.
13. Royston P, Moons KG, Altman DG, Vergouwe Y. Prognosis and prognostic research: developing a prognostic model. BMJ. 2009;338:b604.
14. Rubin DB, Schenker N. Multiple imputation in health-care databases: an overview and some applications. Stat Med. 1991;10(4):585–98.
15. White IR, Royston P, Wood AM. Multiple imputation using chained equations: issues and guidance for practice. Stat Med. 2011;30(4):377–99.
16. van Buuren S, Boshuizen HC, Knook DL: Multiple imputation of missing blood pressure covariates in survival analysis. Stat Med 1999, 18(6):681–94.
17. Hosmer DW, Lemeshow S. Assessing the fit of the model. In: Applied Logistic Regression. second edn. New York: Wiley; 2005. p. 143–202.
18. Steyerberg EW, Bleeker SE, Moll HA, Grobbee DE, Moons KG. Internal and external validation of predictive models: a simulation study of bias and precision in small samples. J Clin Epidemiol. 2003;56(5):441–7.
19. Harrell FE Jr, Lee KL, Mark DB. Multivariable prognostic models: issues in developing models, evaluating assumptions and adequacy, and measuring and reducing errors. Stat Med. 1996;15(4):361–87.
20. Janssen KJ, Vergouwe Y, Kalkman CJ, Grobbee DE, Moons KG. A simple method to adjust clinical prediction models to local circumstances. Can J Anaesth. 2009;56(3):194–201.
21. Toll DB, Janssen KJ, Vergouwe Y, Moons KG. Validation, updating and impact of clinical prediction rules: a review. J Clin Epidemiol. 2008;61(11):1085–94.
22. Kappen TH, Vergouwe Y, van Klei WA, van Wolfswinkel L, Kalkman CJ, Moons KG: Adaptation of clinical prediction models for application in local settings. Med Decis Mak 2012, 32(3):E1-10.
23. Steyerberg EW, Borsboom GJ, van Houwelingen HC, Eijkemans MJ, Habbema JD: Validation and updating of predictive logistic regression models: a study on sample size and shrinkage. Stat Med 2004, 23(16):2567-2586.
24. Lamparelli MJ, Hoque HM, Pogson CJ, Ball AB. A prospective evaluation of the combined use of the modified Alvarado score with selective laparoscopy in adult females in the management of suspected appendicitis. Ann R Coll Surg Engl. 2000;82(3):192–5.
25. Tzanakis NE, Efstathiou SP, Danulidis K, Rallis GE, Tsioulos DI, Chatzivasiliou A, Peros G, Nikiteas NI. A new approach to accurate diagnosis of acute appendicitis. World J Surg. 2005;29(9):1151–6. discussion 1157
26. Kurane SB, Sangolli MS, Gogate AS. A one year prospective study to compare and evaluate diagnostic accuracy of modified Alvarado score and ultrasonography in acute appendicitis, in adults. Indian J Surg. 2008;70(3):125–9.
27. Chong CF, Thien A, Mackie AJ, Tin AS, Tripathi S, Ahmad MA, Tan LT, Ang SH, Telisinghe PU. Comparison of RIPASA and Alvarado scores for the diagnosis of acute appendicitis. Singap Med J. 2011;52(5):340–5.
28. de Castro SM, Unlu C, Steller EP, van Wagensveld BA, Vrouenraets BC: Evaluation of the appendicitis inflammatory response score for patients with acute appendicitis. World J Surg 2012, 36(7):1540-1545.
29. Watters JM. The appendicitis inflammatory response score: a tool for the diagnosis of appendicitis that outperforms the Alvarado score. World J Surg. 2008;32(8):1850.
30. Di Saverio S, Birindelli A, Kelly MD, Catena F, Weber DG, Sartelli M, Sugrue M, De Moya M, Gomes CA, Bhangu A, et al. WSES Jerusalem guidelines for diagnosis and treatment of acute appendicitis. World J Emerg Surg. 2016;11:34.
31. Bhangu A, Soreide K, Di Saverio S, Assarsson JH, Drake FT. Acute appendicitis: modern understanding of pathogenesis, diagnosis, and management. Lancet. 2015;386(10000):1278–87.
32. Soreide K, Korner H, Soreide JA. Diagnostic accuracy and receiver-operating characteristics curve analysis in surgical research and decision making. Ann Surg. 2011;253(1):27–34.
33. Altman DG, Royston P. What do we mean by validating a prognostic model? Stat Med. 2000;19(4):453–73.
34. Held U, Kessels A, Garcia Aymerich J, Basagana X, Ter Riet G, Moons KG, Puhan MA. Methods for handling missing variables in risk prediction models. Am J Epidemiol. 2016;184(7):545–51.
35. Riley RD, Ensor J, Snell KI, Debray TP, Altman DG, Moons KG, Collins GS. External validation of clinical prediction models using big datasets from e-health records or IPD meta-analysis: opportunities and challenges. BMJ. 2016;353:i3140.
36. Di Saverio S, Sibilio A, Giorgini E, Biscardi A, Villani S, Coccolini F, Smerieri N, Pisano M, Ansaloni L, Sartelli M et al: The NOTA study (non operative treatment for acute appendicitis): prospective study on the efficacy and safety of antibiotics (amoxicillin and clavulanic acid) for treating patients with right lower quadrant abdominal pain and long-term follow-up of conservatively treated suspected appendicitis. Ann Surg 2014, 260(1):109-117.
37. Di Saverio S, Sartelli M, Catena F, Birindelli A, Tugnoli G: Renewed interest in acute appendicitis: are antibiotics non-inferior to surgery or possibly clinically superior? What is long-term follow-up and natural evolution of appendicitis treated conservatively with "antibiotics first"? Surg Infect 2016, 17(3):376-377.

30

Performance of imaging studies in patients with suspected appendicitis after stratification with adult appendicitis score

Henna E. Sammalkorpi[1,2*], Ari Leppäniemi[1], Eila Lantto[3] and Panu Mentula[1]

Abstract

Background: Diagnostic scoring is used to stratify patients with suspected appendicitis into three groups: high, intermediate, and low probability of appendicitis. The stratification can be used for selective imaging to avoid the harms of radiation without compromising diagnostic accuracy.
The aim was to study how stratification by Adult Appendicitis Score affects diagnostic performance of imaging studies.

Methods: Analysis of 822 patients who underwent diagnostic imaging for suspected appendicitis was made. Adult Appendicitis Score was used to stratify patients into groups of high, intermediate, and low probability of appendicitis. Diagnostic performance of computed tomography (CT) and ultrasound (US) was compared between these patient groups.

Results: After scoring, pre-test probability of appendicitis ranged from 9-16% in low probability group to 75-79% in high probability group in patients who underwent US or CT. Post-test probability of appendicitis after positive CT was 99, 91, and 75% in high probability, intermediate probability and low probability groups, respectively, $p < 0.001$. After positive US the respective probabilities were 95, 91 and 42%, $p < 0.001$.

Conclusion: Diagnostic imaging has limited value in patients with low probability of appendicitis according to Adult Appendicitis Score.

Keywords: Appendicitis, Imaging, diagnostic, Abdomen, acute, Adult, Ultrasonography, diagnostic, Multidetector computed tomography

Background

CT and US are practical tools in diagnosis of acute appendicitis [1–3]. Lack of guidelines regarding the diagnostic use of imaging may, however, lead to either under- or overuse of these imaging modalities. In many institutions, imaging is mandatory in suspected acute appendicitis [4–6]. Routine CT on all patients with suspected appendicitis induces risks of ionizing radiation and contrast medium as well as increased delay to correct diagnosis and treatment [7–11]. US involves no ionizing radiation, but there is great variance in reported diagnostic performance. The reported sensitivity ranged from 44 to 100% and specificity from 47-99% in a meta-analysis [12]. The aim of avoiding excess radiation has, with good outcomes, led to US utilization as a screening method with additional CT in case of negative or inconclusive finding [1, 4, 6].

In a meta-analysis by van Randen et al. the prevalence of appendicitis was reported to influence the sensitivity and specificity of imaging and benefit less in patient groups with the highest and lowest probabilities of appendicitis [13]. Nevertheless, mandatory imaging for all patients with right lower quadrant abdominal pain is common.

Diagnostic scoring is a simple, free and fast method for stratifying patients according to risk of appendicitis [14, 15]. Diagnostic scoring is recommended in EAES

* Correspondence: henna.sammalkorpi@hus.fi
[1]Department of Gastrointestinal Surgery, Helsinki University Central Hospital, Helsinki, Finland
[2]University of Helsinki, Medical Faculty, Helsinki, Finland
Full list of author information is available at the end of the article

2015 consensus guidelines and WSES 2016 guidelines as a part of diagnostic algorithm for suspected appendicitis [16, 17]. Because of somewhat insufficient discriminating capacities of existing scoring systems, we constructed a novel scoring system, Adult Appendicitis Score (AAS) [18]. The score stratifies patients with suspected appendicitis in three groups according to probability of appendicitis: high, intermediate, and low probability. Instead of replacing imaging, AAS helps to accurately select patients with most uncertain diagnosis to imaging. (Table 1, Fig. 1, www.appendicitisscore.com) Adult Appendicitis Score has been validated and it is now in our hospital part of routine diagnostic work-up of patients suspected of acute appendicitis. In the validation study specificity and sensitivity of high-probability group of the new score were 93.3 and 49.4%, respectively. The negative predictive value of AAS (likelihood of no appendicitis in the low-risk group) was 93% [19].

Diagnostic performance of imaging has not been compared between patient groups of different probability of appendicitis stratified by diagnostic score. Because of potentially high frequency of false positive imaging results, mandatory imaging can induce negative appendectomies in patients with low probability of appendicitis.

This study aimed at evaluating the diagnostic performance of CT and US in patients with different pre-imaging probabilities of appendicitis stratified by Adult Appendicitis Score.

Methods

Patients

We performed an analysis of prospectively collected data of adult (≥16 years) patients at the emergency department. The data were collected in two periods (2011 and 2014–2015). All patients with acute right lower abdominal quadrant pain and/or suspected acute appendicitis were included in the original data collection. For the current study all patients that underwent diagnostic imaging for suspected appendicitis were included. The first data collection was originally for the construction, and the second for the validation of the new diagnostic score. Patients and methods for the first data collection are described in more detailed fashion in the original article of the construction of the score [18]. During the first data collection there were no guidelines of diagnostic work-up of patients with suspected acute appendicitis. Imaging was at all times available and performed at each surgeon's discretion.

In the beginning of the second study period, the AAS was introduced into emergency room routine to guide the diagnostic work-up of patients suspected of acute appendicitis. With the help of AAS patients were stratified in three groups of different probabilities for appendicitis - high, intermediate and low probability. A recommendation according to scoring was provided as follows: High-probability patients could be operated on without further examinations whereas low-probability patients could be discharged. Patients in the intermediate-probability group should undergo diagnostic imaging. This way diagnostic scoring, instead of replacing imaging, helps to accurately select patients with most uncertain diagnosis to imaging [18]. Scoring was performed with a web application that calculated the score and suggested further action based on the scoring result. (Figure 1) Scoring was mandatory, but adherence to the associated guidelines was not controlled. Each surgeon responsible for the patient was able to perform diagnostic imaging regardless of the scoring result.

Both data collections were performed at the emergency department by the surgeons on duty. Additional data was retrieved from patient databases. The collected data included all variables required for scoring, patient demographics, results of possible diagnostic imaging, surgery, histological analysis of appendix, final diagnosis, timing of surgery, delay to diagnosis and surgery, and possible complications. The patients' medical records were reviewed after a minimum of one month after hospital discharge for possible misdiagnosis and complications.

At surgeries for suspected appendicitis, the appendix was at all times removed, and the final diagnosis of appendicitis was invariably based on histological analysis showing transmural neutrophilic inflammation of appendix.

Table 1 Adult Appendicitis Score

Symptoms and findings		Score
Pain in RLQ		2
Pain relocation		2
RLQ tenderness	Women, age 16-49	1
	All other patients	3
Guarding	mild	2
	moderate or severe	4
Laboratory tests		
Blood leukocyte count (x10^9)	> = 7.2 and <10.9	1
	> = 10.9 and <14.0	2
	> = 14.0	3
Proportion of neutrophils (%)	> = 62 and < 75	2
	> = 75 and < 83	3
	> = 83	4
CRP (mg/l), symptoms < 24 h	> = 4 and <11	2
	> = 11and <25	3
	> = 25 and <83	5
	> = 83	1
CRP (mg/l), symptoms > 24 h	> = 12 and <53	2
	> = 53 and <152	2
	> = 152	1

RLQ, right lower abdominal quadrant

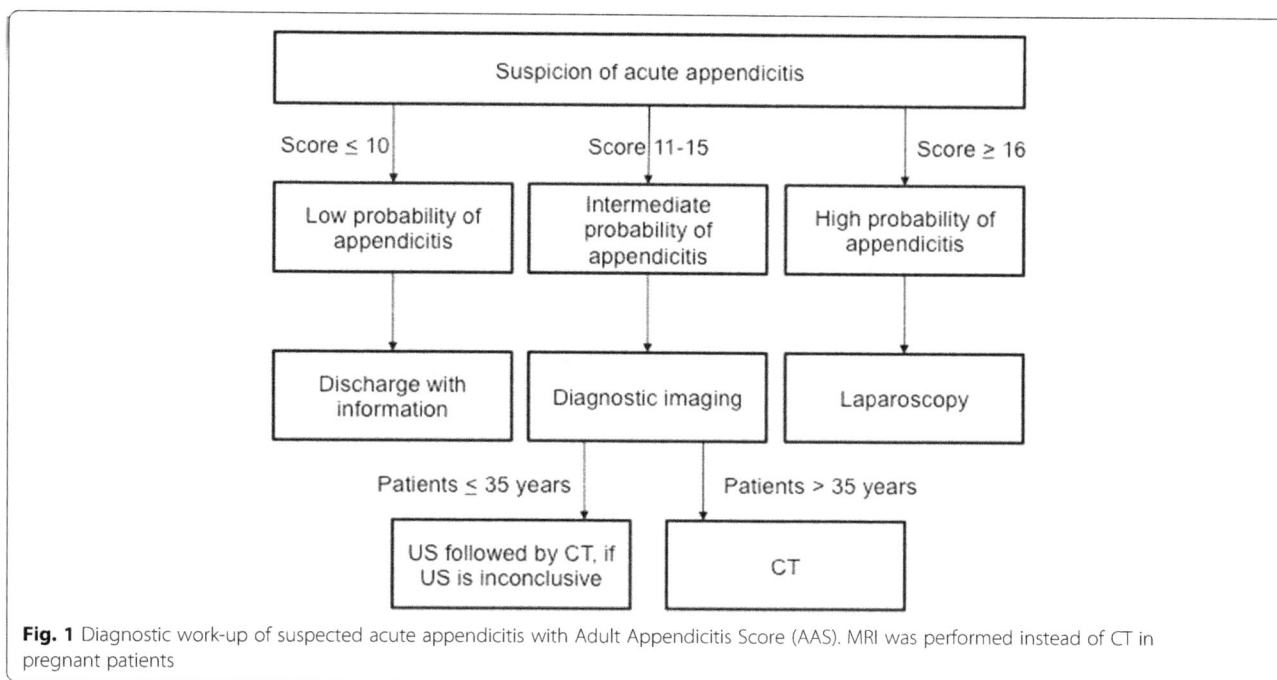

Fig. 1 Diagnostic work-up of suspected acute appendicitis with Adult Appendicitis Score (AAS). MRI was performed instead of CT in pregnant patients

Imaging procedures

In patients of age 35 or less and all pregnant patients, US was recommended as a primary imaging modality, CT (or MRI in pregnant patients) was recommended in case of negative or inconclusive US.

US examinations were performed by radiology residents with minimum experience of 2 years or attending radiologists with a possibility to consult a more experienced colleague. A general survey of the abdomen and pelvis was done using the graded compression technique with convex 3.5 – 5 MHz probe and linear 6–12 MHz probe (GE Logic 9E, GE Healthcare, Wisconsin, USA). Inconclusive US reports were classified as negative for appendicitis in this study.

CT scans were performed by using 128 multi-detector row scanner with automatic tube current and tube voltage modulation (Somatom Definition AS+, Siemens Medical Systems, Erlangen, Germany). Patients underwent an abdominopelvic CT protocol with intravenous contrast-enhancement (iohexol, Omnipaque 350 mgI/ml, GE Healthcare, Oslo, Norway, bolus 1,5 ml/kg body weight at 3 ml/s flow rate) in portal venous phase. Patients with known renal failure or hypersensitivity to contrast media underwent unenhanced CT. CT parameters were as follows: reference mAs 110, reference kV 120, collimation 128 x 0,6 mm, rotation time 0,5 s. Data was reconstructed at 3 mm axial, coronal and sagittal slices and analysed using PACS workstations by a staff radiologist during working hours and by a radiologic resident after hours. These original reports contributing to surgeons' decision-making were used in study analysis.

Effective dose of low dose CT was 3.2 mSv in women and 2.6 mSv in men.

Non-compressible appendix larger than 6 mm in diameter with or without appendicolith together with local transducer tenderness, and peri-appendiceal fat infiltration were criterion for acute appendicitis in ultrasound.

On CT, increased appendiceal diameter (greater than 6 mm), with or without appendicolith together with appendiceal wall thickening, increased wall enhancement, and peri-appendiceal fat infiltration were criteria for acute appendicitis.

Statistical analysis

Statistical analysis was performed using SPSS® version 22 (IBM, Armonk, New York, USA). AAS was calculated for all patients. The pre-test probability (probability of appendicitis in patients undergoing imaging) and post-test probabilities (probability of appendicitis in patients with positive or negative imaging result) of acute appendicitis as well as accuracy, specificity, sensitivity, likelihood ratios, and diagnostic odds ratio for US and CT were calculated. Diagnostic performance of MRI was left outside further analysis because of small amount of patients.

These results were compared between patient groups of different prevalence of acute appendicitis stratified by AAS.

Results

All patients

Diagnostic imaging was performed on 822 (53%) of 1545 patients with suspected acute appendicitis. 892 (58%) of

1545 patients with suspected appendicitis had appendectomy, out of which 121 (13.6%) were not inflamed. Of all patients that underwent diagnostic imaging, 368 (45%) had appendicitis. CT was performed to 489 (32%), US to 497 (32%), and magnetic resonance imaging (MRI) to 14 (1%) patients. (Table 2).

Pre-test probability of appendicitis in all patients that underwent CT was 257 of 489 (52.6%). The overall sensitivity and specificity of CT were 98.4 and 92.2%, respectively. The observed post-test probability for positive CT was 253 of 260 (97.3%) and for negative CT 4 of 229 (1.75%). The accuracy of CT (the proportion of correct (true positive or true negative) imaging results) 478 of 489 (97.8%).

Pre-test probability of appendicitis in all patients that underwent US was 177 of 497 (36.6%). The overall sensitivity and specificity of US were 48.6 and 94.4%, respectively. The post-test probability for positive US was 86 of 104 (82.7%), and for negative US 91 of 393 (23.2%). The overall accuracy of US was 388 of 497 (78.1%). (Tables 2-4).

High probability group (AAS ≥16)
In the group of high probability of acute appendicitis there were 439 patients of whom 386 (88%) had appendicitis. CT was performed to 114 (26%) patients. In patients that underwent CT pre-test probability of acute appendicitis was 90 of 114 (78.9%). The post-test probability for appendicitis was for a positive test 90 of 91 (98.9%) and for a negative test 0 of 23 (0%). The accuracy of CT was in this group 113 of 114 (99.1%). (Table 3, Table 4, Fig. 2).

US was performed to 52 (12%) patients. Pre-test probability of appendicitis in patients that underwent US was 41 of 52 (75.0%). The post-test probability for appendicitis was for a positive US 19 of 20 (95%) and for a negative 22 of 32 (68.8%). The accuracy of US was in this group 29 of 52 (55.8%) (Tables 2-4, Fig. 2).

Intermediate probability group (AAS 11-15)
In the group of intermediate probability of acute appendicitis there were 596 patients of whom 304 (51%) had appendicitis. CT was performed to 276 (46%) patients. Pre-test probability of appendicitis in patients that underwent CT was 138 of 276 (50%). The post-test probability for appendicitis was for a positive test 135 of 148 (91.2%) and for a negative 3 of 128 (2.3%). The accuracy of CT was in this group 260 of 276 (94.2%). (Tables 2-4, Fig. 2).

US was performed to 258 (43%) patients in the intermediate probability group. Pre-test probability of appendicitis in patients that underwent US was 122 of 258 (47.3%). The post-test probability for appendicitis was for a positive US 59 of 65 (90.8%) and for a negative 69 of 193 (32.6%). The accuracy of US was in this group 189 of 258 (73.3%). (Tables 2-4, Fig. 2).

Low probability group (AAS ≤10)
In the group of low probability for appendicitis there were 510 patients of whom 34 (7%) had appendicitis. CT was performed to 99 (19%) patients. Pre-test probability of appendicitis in patients that underwent CT was 16 of 99 (16.2%). The post-test probability for appendicitis was for a positive CT 15 of 20 (75.0%) and for a negative 1 of 79 (1.3%). The accuracy of CT was in this group 93 of 99 (93.9%). (Tables 2-4, Fig. 2).

US was performed to 187 (37%) patients in the low probability group. Pre-test probability of appendicitis in patients that underwent US was 17 of 187 (9.1%). The post-test probability for appendicitis was for a positive US 8 of 19 (42.1%) and for a negative 9 of 168 (5.4%). The accuracy of US was in this group 167 of 187 (89.3%). (Tables 2-4, Fig. 2).

Diagnostic performance of imaging related to prevalence of appendicitis
There was statistically significant difference between the different score groups in observed post-test probability after positive imaging result (the proportion of true positive compared to false positive imaging results). (Figure 2) In the low-probability patients, there were 15 true positive and 5 false positive CT examinations (post-test probability after positive test 75%). In the intermediate-probability patients the post-test probability was 135 of 148 (91%), and in the high-probability group 90 of 91 (99%) ($p < 0.001$, chi-square test). (Tables 3 and 4, Fig. 2).

In the low probability group, there were 8 true positive and 11 false positive US examinations and post-test

Table 2 Prevalence of appendicitis in patients that underwent either no diagnostic imaging, US, CT or MRI

Probability of appendicitis	All patients[a]	No imaging[a]	CT[a]	US[a]	MRI[a]
All patients	724/1545 (46.9%)	356/723 (49.2%)	257/489 (52.6%)	177/497 (35.6%)	5/14 (35.7%)
High (AAS ≥16)	386/439 (87.9%)	261/282 (92.6%)	90/114 (78.9%)	41/52 (78.8%)	1/2 (50%)
Intermediate (AAS 11-15)	304/596 (51.0%)	89/172 (51.7%)	138/276 (50.0%)	122/258 (47.3%)	2/8 (25%)
Low (AAS ≤10)	34/510 (6.7%)	6/269 (2.2%)	16/99 (16.2%)	17/187 (9.1%)	2/4 (50%)

[a]Numbers show patients with appendicitis/total amount of patients in each group (%)
AAS, Adult Appendicitis Score

Table 3 Diagnostic performance of US and CT

Probability of appendicitis according to AAS	Sensitivity	Specificity	LR+	LR-	DOR
US					
All patients	48.6%	94.4%	8.646	0.545	15.86
High (AAS ≥16)	46.3%	90.9%	5.098	0.590	8.636
Intermediate (AAS 11–15)	48.4%	95.6%	10.971	0.540	20.291
Low (AAS ≤10)	47.1%	93.5%	7.274	0.566	12.848
CT					
All patients	98.4%	92.2%	12.615	0.017	742.06
High (AAS ≥16)	100.0%	95.8%	23.98	0	Infinite
Intermediate (AAS 11–15)	97.8%	90.6%	10.385	0.024	432.69
Low (AAS ≤10)	93.8%	94.0%	15.573	0.067	234.00

AAS, Adult Appendicitis Score, *LR+*, positive likelihood ratio, *LR*, negative likelihood ratio, DOR diagnostic odds ratio

probability of appendicitis after positive US was 42%. In the intermediate and high probability patients the post-test probability was 59 of 65 (90.8%) and 19 of 20 (95%), respectively ($p < 0.001$, chi-square test).

Other diagnostic findings
In high probability group 18 (16%) patients had other specific diseases and 6 (5%) did not have diagnostic findings on CT scan. In the intermediate probability group and low probability group the rate of other diagnosis on CT were 33 and 35%, respectively. On the contrary US found other diagnosis only in 4 (7%) patients and 26 (50%) did not have diagnostic findings on US in high probability group. Other specific diagnoses were found with US in 19 (7%) and 18 (10%) patients in intermediate and low probability groups, respectively.

Prevalence of appendicitis in patients managed without imaging
Seven hundred twenty-three (47%) patients included into prospective data collection did not undergo diagnostic imaging. Among these patients, in high probability group

261 (92.6%) out of 282 patients, in intermediate probability group 89 (51.7%) out of 172 patients, and in low probability group 6 (2.2%) out of 269 patients had appendicitis.

Discussion
This study shows that, based on the clinical score, in patients with most improbable appendicitis (AAS ≤10), screening with US adds little benefit and can even be harmful because of considerable amount of false positive imaging results. There were more false than true positive results in US in this group, leading to a negative appendectomy rate of 58% after US in this group. When the low-probability patients underwent CT, 25% of positive results were false. In every 20 CT examinations in the low-probability group there were 3 true and 1 false positive results, leading to negative appendectomy rate of 25%. Hence only 15% of patients in low probability group had benefit from CT, whereas 85% were exposed to ionizing radiation without significant benefit in diagnosis. In the low probability group, there were no patients with perforated appendix and peritonitis. To avoid false positive imaging results and high rate of negative

Table 4 Pre- and post-test probabilities of appendicitis, patients who underwent US or CT

Probability of AA according to AAS	Pre-test probability of AA	Post-test probability of AA, positive test	Post-test probability of AA, negative test
US			
All patients, n = 497	177/497 (37%)	86/104 (83%)	91/393 (23%)
High, n = 52	41/52 (75%)	19/20 (95%)	22/32 (69%)
Intermediate, n = 258	122/258 (47%)	59/65 (91%)	63/193 (33%)
Low, n = 187	17/187 (9%)	8/19 (42%)	9/168 (5.4%)
CT			
All patients, n = 489	257/489 (53%)	253/260 (97%)	4/229 (1.8%)
High, n = 114	90/114 (79%)	90/91 (99%)	0/23 (0%)
Intermediate, n = 276	138/276 (50%)	135/148 (91%)	3/128 (2.3%)
Low, n = 99	16/99 (16%)	15/20 (75%)	1/79 (1.3%)

AA, Acute appendicitis, *AAS*, Adult Appendicitis Score

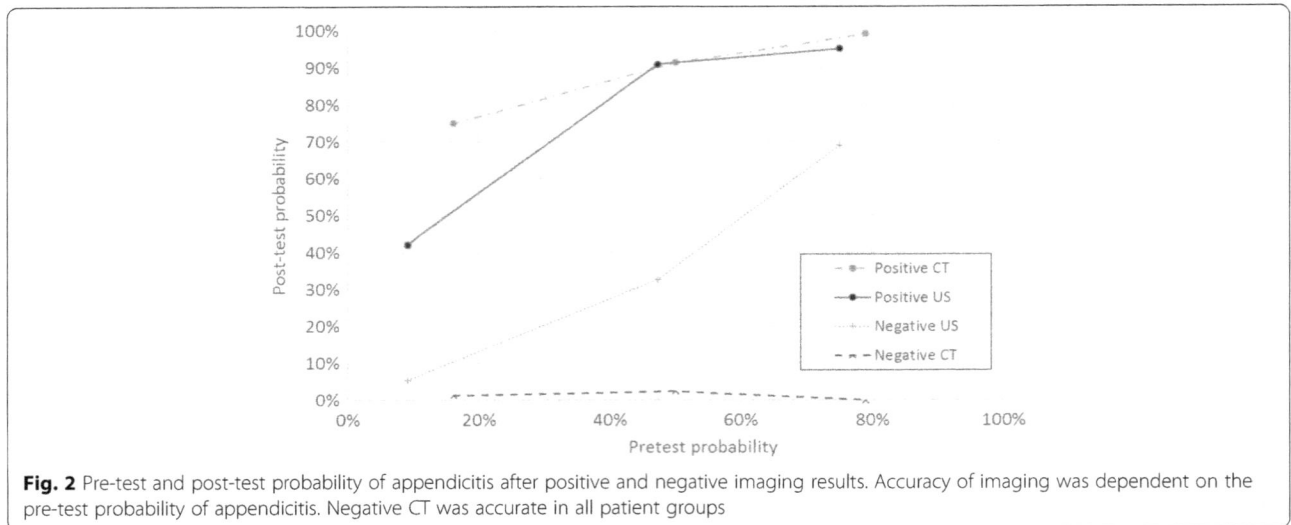

Fig. 2 Pre-test and post-test probability of appendicitis after positive and negative imaging results. Accuracy of imaging was dependent on the pre-test probability of appendicitis. Negative CT was accurate in all patient groups

appendectomies, we suggest that patients with low AAS and equivocal diagnosis would undergo clinical observation instead of immediate imaging. In this group patients have vague symptoms and part of the patients probably have appendicitis that would resolve spontaneously during the follow-up [20, 21].

CT, with excellent diagnostic performance, is the best method for excluding appendicitis in the high probability patients when there is disagreement between scoring and the clinical evaluation. In the high probability group, scoring alone had in our study of the validation of AAS specificity of 93.3%, and hence we do not recommend routine imaging in this group. Also, in high probability group, patients who did not have diagnostic imaging the probability of appendicitis was 93%, which was higher than post-test probability of appendicitis after positive CT scan in intermediate probability group. However, in these patients, diagnostic performance of US is good and of CT excellent and imaging should be performed without hesitation when there is clinical suspicion of other diagnosis than appendicitis. In young patients, to avoid radiation, US should be the primary imaging modality. However, US has limited value in finding other diagnosis, and thus CT is usually needed when US is negative or inconclusive.

In meta-analysis by Parker et al. of cost and radiation savings of partial substitution of US for CT, the sensitivity and specificity of CT were 93.4 and 95.3% respectively [2]. In the meta-analysis by van Randen et al. the prevalence of appendicitis was related to post-test probability in three different populations. The analysis showed that the added value of imaging in suspected appendicitis depends on the pre-test probability of appendicitis. The respective mean sensitivity and specificity of CT were 91 and 91% [13]. In our study, the sensitivity of CT was in all patients 98.4% and specificity 97.0%. Alike in the

meta-analysis by van Randen, the post-test probability after positive CT was related to the prevalence of appendicitis and differed significantly in different risk groups.

In the meta-analysis by Parker et al. the sensitivity of US was 87.5% and specificity 92.7%. In the meta-analysis by van Randen et al. mean sensitivity and specificity of US were 78 and 83% respectively. In our study the sensitivity of US in all patients was 48.6% and specificity 94.4%. In both the meta-analysis by van Randen et al. and the current study the post-test probability of appendicitis after positive US decreased dramatically along decreasing prevalence of appendicitis.

Spontaneously resolving appendicitis is a phenomenon that has been described in surgical and radiological literature [20, 22–24]. Despite the increased diagnostic accuracy of appendicitis, we are currently not able to recognize patients with resolving appendicitis in the early phase of disease. The patients with spontaneous resolution of appendicitis probably have milder, nonspecific symptoms. This is supported by the studies by Decadt et al. and Morino et al. in which patients with non-specific abdominal pain were randomized to either early laparoscopy or close observation. In both studies in the laparoscopy groups, there were significantly more patients with acute appendicitis than in the observation groups [25, 26]. In suspected appendicitis, if imaging is mandatory, prevalence of uncomplicated appendicitis increases because patients with possible spontaneous resolution of appendicitis undergo surgery [27, 28]. Hence, diagnostic guidelines with conditional imaging aid to prevent surgery for patients with resolving appendicitis.

We have implemented the AAS scoring system to guide the diagnostic work-up of patients with suspected acute appendicitis. The aim of scoring is not to replace imaging. In contrary, scoring helps to avoid under- and overuse of imaging studies by targeting these investigations to patients with most equivocal diagnosis. All patients with suspected appendicitis were included in the study. Some patients, however, should be excluded from the routine diagnostic work-up. Pregnant patients should invariably undergo imaging in case of suspected appendicitis because of increased negative appendectomy rate and high risk of fetal loss after surgery [29, 30]. CT should in pregnant patients be replaced with MRI to avoid ionizing radiation [31]. Patients with clinical suspicion of appendiceal abscess should undergo CT examination. In these patients, CT, in addition to being the most accurate imaging method, also benefits in planning the treatment. In immunosuppressed patients, threshold of imaging should be low. Immunosuppression alters laboratory results and can mask the typical clinical signs and symptoms of appendicitis.

In this study, US was performed and CT reported by radiology residents and attending radiologists with varying experience. Hence this study describes well the real-life situation in the emergency setting. The preliminary reports by on-call residents are in our hospital re-evaluated next morning by a staff radiologist. However, the re-evaluation is rarely performed before the decision of treatment is made.

In the Netherlands, the national guidelines recommend mandatory imaging in suspected acute appendicitis. The primary imaging modality is US followed by CT in case of inconclusive US. With this protocol, excellent results have been published [5, 6]. In a study by Atema et al., immediate CT was compared to conditional CT after negative or non-diagnostic US [4]. The amount of CT examinations was halved with the conditional strategy, but resulted in more false positive imaging results. In our study, false positive imaging results lead to high rate of negative appendectomy in the low probability patients. We suggest that scoring would be implemented in the diagnostic work-up to exclude from the mandatory imaging protocol the low-probability patients with frequent false positive findings in imaging.

There was no cost-benefit analysis involved in this study. However, previous research suggests that mandatory imaging is cost-beneficial, and that conditional CT has cost benefits when CT is partially replaced with US [2, 5]. In the light of present study, excluding the patients with least probable appendicitis from mandatory imaging can further increase these benefits.

Limitations

Adult Appendicitis Score is novel, and no large external validation studies have been published yet. More studies would strengthen the validation of the score. Another potential limitation of this study is that only part of patients suspected of appendicitis was imaged. Because patients underwent imaging at surgeons' discretion, potential verification bias exists.

Conclusions

In conclusion, this study shows that diagnostic performance of CT and US depends on pre-test probability of appendicitis. Adult Appendicitis Score (online calculator available on www. appendicitisscore.com) can be used in patients with suspected appendicitis to guide selective use of imaging studies. Patients with low probability of appendicitis according to scoring have limited value from diagnostic imaging.

Abbreviations
AA: Acute appendicitis; AAS: Adult Appendicitis Score; CT: Computed tomography; DOR: diagnostic odds ratio; LR: negative likelihood ratio; LR+: positive likelihood ratio; MRI: Magnetic resonance imaging; US: Ultrasound

Acknowledgements
Not applicable.

Funding
The study was financially supported by the Martti I. Turunen's foundation (personal research grant for the corresponding author).

Author contributions
HS, PM, and AL designed the study. HS collected, analyzed, and interpreted the data together with PM. HS wrote the manuscript except for the part describing radiological methods which was written by EL. All four authors revised the manuscript. All authors read and approved the final manuscript.

Competing interest
The authors declare that there are no competing interests.

Author details
[1]Department of Gastrointestinal Surgery, Helsinki University Central Hospital, Helsinki, Finland. [2]University of Helsinki, Medical Faculty, Helsinki, Finland. [3]Department of Radiology, Helsinki University Central Hospital, Helsinki, Finland.

References
1. Boonstra PA, van Veen RN, Stockmann HB. Less negative appendectomies due to imaging in patients with suspected appendicitis. Surg Endosc. 2015;29:2365–70.
2. Parker L, Nazarian LN, Gingold EL, Palit CD, Hoey CL, Frangos AJ. Cost and radiation savings of partial substitution of ultrasound for CT in appendicitis evaluation: a national projection. AJR Am J Roentgenol. 2014;202:124–35.
3. Kim K, Kim YH, Kim SY, et al. Low-dose abdominal CT for evaluating suspected appendicitis. N Engl J Med. 2012;366:1596–605.
4. Atema JJ, Gans SL, Van Randen A, et al. Comparison of imaging strategies with conditional versus immediate contrast-enhanced computed tomography in patients with clinical suspicion of acute appendicitis. Eur Radiol. 2015;25:2445–52.
5. Lahaye MJ, Lambregts DM, Mutsaers E, et al. Mandatory imaging cuts costs and reduces the rate of unnecessary surgeries in the diagnostic work-up of patients suspected of having appendicitis. Eur Radiol. 2015;25:1464.1470.
6. van Rossem CC, Bolmers MD, Schreinemacher MH, van Geloven AA, Bemelman WA, Snapshot Appendicitis Collaborative Study G. Prospective

nationwide outcome audit of surgery for suspected acute appendicitis. Br J Surg. 2016;103:144–51.

7.   Rogers W, Hoffman J, Noori N. Harms of CT scanning prior to surgery for suspected appendicitis. Evid Based Med. 2015;20:3–4.

8.   Lee SL, Walsh AJ, Ho HS. Computed tomography and ultrasonography do not improve and may delay the diagnosis and treatment of acute appendicitis. Arch Surg. 2001;136:556–62.

9.   Sammalkorpi HE, Leppäniemi A, Mentula P. High admission C-reactive protein level and longer in-hospital delay to surgery are associated with increased risk of complicated appendicitis. Langenbecks Arch Surg Vol. 2015;400:221–8.

10. Lehtimaki T, Juvonen P, Valtonen H, Miettinen P, Paajanen H, Vanninen R. Impact of routine contrast-enhanced CT on costs and use of hospital resources in patients with acute abdomen. Results of a randomised clinical trial. Eur Radiol. 2013;23:2538–45.

11. Pritchett CV, Levinsky NC, Ha YP, Dembe AE, Steinberg SM. Management of acute appendicitis: the impact of CT scanning on the bottom line. J Am Coll Surg. 2010;210(699–705):705–697.

12. Pinto F, Pinto A, Russo A, et al. Accuracy of ultrasonography in the diagnosis of acute appendicitis in adult patients: review of the literature. Crit Ultrasound J. 2013;5 Suppl 1:S2.

13. van Randen A, Bipat S, Zwinderman AH, Ubbink DT, Stoker J, Boermeester MA. Acute appendicitis: meta-analysis of diagnostic performance of CT and graded compression US related to prevalence of disease. Radiology. 2008;249:97–106.

14. Andersson M, Andersson RE. The appendicitis inflammatory response score: a tool for the diagnosis of acute appendicitis that outperforms the alvarado score. World J Surg. 2008;32:1843–9.

15. Kollar D, McCartan DP, Bourke M, Cross KS, Dowdall J. Predicting acute appendicitis? a comparison of the alvarado score, the appendicitis inflammatory response score and clinical assessment. World J Surg. 2015;39:104–9.

16. Gorter RR, Eker HH, Gorter-Stam MA, et al. Diagnosis and management of acute appendicitis. EAES consensus development conference 2015. Surg Endosc. 2016. doi:10.1007/s00464-016-5245-7.

17. Di Saverio S, Birindelli A, Kelly MD, et al. WSES jerusalem guidelines for diagnosis and treatment of acute appendicitis. World J Emerg Surg. 2016;11:34.

18. Sammalkorpi H, Mentula P, Leppäniemi A, Sammalkorpi H, Mentula P, Leppäniemi A. A new adult appendicitis score improves diagnostic accuracy of acute appendicitis–a prospective study. BMC Gastroenterol. 2014;14:114.

19. Sammalkorpi H, Mentula P, Savolainen H, Leppäniemi A. The introduction of Adult Appendicitis Score reduced negative appendectomy rate. Scandinavian Journal of Surgery. 2016 in press

20. Andersson RE. The natural history and traditional management of appendicitis revisited: spontaneous resolution and predominance of prehospital perforations imply that a correct diagnosis is more important than an early diagnosis. World J Surg. 2007;31:86–92.

21. Di Saverio S, Birindelli A, Piccinini A, Catena F, Biscardi A, Tugnoli G. How reliable is alvarado score and its subgroups in ruling Out acute appendicitis and suggesting the opportunity of nonoperative management or surgery? Ann Surg. 2016. doi:10.1097/sla.0000000000001548.

22. Ciani S, Chuaqui B. Histological features of resolving acute, non-complicated phlegmonous appendicitis. Pathol Res Pract. 2000;196:89–93.

23. Cobben LP, de Van Otterloo AM, Puylaert JB. Spontaneously resolving appendicitis: frequency and natural history in 60 patients. Radiology. 2000;215:349–52.

24. Barber MD, McLaren J, Rainey JB. Recurrent appendicitis. Br J Surg. 1997;84:110–2.

25. Decadt B, Sussman L, Lewis MP, et al. Randomized clinical trial of early laparoscopy in the management of acute non-specific abdominal pain. Br J Surg. 1999;86:1383–6.

26. Morino M, Pellegrino L, Castagna E, Farinella E, Mao P. Acute nonspecific abdominal pain: a randomized, controlled trial comparing early laparoscopy versus clinical observation. Ann Surg. 2006;244:881–6. discussion 886–888.

27. Andersson RE. Resolving appendicitis is common: further evidence. Ann Surg. 2008;247:553. author reply 553.

28. Rao PM, Rhea JT, Rattner DW, Venus LGAS, Novelline RA. Introduction of appendiceal CT: impact on negative appendectomy and appendiceal perforation rates. Ann Surg. 1999;229:344–9.

29. Ito K, Ito H, Whang EE, Tavakkolizadeh A. Appendectomy in pregnancy: evaluation of the risks of a negative appendectomy. Am J Surg. 2012;203:145–50.

30. McGory ML, Zingmond DS, Tillou A, Hiatt JR, Ko CY, Cryer HM. Negative appendectomy in pregnant women is associated with a substantial risk of fetal loss. J Am Coll Surg. 2007;205:534–40.

31. Konrad J, Grand D, Lourenco A. MRI: first-line imaging modality for pregnant patients with suspected appendicitis. Abdom Imaging. 2015;40:3359–64.

31

The abdominal wall hernia in cirrhotic patients

Giuseppe Salamone[*†], Leo Licari[†], Giovanni Guercio, Sofia Campanella, Nicolò Falco, Gregorio Scerrino, Sebastiano Bonventre, Girolamo Geraci, Gianfranco Cocorullo and Gaspare Gulotta

Abstract

Background: The incidence rate of abdominal wall hernia is 20–40% in cirrhotic patients. A surgical approach was originally performed only if complication signs and symptoms occurred. Several recent studies have demonstrated the usefulness of elective surgery. During recent decades, the indications for surgical timing have changed.

Methods: Cirrhotic patients with abdominal hernia who underwent surgical operation for abdominal wall hernia repair at the Policlinico "Paolo Giaccone" at Palermo University Hospital between January 2010 and September 2016 were identified in a prospective database, and the data collected were retrospectively reviewed; patients' medical and surgical records were collected from charts and surgical and intensive care unit (ICU) registries. Postoperative morbidity was determined through the Clavien-Dindo classification. Cirrhosis severity was estimated by the Child-Pugh-Turcotte (CPT) score and MELD (model of end-stage liver disease) score. Postoperative mortality was considered up to 30 days after surgery. A follow-up period of at least 1 year was used to evaluate hernia recurrence.

Results: The univariate and multivariate analyses demonstrated the unique independent risk factors for the development of postsurgical morbidity (emergency surgery (OR 6.42; p 0.023), CPT class C (OR 3.72; p 0.041), American Society of Anesthesiologists (ASA) score $\geq$ 3 (OR 4.72; p 0.012) and MELD $\geq$ 20 (OR 5.64; p 0.009)) and postsurgical mortality (emergency surgery (OR 10.32; p 0.021), CPT class C (OR 5.52; p 0.014), ASA score $\geq$ 3 (OR 8.65; p 0.018), MELD $\geq$ 20 (OR 2.15; p 0.02)).

Conclusions: Concerning abdominal wall hernia repair in cirrhotic patients, the worst outcome is associated with emergency surgery and with uncontrolled disease. The correct timing of the surgical operation is elective surgery after ascites drainage and albumin/electrolyte serum level and coagulation alteration correction.

Keywords: Abdominal wall hernia, Cirrhosis, Surgery, Emergency, Risk factors

Background

The overall incidence of abdominal wall hernias is approximately 14%; it increases to 20% in cirrhotic patients and might be up to 40% in cases of major ascites [1, 2]. Factors such as weakness of the fascia and of the abdominal muscles due to malnutrition state and enlargement of pre-existing openings in the fascia promoted by increased abdominal pressure as a result of ascites formation are important contributors to the development of the hernias [3, 4]. The watch-and-wait policy was commonly accepted in the past because of the high perioperative morbidity and

mortality that cirrhotic patients encountered. A surgical approach was then performed only if complication signs and symptoms occurred. However, the recommendations have changed during the last decade [5–7]. Previous retrospective studies [8] demonstrated that conservative treatment of abdominal wall hernias in cirrhotic patients is associated with considerable morbidity and mortality. Optimizing the patients with liver cirrhosis before elective hernia repair is critical for minimizing postoperative complications and reducing recurrence.

Moreover, it is commonly accepted that abdominal wall hernia repair should ideally be performed during liver transplantation or during liver function improvement.

In candidates for liver transplantation, the surgical operation should be performed during transplantation

* Correspondence: lele.licari@gmail.com
†Salamone Giuseppe and Licari Leo contributed equally to this work.
Department of Surgical, Oncological and Oral Science, University of Palermo, Policlinico P. Giaccone. Via Liborio Giuffré 5, 90127 Palermo, Italy

unless the patient presents with significant symptoms or hernia complications or if the perspective to be transplanted exceeds 3–6 months [9].

Several studies have demonstrated that elective surgery in cirrhotic patients could be safe, even when refractory ascites or advanced cirrhosis is diagnosed, if it is performed in a high-volume liver center [9–11]. Early elective hernia repair in these patients should be advocated considering the hepatic reserve and the patient's condition. The study herein analyzed the characteristics of cirrhotic patients who underwent abdominal wall hernia repair and investigated the risk factors for postoperative morbidity and mortality.

Methods

Cirrhotic patients with abdominal hernia who underwent surgical operation for abdominal wall hernia repair at the Policlinico "Paolo Giaccone" at Palermo University Hospital between January 2010 and September 2016 were identified in a prospective database, and the data collected were retrospectively reviewed; patients' medical and surgical records were collected from charts and the surgical and ICU registries.

The diagnosis of abdominal wall hernia was obtained after physical examination and US/CT scan execution.

Cirrhosis was documented by anamnestic data and confirmed through clinical, laboratory, and radiological findings.

Postoperative morbidity was determined through the Clavien-Dindo classification; classes III to V events were considered major complications. Cirrhosis severity was estimated by the Child-Pugh-Turcotte (CPT) score and MELD score calculated at the time of the surgical procedure.

Postoperative mortality was considered up to 30 days after surgery [12–14]. A follow-up period of at least 1 year was used to evaluate hernia recurrence, as diagnosed with physical examination and US/CT scan.

Patients with refractory ascites underwent paracentesis, albumin and serum electrolytes were replaced, nutritional support was guaranteed, and coagulation disorders were corrected pre- and postoperatively when indicated.

Abdominal wall hernias were repaired with the direct suture repair surgical technique when the defect did not exceed 3 cm or in cases of a contaminated/dirty surgical field; otherwise, the mesh-repair technique was adopted with sublay retromuscular positioning of a polyester mesh fixed at the posterior fascia of the rectus abdominis muscle with non-reabsorbable sutures. Indirect inguinal hernias were repaired with the plug- and mesh-mediated technique using a polypropylene plug fixed in the internal inguinal ring at the conjoint tendon and Cooper ligament; the polypropylene mesh was then positioned under the aponeurosis of the external oblique muscle (Trabucco

technique). Direct inguinal hernias were repaired by performing the Lichtenstein technique after sac isolation and inversion into the preperitoneal space, preserving the integrity of the peritoneal sac. Patients with a diagnosis of recurrent abdominal wall hernia were not enrolled in the database. All surgical operations were performed via laparotomy.

Patient characteristics are shown in Table 1.

Twenty-six patients (22%) were operated on under general anesthesia; 83 patients (71%) underwent the surgical operation under local anesthesia, and eight patients (7%) had spinal anesthesia. Details regarding the distribution of the type of hernia, anesthesia regimen used for each surgical operation and mesh usage are shown in Table 1.

Statistical analyses

Data were analyzed using Excel 2013 and IBM SPSS software, version 21. The median was obtained for continuous variables. Comparisons of continuous variables were made using Student's t test or the Mann-Whitney test, where appropriate. Comparisons of categorical variables were made with the chi-squared (χ^2) test or Fisher's exact test. The statistical significance level was set to p value < 0.05.

Univariate analysis for morbidity and survival was performed; the clinical variables included were emergency, CPT, ASA score, ascites, prosthesis use, MELD score, age, sex, and general anesthesia; the type of hernias was evaluated in the univariate analysis to identify possible risk factors for postoperative morbidity. The variables with p values < 0.05 in the univariate analysis were included in the multivariate logistic regression, considering odds ratios with 95% confidence intervals and p values < 0.05.

Results

Between January 2010 and September 2016, 117 cirrhotic patients were identified as undergoing abdominal wall hernia repair. Forty-one patients (35% of the cirrhotic patients with abdominal wall hernia) were treated in emergency situations. The median pre-operative MELD score was 13. The MELD score rate ≥ 20 in elective and emergency surgery was 20% and 41% respectively (Table 1). The minimal follow-up time was 1 year. Mesh positioning was performed in 76 cases, of which 21 were in the emergency group. Emergency criteria were perforation ($n = 4$), incarceration ($n = 27$), strangulation ($n = 7$), and skin ulceration ($n = 3$).

Six patients had bilateral inguinal hernia, 30 had monolateral inguinal hernia, 60 had umbilical hernia, and 21 had incisional hernia.

Death occurred in 27 patients within 30 days after surgery and in 22 after emergency surgical operations; the causes of death were MOF due to sepsis after infection of the ascites ($n = 16$) and major ascites for decompensated

Table 1 Characteristics of the population

Variables		Population (n = 117)	Elective surgery (n = 76)	Emergency surgery (n = 41)
Age		60 (53–81)	60 (53–81)	65 (60–81)
Male		100 (86%)	66 (88%)	34 (82%)
Mean BMI		25	27	24
Poorly controlled ascites (n of patients)		41	14	27
CPT:	A (n of patients)	41 (35%)	41 (54%)	0
	B (n of patients)	27 (23%)	23 (30%)	4 (10%)
	C (n of patients)	49 (42%)	12 (16%)	37 (90%)
Mean pre-operative MELD score		13	12	16
n of patients with MELD score ≥ 20		32 (27%)	15 (20%)	17 (41%)
Mesh use		76 (65%)	55 (47%)	21 (18%)
Mean in-hospital stay (days)		10	7	16
Post-operative ICU (n of patients)		23 (20%)	8 (10%)	15 (36%)
Mean ICU stay (days)		7	2	10
Death		27 (23%)	5 (6.6%)	22 (53.6%)
Clavien-Dindo score	I	27	27	0
	II	22	22	0
	III	31	22	9
	IV	10	0	10
	V	27	5	22
ASA score < 3		29 (25%)	29 (38%)	0 (0%)
ASA score ≥ 3		88 (75%)	47 (62%)	41 (100%)
Bilateral hernia		6	4	2
Mesh use		6	4	2
General anesthesia		1 (20%)	0	1
Spinal anesthesia		5 (80%)	4	1
Monolateral hernia		30	19	11
Mesh use		30	19	11
General anesthesia		1 (3%)	0	1
Local anesthesia		26 (87%)	16	10
Spinal anesthesia		3 (10%)	3	0
Umbilical hernia		60	37	23
Mesh use		19	16	3
General anesthesia		3 (5%)	0	3
Local anesthesia		57 (95%)	37	20
Incisional hernia		21	16	5
Mesh use		21	16	5
General anesthesia		21 (100%)	16	5

cirrhosis (n = 6) with ascites leakage. In the elective group, death occurred after postoperative heart attack (n = 1), major ascites for decompensated cirrhosis (n = 2), and acute kidney failure (n = 2).

Emergency patients also presented with a markedly higher number of perioperative class III–V complications according to the Clavien-Dindo classification.

The median in-hospital stay was 10 days. Longer median hospital (16 vs. 7 days) and intensive care unit (10 vs. 2 days) stays were observed in the emergency patient group. Two hernia recurrences (monolateral indirect inguinal hernia—P2L according to European Hernia Society (EHS) classification—treated with Trabucco mesh repair and umbilical hernia treated with direct suture repair) were identified in the emergency group during the follow-up period; the umbilical hernia was then electively treated with the mesh-mediated pre-peritoneal open technique; the recurrent inguinal hernia was then electively treated by identifying the sac and the defect. The defect was diagnosed in the canal's posterior wall, describing a direct recurrent inguinal hernia, perhaps from displacement of the mesh from the pubic tubercle surface, where it was first anchored; a plug was then positioned in the defect after hernia inversion inside the abdominal cavity, reconstructing the anatomy of the inguinal canal.

The univariate analysis conducted to identify if the type of hernia could represent a risk factor for postoperative morbidity showed a considerable p value for bilateral inguinal hernia ($p < 0.01$) and incisional hernia ($p < 0.01$) (Table 2) not confirmed on the multivariable analysis. In the same way, we demonstrated that general anesthesia had a considerable p value in the univariate analysis for morbidity ($p = 0.009$) and mortality ($p = 0.008$) not confirmed on the multivariable analysis (Table 2).

The variables with p values < 0.05 in the univariate analysis were included in the multivariate logistic regression. The multivariate analysis conducted showed that emergency surgery, CPT class C, ASA score ≥ 3, and

MELD ≥ 20 were unique independent risk factors for the development of postsurgical morbidity (Table 2) and mortality (Table 3).

Discussion

Traditionally, hernia repair in the presence of advanced cirrhosis and ascites has resulted in high rates of morbidity and mortality, prompting many surgeons to avoid elective repair and to operate only when complications develop. In 1960, Baron reported a mortality of 31% in a case series of 16 patients who underwent umbilical hernia repair and who had cirrhosis. O'Hara et al. reported a morbidity rate of 22% and a mortality of 16% in emergency surgery; these data suggest that surgical repair should be performed in uncomplicated hernias. The risk of treating complicated hernia conservatively heavily outweighs the risk of surgical repair. Non-operative management of complicated hernias with antibiotics and dressing changes might result in mortality rates in the range of 60–88%. Therefore, complicated umbilical hernias in cirrhotic patients should be repaired emergently [15].

The complications related to surgical operations of abdominal wall hernias are high in cirrhotic patients, as much of the impact of abdominal hernia presence is on QoL. In recent decades, the indications for surgical timing and management have changed. The watch-and-wait strategy has been abandoned in favor of elective surgery. However, the indications for surgical repair of abdominal wall hernias in cirrhotic patients remain a controversial challenge.

Table 2 Univariate and multivariate logistic regression analyses for morbidity

	OR	95% CI	p
Univariate			
Emergency	11.62	3.23–40.76	0.026
CPT C	10.49	2.16–32.43	0.003
ASA score ≥ 3	9.43	2.01–25.57	0.001
Ascites	0.76	0.23–50.78	0.114
Mesh use	0.54	0.57–70.87	0.214
MELD score ≥ 20	2.06	2.41–22.76	0.017
Age > 60	1.53	0.12–56.19	0.421
Male	1.54	0.09–12.93	0.769
Bilateral inguinal hernia	7.62	5.32–30.11	0.009
Monolateral inguinal hernia	3.23	0.82–11.41	0.11
Umbilical hernia	0.76	0.98–45.71	0.23
Incisional hernia	1.82	2.92–7.34	0.009
General anesthesia	4.32	2.76–80.91	0.009
Multivariate			
Emergency	6.42	1.76–40.53	0.023
CPT C	3.72	1.23–37.28	0.041
ASA score ≥ 3	4.72	3.41–45.81	0.012
MELD score ≥ 20	5.64	1.71–23.67	0.009
Bilateral inguinal hernia	4.12	0.42–46.71	0.17
Incisional hernia	6.75	0.67–52.86	0.26
General anesthesia	2.87	0.12–34.22	0.12

Table 3 Univariate and multivariate logistic regression analyses for mortality

	OR	95% CI	p
Univariate			
Emergency	21.76	4.26–31.53	0.003
CPT C	3.56	13.21–76.32	0.001
ASA score ≥ 3	10.31	3.54–16.32	0.001
Ascites	2.45	0.22–67.21	0.51
Mesh use	1.21	0.86–14.32	0.41
MELD score ≥ 20	1.69	2.02–23.63	0.017
Age > 60	2.47	0.63–45.61	0.21
Male	0.12	0.03–10.45	0.53
General anesthesia	2.43	5.28–43.61	0.008
Multivariate			
Emergency	10.32	3.66–47.82	0.021
CPT C	5.52	1.67–32.45	0.014
ASA score ≥ 3	8.65	3.65–87.23	0.018
MELD score ≥ 20	2.15	2.71–32.68	0.002
General anesthesia	7.22	4.71–13.65	0.23

Expectant treatment of cirrhotic patients with abdominal wall hernia and ascites is associated with an increased rate of complications, such as incarceration, evisceration, ascites drainage, and peritonitis. These complications require emergency surgical treatment, which carries increased risk of morbidity and mortality. Conversely, elective hernia correction might be performed with fewer complications and is therefore advocated [9].

It has been demonstrated that the improved complication rates associated with modern surgical techniques and perioperative care justify the consideration of an early repair before complications occur. Kirkpatrick and Schubert reported improved outcomes and lower mortality in patients treated after 1975 than in patients treated prior to 1975. A review by Maniatis and Hunt of papers published between 1956 and 1990 found a mortality rate of only 2% in the non-emergency setting, whereas the mortality rate was 14% with repair due to complications carried out as an emergency [16].

The data proposed suggest that emergency, CPT-C, ASA score ≥ 3, and MELD score ≥ 20 are risk factors for postoperative morbidity and mortality. In contrast, elective surgery appears to be successful and to be associated with lower mortality rate. Scientific reports indicate that adequate preparation of cirrhotic patients, with control of ascites, albumin and electrolytes serum levels, nutritional support, and coagulation patterns, allows for the success of elective surgery [16, 17].

The mortality rates for elective and emergency patients reported by our series were, respectively, 6.6 and 53.6%. A reported mortality rate higher than that in the data published in the international literature can be explained not only by the high rate of MELD score ≥ 20 in the two groups (20 and 41%, respectively), but also by the high rate of CPT class C and ASA score ≥ 3 that are respectively 16 and 62% in elective surgery group, 90 and 100% in emergency surgery group, as reported in Table 1.

Ascites control is essential to reducing perioperative complications and recurrence.

In the past, there was a considerable lack of evidence regarding how severe liver dysfunction must be to preclude operative repair. There did not appear to be any reliable, commonly accepted methods to determine whether the cirrhosis was too severe to allow for elective repair or was mild enough that the risk of major complications was low enough to justify the repair [16].

It has now been demonstrated that the CPT score and MELD score are the best ways to identify the severity of liver illness; these scores adequately correlate with prognostic evaluations of postoperative morbidity and mortality in cirrhotic patients.

Recently, although the MELD score was optimized for liver transplantation patients, it appears to be the most objective means to evaluate the surgical risk in cirrhotic patients. It has been demonstrated that a MELD score between 8 and 14 predicts poor surgical outcomes. Moreover, the worst outcome for abdominal surgery is described when the MELD score is above 20 [18–26]. The median pre-operative MELD score in our series was 13.

According to the multivariate analysis, elective surgery is preferable concerning the timing for hernia repair. Emergency surgery is strongly associated with a higher incidence of postoperative morbidity and mortality.

Refractory ascites is frequently associated with urgency even if it does not represent a risk factor in the multivariate analysis. Refractory ascites is surely considered a direct cause of a complicated hernia because of the increased abdominal pressure. This complication is also correlated with skin ulceration, risk of SSI, and ascites leaks.

Conclusions

The results of the data analysis show that performing the surgical operation of abdominal wall hernia repair in cirrhotic patients emergently is related to higher postoperative morbidity and mortality rates. This finding suggests that the correct timing of the surgical operation is elective surgery in controlled liver disease, monitoring the disease with the CPT score and the MELD score. An ASA score ≥ 3 is also a risk factor for postoperative morbidity and mortality. All these risk factors should be considered in the prognostic evaluation of cirrhotic patients who require surgical operation for abdominal wall hernia repair. Furthermore, pre-operative refractory ascites should be managed with paracentesis and albumin/electrolytes serum level and coagulation alteration with appropriate correction.

Acknowledgements
We thank Dr. Comelli Albert, Department of Industrial and Digital Innovation, Policlinico P. Giaccone, University of Palermo, who performed the statistical analysis.
The first and the second authors (Salamone G and Licari L) contributed to the writing of the manuscript in equal measure and should both therefore be considered first authors.

Authors' contributions
GS, LL, and GG conceived of and designated the study. LL, SC, NF, GG, GS, SB, and GC analyzed and interpreted the patient data. GS and LL were major contributors in writing the manuscript. GC and GG supervised the manuscript, discussed the results, and commented on the manuscript. GS and LL contributed to the design and implementation of the research, to the analysis of the results, and to the writing of the manuscript. All authors read and approved the final manuscript.

Permissions

Competing interests
The authors declare that they have no competing interests.

References
1. Belghiti J, Durand F. Abdominal wall hernias in the setting of cirrhosis. Semin Liver Dis. 1997;17:219–26.
2. Carbonell AM, Wolfe LG, DeMaria EJ. Poor outcomes in cirrhosis-associated hernia repair: a nationwide cohort study of 32,033 patients. Hernia. 2005;9:353–7.
3. Shlomovitz E, Quan D, Etemad-Rezai R, McAlister VC. Association of recanalization of the left ombilical vein with umbilical hernia in patients with liver disease. Liver Transpl. 2005;11:1298–9.
4. Garrison RN, Cryer HM, Howard DA, Polk HC. Classification of risk factors for abdominal operations in patients with hepatic cirrhosis. Ann Surg. 1984;199:648–55.
5. Leonetti JP, Aranha GV, Wilkinson WA, et al. Umbilical herniorrhaphy in cirrhotic patients. Arch Surg. 1984;119:442–5.
6. O'Hara ET, Oliai A, Patek AJ, Nabseth DC. Management of umbilical hernias associated with hepatic cirrhosis and ascites. Ann Surg. 1975;181:85–7.
7. Arroyo A, García P, Pérez F, et al. Randomized clinical trial comparing suture and mesh repair of umbilical hernia in adults. Br J Surg. 2001;88:1321–3.
8. Gray SH, Vick CC, Graham LA, et al. Umbilical herniorrhapy in cirrhosis: improved outcomes with elective repair. J Gastrointest Surg. 2008;12:675–81.
9. Coelho JCU, Claus CMP, Campos ACL, et al. Umbilical hernia in patients with liver cirrhosis: a surgical challenge. World J Gastrointest Surg. 2016;8(7):476–82.
10. Andraus W, Sepulveda A, Pinheiro RS, et al. Management of uncommon hernias in cirrhotic patients. Transplant Proc. 2010;42:1724–8.
11. Park JK, Lee SH, Yoon WJ, et al. Evaluation of hernia repair operation in child-turcotte-pugh class c cirrhosis and refractory ascites. J Gastroenterol Hepatol. 2007;22:377–82.
12. Pugh RN, Murray-Lyon IM, Dawson JL, et al. Transection of the oesophagus for bleeding oesophageal varices. Br J Surg. 1973;60:646–9.
13. Kamath PS, Wiesner RH, Malinchoc M, et al. A model to predict survival in patients with end-stage liver disease. Hepatology. 2001;33:464–70.
14. Green SB. How many subjects does it take to do a regression analysis? Multivar Behav Res. 1991;26:499–510.
15. McKay A, Dixon E, Bathe O, Sutherland F. Umbilical hernia repair in the presence of cirrhosis and ascites: results of a survey and review of the literature. Hernia. 2009;13(5):461–8.
16. Belyansky I, Tsirline VB, Klima DA, et al. Prospective, comparative study of postoperative quality of life in tep, tapp, and modified lichtenstein repairs. Ann Surg. 2011;254:709–14. Discussion 714–705
17. Hansen JB, Thulstrup AM, Vilstup H, Sørensen HT. Danish nationwide cohort study of postoperative death in patients with liver cirrhosis undergoing hernia repair. Br J Surg. 2002;89:805–6.
18. Hurst RD, Butler BN, Soybel DI, Wright HK. Management of groin hernias in patients with ascites. Ann Surg. 1992;216:696–700.
19. Eker HH, van Ramshorst GH, de Goede B, et al. A prospective study on elective umbilical hernia repair in patients with liver cirrhosis and ascites. Surgery. 2011;150:542–6.
20. Hur YH, Kim JC, Kim DY, Kim SK, Park CY. Inguinal hernia repair in patients with liver cirrhosis accompanied by ascites. J Korean Surg Soc. 2011;80(6):420–5.
21. Farnsworth N, Fagan SP, Berger DH, Awad SS. Child-Turcotte-Pugh versus MELD score as a predictor of outcome after elective and emergent surgery in cirrhotic patients. Am J Surg. 2004;188:580–3.
22. Befeler AS, Palmer DE, Hoffman M, et al. The safety of intra-abdominal surgery in patients with cirrhosis: model for end-stage liver disease score is superior to Child-Turcotte-Pugh classification in predicting outcome. Arch Surg. 2005;140:650–4. discussion 655
23. Teh SH, Nagorney DM, Stevens SR, et al. Risk factors for mortality after surgery in patients with cirrhosis. Gastroenterology. 2007;132:1261–9.
24. Arif R, Seppelt P, Schwill S, et al. Predictive risk factors for patients with cirrhosis undergoing heart surgery. Ann Thorac Surg. 2012;94:1947–52.
25. Neeff H, Mariaskin D, Spangenberg HC, et al. Perioperative mortality after non-hepatic general surgery in patients with liver cirrhosis: an analysis of 138 operations in the 2000s using child and meld scores. J Gastrointest Surg. 2011;15:1–11.
26. Maniatis AG, Hunt CM. Therapy for spontaneous umbilical hernia rupture. Am J Gastroenterol. 1995;90:310–2.

32

The rate of success of the conservative management of liver trauma in a developing country

S. Buci[1]* (iD), M. Torba[1], A. Gjata[2], I. Kajo[3], Gj. Bushi[1] and K. Kagjini[1]

Abstract

Background: The conservative treatment of liver trauma has made important progress over the last 10 years at the Trauma University Hospital in Tirana, Albania. The percentage of success was 58.7%. The aims of this study were to analyze the conservative treatment of liver trauma and to compare the results with those in the literature.

Methods: This study was conducted prospectively from January 2009 to December 2012. We analyzed 173 patients admitted to our hospital with liver trauma. Liver injuries were evaluated according to the American Association for the Surgery of Trauma and the World Society of Emergency Surgery classification, while the anatomic gravity of the associated injuries was defined using the Injury Severity Score system. The potential mortality was estimated with the Revised Trauma Score.

Results: Out of the 173 patients with liver trauma, 83.2% were male. The main cause of liver trauma was motor vehicle crashes (50.9%). Blunt trauma was the cause of liver injury in 129 cases (74.6%), and penetrating trauma occurred in 44 cases (25.4%). Initially, the decision was to manage 88 cases (50.9%) via the conservative approach. Of these, 73 cases (42.2%) were successfully treated with conservative treatment, while in 15 cases (17.2%), this approach failed. The success rate of conservative treatment by grade of injuries was as follows: grade I (38.4%), grade II (30.1%), grade III (28.8%), and grade IV (2.7%). The likelihood of the success of conservative treatment had a significant correlation with the grade of the liver injury ($p < 0.00001$), associated intra-abdominal injuries ($p = 0.00051$), and complications ($z = 2.3169$, $p = 0.02051$). The overall mortality rate of liver trauma was 13.2%.

Conclusions: The likelihood of success in using conservative treatment had a significant correlation with the grade of liver injury and associated intra-abdominal injuries. The limited hospital resources and low level of consensus on conservative treatment had a negative impact on the level of success.

Keywords: Liver trauma, Grade of injuries, Conservative treatment, Success

Background

Currently, the conservative management of liver trauma is considered the "Gold Standard." More than 80% of patients with non-severe liver injuries are treated successfully without surgery [1–4]. Nance and Cohn support the use of conservative treatment in hemodynamically stable patients who do not exhibit signs of peritoneal irritation [5]. In Albania, the conservative treatment of liver trauma has made important progress over the last decade. The diagnostic and therapeutic strategy for liver injury depends on the hemodynamic status of the traumatized patients and the associated injuries.

The World Society of Emergency Surgery (WSES) liver trauma classification considers not only the anatomic American Association for the Surgery of Trauma (AAST) classification but also, more importantly, the hemodynamic status and the associated injuries [6] (Table 1).

The abdominal echography procedure is essential in the emergency department for patients with hemodynamic instability. Currently, computerized tomography is the preferred method to evaluate blunt liver trauma in hemodynamically stable patients or in patients who have been stabilized after an initial fluid resuscitation [7].

* Correspondence: buciskender@gmail.com
[1]Service of General Surgery, Trauma University Hospital, Tirana, Albania
Full list of author information is available at the end of the article

Table 1 WSES liver trauma classification

	WSES grade	Blunt/penetrating (stab/guns)	AAST	Hemodynamic	CT scan	First-line treatment
Minor	WSES grade I	B/P	I–II	Stable		
		SW/GSW				
Moderate	WSES grade II	B/P	III	Stable	Yes	NOM*
		SW/GSW			Local Exploration in SW	Serial Clinical/Laboratory/ Radiological Evaluation
Severe	WSES grade III	B/P	IV–V	Stable		
		SW/GSW				
	WSES grade IV	B/P	I–VI	Unstable	No	OM
		SW/GSW				

SW stab wound, *GSW* gunshot wound, *OM* operative management, * *NOM* non-operative management

The conservative treatment of liver injury can be initiated when there is a possibility of monitoring the traumatized patient clinically, biologically, and radiologically in the correct manner and when there is a close collaboration between surgeons, intensivists, and radiologists. The failure of conservative treatment occurs in 15% of cases, often in patients with extrahepatic injuries or white laparotomy [8, 9].

The objectives of this study were to analyze the conservative management of liver trauma, the likelihood for success, and the causes of failure and to compare the results with those in the literature.

Methods

This is a prospective study performed from January 2009 to December 2012. We analyzed 173 patients with hepatobiliary trauma who were admitted to the Trauma University Hospital, Tirana, Albania. Liver injuries were evaluated according to AAST and WSES classifications via ultrasonography and CT scan. The anatomic gravity of the associated injuries was defined using the Injury Severity Score (ISS) system. The potential mortality was estimated using the Revised Trauma Score (RTS). A simple ordinary least square regression (OLS) of several factors on the success of conservative treatment of trauma injury patient reveals the results of the following table. For this analysis, the variables are Surviv (whether the patient survives the treatment of the injury [No = 0; Yes = 1]); Age (age of the patient [6–15 years old = 1; 16–25 years old = 2; 26–35 years old = 3; 36–45 years old = 4; 46–55 years old = 5; 56–65 years old = 6; 66–75 years old = 7]); Gender (gender [Male = 1; Female = 0]); Cinjur (if only the liver is injured, then the value is 0. For all other combinations, like the liver and head and the liver and thorax, the variable takes the value of 1); Grade (grade [the six-grade scale standard is used: Minor = 1; Moderate = 2; Serious = 3; Severe = 4; Critical = 5; Un-survivable = 6]); Conserv (conservative treatment of the patient [Yes = 1; No = 0]); Interv (the patient

is treated with an intervention [Yes = 1; No = 0]); ISS (anatomical; the higher the number, the more severe the injury); and RTS (psychological; the lower the number, the more severe the condition of the patient).

Treatment for each patient was chosen based on the set of indicators for laparotomy and under the consideration for conservative treatment. The indicators were (1) hemodynamic stability, (2) presence/absence of peritoneal irritation signs, (3) identification and evaluation of CT scan grade of liver injuries, (4) hemoperitoneum <500 ml, and (5) the absence of injury to cavitare organs [10, 11], based on the algorithm for the non-operative management of blunt hepatic trauma [12].

Based on these criteria, patients were divided into two main groups: group A (including 88 patients who met the conditions for conservative treatment) and group B (including 85 patients who had indications for immediate laparotomy).

Results

The average age of patients with hepatic trauma was 23.4 years old (ranging from 6 to 75), including 83.2% male and 16.8% female patients.

In our study, blunt trauma was the cause of liver injury in 129 cases (74.6%), while penetrating trauma occurred in 44 cases (25.4%).

The causes of hepatic trauma were motor vehicle crashes in 88 cases (50.9%), falls from height in 32 cases (18.4%), gunshot wounds in 24 cases (13.8%), sharp tools in 19 cases (11%), direct blows in 8 cases (4.7%), iatrogenic in 1 case (0.6%), and hepatic trauma from an electrical arc in 1 case (0.6%) (Tables 2 and 3).

Alanine aminotransferase (ALT) >100 U/l and aspartate aminotransferase (AST) >200 U/l were found in 96 patients (55.5%), and ALT >1000 U/l and AST >1100 U/l were found in 2 patients (1.6%).

Diagnostic peritoneal lavage (DPL) was used in10 patients (5.6%). In 6 patients, we found intestine leak.

Table 2 Hemodynamic status

Initial hemodynamic status	No. of patients	Percentage
Hemodynamic instability	47	27.1
Stabilized after intravenous liquid administration	84	48.6
Hemodynamic stability	42	24.3

Table 4 Hepatic injuries according to AAST grade

Grade	Number of cases	Percentage
I	36	20.8
II	60	34.7
III	47	27.2
IV	21	12.1
V	8	4.6
VI	1	0.6

In our study, 62 patients (35.9%) were transfused with 1 unit of blood, 41 (23.8%) were transfused with 2 units, 30 (17.9%) were transfused with 3 units, 22 (12.8%) were transfused with 4 units, and 17 (9.6%) were transfused with more than 4 units (Table 4).

The injury frequencies, according to the Couinaud segment, were as follows: I segment ($n = 8$) 2.5%, II segment ($n = 10$) 3.1%, III segment ($n = 16$) 5%, IV segment ($n = 32$) 10%, V segment ($n = 49$) 15.3%, VI segment ($n = 76$) 23.8%, VII segment ($n = 65$) 20.3%, and VIII segment ($n = 64$) 20%.

The frequency of liver injury according to the WSES were WSES grade I ($n = 65$) 37.6%, WSES grade II ($n = 55$) 31.8%, WSES grade III ($n = 6$) 3.5%, and WSES grade IV ($n = 47$) 27.1%.

Isolated hepatic injuries were detected in 45 cases (26.1%), and combined hepatic injuries were present in 128 cases (73.9%).

Hepatic injuries were associated with intra-abdominal hollow organ injuries in 33 cases (19.1%) and with parenchymal injuries in 31 cases (17.9%) (Table 5).

Hepatic injuries were associated with extra-abdominal injuries, including the head in 27 cases (15.6%), the thorax and diaphragm in 80 cases (46.2%), the heart in 2 cases (1.2%), the vertebral column in 3 cases (1.7%), pelvic fracture in 12 cases (6.9%), and limb fractures in 19 cases (11%) (Tables 6 and 7).

In group A (conservative treatment of 88 patients), 73 patients (42.2%) benefitted from successful conservative treatment. Unsuccessful conservative treatment due to further complications was seen in 15 patients (17.2%). In patients with isolated liver injuries, conservative treatment was successful in 27 cases (58.7%).

In group B, 100 patients underwent laparotomy. An immediate laparotomy was performed in 85 patients (49.1%), a laparotomy for hepatic injury was performed in 30 patients (30%), laparotomy for extrahepatic injury was performed in 70 patients (70%), perihepatic packing was performed in 10 patients (11.7%), and relaparotomy

was performed in 6 patients (7%). Extrahepatic injuries included the stomach ($n = 10$, 12.3%), the small intestine and duodenum ($n = 12$, 14.8%), the large intestine and rectum ($n = 9$, 11.1%), the spleen ($n = 16$, 19.7%), the kidneys ($n = 12$, 14.8%), the pancreas ($n = 4$, 4.9%), the diaphragm ($n = 35$, 43.2%), the intra-abdominal esophagus ($n = 1$, 1.2%), the cholecyst ($n = 3$, 3.7%), and the urinary bladder ($n = 2$, 2.5%).

We observed that 10.9% of the patients who were treated in a conservative manner had an ISS of ≥20. We also observed that in this group of patients, 86.3% had an RTS of >5 (Tables 8, 9, 10, and 11).

The chances of successful conservative treatment significantly depend on the grade of liver injury ($p < 0.00001$). There is also a statistically significant connection between the successful conservative treatment of liver trauma and a combination of injuries with other organs (p value = 0.00051) and complications ($z = 2.3169$, $p = 0.02051$) (Table 12).

The OLS shows that the patient age, gender, combined injury, and grade of injury (anatomical, physiological, and locational) account for more than 30% of the variation in the success of conservative treatment (as seen with an adjusted R-squared = 0.319). From the variables under consideration, it is clear that patient age, combination of injuries with other organs besides the liver,

Table 3 Hematocrit level (at the time of arrival in the ER)

Initial hematocrit level	No. of patients	Percentage
Up to 37	124	71.7
37-30	34	19.7
Under 30	15	8.6

Table 5 The mechanism of trauma and associated abdominal injuries

Organ	Blunt trauma	Penetrating trauma	Total	Percentage
Spleen	14	2	16	9.2
Kidneys	9	3	12	6.9
Pancreas	2	2	4	2.3
Stomach	3	7	10	5.8
Small intestine + duodenum	3	9	12	6.9
Large intestine + rectum	3	6	9	5.2
Diaphragm	8	27	35	20.2
Esophagus	0	1	1	0.6
Urinary bladder	1	0	2	1.2
Total	43	57	100	58.3

Table 6 Success of conservative management according to AAST grade

Grade	Number of cases	Percentage
I	28	38.4
II	22	30.1
III	21	28.8
IV	2	2.7
V	0	0
VI	0	0

grade of injury, and RTS (psychological trauma) are statistically important. This is verifiable from the above table that presents both the *p* values and the *t* values.

The overall mortality rate of liver trauma was 13.2%.

Discussion

Our study demonstrated that liver injuries occurred in 17% of patients with abdominal trauma. Shanmuganathan et al. have reported that liver injuries occurred in 20% of patients with blunt abdominal trauma [13]. We found that male to female ratio was 5:1. Beel et al. found that the male to female ratio varies from 15:1 [14]. Approximately 15–20 years ago, all traumatic liver injuries were treated surgically, but in 50–80% of cases, no active bleeding was found [15, 16]. We also found liver injuries with no active bleeding during laparotomy for associated injuries.

In our study, the hemodynamic status was the main criterion in determining the therapeutic approach. Approximately 85% of patients with blunt liver trauma are hemodynamically stable or stabilize after receiving intravenous liquids [17], which corresponds with the findings in our study. Richardson et al. commented that many experienced surgeons in trauma surgery apply surgical treatment in hemodynamically stable patients and they have concluded that conservative treatment has a positive impact on patient survival [18]. In hemodynamically stable patients, a helical CT examination with oral and venous contrast was performed to determine the grade of the liver injury, the amount of hemoperitoneum, the presence of pseudoaneurysms, and the presence of other intraperitoneal injuries.

Hemoperitoneum was observed in repeated ultrasound examinations, and in some cases, re-evaluation was done via CT scan. Malhotra et al. reports that a large amount of hemoperitoneum (when blood is present in the lateral

Table 7 Management according the WSES grade

WSES	Conservative	Laparotomy
WSES grade I	50 (76.9%)	15 (23.1%)
WSES grade II	21 (38.2%)	34 (61.8%)
WSES grade III	2 (33.3%)	4 (66.7%)
WSES grade IV	0 (0%)	47 (100%)

Table 8 The causes of failure of conservative treatment

Complications	No. of patients	Percentage
Secondary hemorrhage	3	3.4
Biliary peritonitis	2	2.3
Intrahepatic biloma	1	1.1
Extrahepatic biloma	2	2.3
Hollow organ injuries	2	2.3
Liver compartment syndrome	1	1.1
Gangrenous cholecystitis	2	2.3
Peritoneal inflammatory syndrome	2	2.3
Total	15	17.2

channels, the perihepatic space, and the Douglas pouch) is a significant risk factor for the failure of conservative treatment [19]. Due to limited resources for transfusion in our hospital, we interrupted conservative treatment in patients who had a considerable need for transfusion and when the amount of hemoperitoneum was determined to be progressively increasing.

From group A of 88 patients selected for conservative management, 15 patients showed complications that necessitated surgery. Group B consisted of 85 patients who underwent immediate laparotomy due to the following indications: hemodynamic instability, associated intra-abdominal injuries, and penetrating trauma. It is worth emphasizing that a case with penetrating liver trauma caused by hunting rifle wounds was managed conservatively. Ten patients underwent perihepatic packing; of these, a second laparotomy was performed in 6 patients and 4 patients did not survive.

In our study, we found that gunshot wounds and wounds caused by sharp tools had an incidence of 24.8%.

This percentage was significant and contributed to a reduction in the number of patients managed conservatively. The gunshot wounds were penetrating in 35–70% of cases [20], and the wounds caused by sharp tools were not penetrating in 35–61% of cases [21, 22].

Diagnostic peritoneal lavage (DPL) is another valid tool to determine the presence or nature of intraperitoneal liquids. We used this procedure in a few cases. DPL, described by Root in 1965, remains an important tool in the

Table 9 Complications of conservative treatment of patients with combined liver trauma according to some authors

Complications	References	Our study (%)
Secondary hemorrhage	5% [30]	3.4
Missed injuries	3–5% [28, 35]	2.3
Hemobilia	0.3–1.2% [36, 37]	1
Bilhemia	0.2–1% [38]	1
Bile leakage	3–20%	6.8

Table 10 Comparative data on secondary indications for surgical treatment after an initial determination to perform conservative treatment

Secondary indications for surgical treatment	Letoublon et al. (186 patients) (%)	Our study (173 patients) (%)
Peritoneal inflammatory syndrome	5.5	2.3
Secondary hemorrhage	1	3.4
Liver compartment syndrome	1	1.1
Hollow organ injuries	1	2.3
Biliary peritonitis	0.5	2.3
Extrahepatic biloma	0	2.3
Post-traumatic cholecystitis	0	2.3
Intrahepatic biloma	0	1.1
Bilothorax	0.5	0
Abdominal compartment syndrome	1	0
Post-traumatic pancreatitis	0.5	0

hands of surgeons, especially in the absence of minimally invasive equipment. DPL has a very high sensibility and specificity rate for intraperitoneal injuries, 95 and 99%, respectively. However, this procedure is associated with complications in 0.8–1.7% of cases [23].

Our study showed that conservative treatment turned out to be successful in 42.2% of patients with combined hepatic trauma and in 58.7% of patients with isolated hepatic trauma. These percentages recorded in our study are lower than those reported elsewhere. It is our view that these differences are related to two factors: (1) a low level of consensus for conservative management and (2) limited hospital resources (limited interventional radiology procedures). Conservative treatment failed in 17.2% of cases. In some studies, it has been reported that

Table 11 Frequencies of several variables for both treatment modes (conservative and laparotomy)

Variable	Conservative	Laparotomy
Male	61 (42.4%)	83 (57.6%)
Female	12 (41.4%)	17 (58.6%)
>55 years old	8 (57.1%)	6 (42.9%)
<55 years old	65 (40.9%)	94 (59.1%)
ISS >20	8 (8.8)	83 (91.2%)
ISS <20	65 (79.3%)	17 (20.7%)
RTS >5	63 (63.6%)	36 (36.4%)
RTS <5	10 (13.5%)	64 (86.5%)
≤Grade IV	73 (42.1%)	100 (57.9%)
>Grade IV	0 (0%)	9 (100%)
Complications	15 (20.5%)	11 (11%)
Mortality	1 (1.4%)	12 (12%)

Table 12 OLS, "success of the conservative management" as the dependent variable

Variables	Coefficient	Std. error	t ratio	p value
Const	−0.233669	0.311065	−0.7512	0.4536
Age	0.0493656	0.0196583	2.5112	0.0130
Gender	0.0253333	0.0731743	0.3462	0.7296
Cinjur	0.136536	0.0745459	1.8316	0.0688
Grade	0.0414623	0.0336495	1.2322	0.2196
Resec	−0.151871	0.134283	−1.1310	0.2597
ISS	−0.0124758	0.0027189	−4.5885	<0.0001
RTS	0.0892609	0.0315478	2.8294	0.0052
Mean dependent var.	0.445087	S.D. dependent var.		0.498418
Sum-squared resid.	27.91268	S.E. of regression		0.411300
R-squared	0.346740	Adjusted R-squared		0.319026

the efficacy of conservative management of liver trauma in hemodynamically stable patients is between 87 and 98%, and the failure rate is between 10 and 25% [24, 25].

Injuries that were grade III or worse added substantially to the failure of conservative management. We had only two patients with grade IV liver injury that were successfully managed conservatively. Malhotra et al. found that in 14% of patients with grade IV injuries and 22.6% of patients with grade V injuries, conservative treatment was not successful, and the failure rate in patients with grades I, II, and III injuries was 3–7 and 5% [19]. The likelihood of the success of conservative treatment had a significant correlation with the grade of liver injury. The coefficient of grade injury was −2.6, which means that for every increase in the grade of the injury, the likelihood of the success of conservative treatment drops to 2.6. In addition, the success of conservative treatment had a significant correlation with associated intra-abdominal injuries. Other factors were statistically insignificant in the success of the conservative treatment.

The failure of the conservative treatment was often attributed to the deterioration of hemodynamic parameters, bile leakage, and the presence of overlapping septic complications. Durham et al. and Hammond et al. have reported that secondary hemorrhage occurs in less than 5% of cases treated conservatively [26, 27]. We observed that the failure of conservative treatment due to secondary hemorrhage occurred in 3% of cases. Buckman et al. showed that bile leakage can occur in 3–20% of patients who are managed conservatively [28, 29]. The frequency of hemobilia, as reported by Croce et al. and Walt et al., ranges from 0.3 to 1.2% [28, 30]. A rare complication, such as bilhemia, occurs in less than 1% of patients with hepatic trauma [31]. Bilhemia is determined by the presence of pseudoaneurysm (that is found in angio CT), increased bilirubin level, and a normal level of liver enzymes (ALT,

AST). We found the same frequency of bilhemia and hemobilia. Subcapsular hematoma should be surgically treated only for two reasons: (1) to increase the value of ALT and AST and (2) if the patient has Budd-Chiari syndrome [32, 33]. In our study, only one patient underwent surgical intervention due to increases in ALT and AST values.

The incidence of failure of conservative treatment due to associated intra-abdominal injuries has been reported to be between 0.5 and 3.5% [11, 34], whereas in our study, the failure rate with associated intra-abdominal injuries was 2.3%.

Conclusions

The likelihood of the success of conservative treatment has a significant correlation with the grade of liver injury and associated intra-abdominal injuries. Limited hospital resources and the low level of consensus for non-surgical management have a negative impact on the outcome. The main causes of failure are secondary hemorrhage and bile leakage.

Acknowledgements
The authors are very grateful to the staff of the Trauma University Hospital in Tirana, who have been generous and supportive throughout the conduction of this research.

Funding
This research did not use any internal or external funds.

Authors' contributions
BS designed the study and methodology, participated in gathering the data, and conducted the analysis. TM provided the literature review, participated in the data collection, and contributed to the statistical analysis. GA participated in the methodology and provided insights for the WSES classification system. KI evaluated the diagnosis and complications and provided important insights for the data classification. BG contributed to the data collection and provided systematic assistance in crafting the analysis. KK contributed to the data classification and the interpretation of the results. All authors read and approved the final manuscript.

Competing interests
The authors declare that they have no competing interests.

Author details
[1]Service of General Surgery, Trauma University Hospital, Tirana, Albania. [2]Department of Surgery, UHC "Mother Teresa", Tirana, Albania. [3]Department of Internal Medicine, Trauma University Hospital, Tirana, Albania.

References
1. Petrowsky H, Raeder S, Zuercher L, et al. A quarter century experience in liver trauma: a plea for early computed tomography and conservative management for all hemodynamically stable patients. World J Surg. 2012;36: 247–54.
2. Leppäniemi AK, Mentula PJ, Streng MH, et al. Severe hepatic trauma: nonoperative management, definitive repair, or damage control surgery? World J Surg. 2011;35:2643–9.
3. Polanco PM, Brown JB, Puyana JC, et al. The swinging pendulum: a national perspective of nonoperative management in severe blunt liver injury. J Trauma Acute Care Surg. 2013;75:590–5.
4. Piper GL, Peitzman AB. Current management of hepatic trauma. Surg Clin North Am. 2010;90:775–85.
5. Pruvot F, Meaux F, Truant S, et al. Traumatismes graves fermés du foie: à la recherche de critères décisionnels pour le choix du traitement non opératoire. À propos d'une série de 88 cas. Ann Chir. 2005;130:70–80.
6. Coccolini F, Catena F, Moore EE, et al. WSES classification and guidelines for liver trauma. World J Emerg Surg. 2016;10(11):50. eCollection 2016.
7. Fabian TC, Bee TK. Ch 32. Liver and biliary tract. In: Feliciano DV, Mattox KL, Moore EE, editors. Trauma. 6th ed. Pennsylvania Plaza: The McGraw-Hill Companies, Inc; 2008. p. 637–58.
8. Velmahos G, Toutouzas K, Radin R, et al. High success with nonoperative management of blunt hepatic trauma: the liver is a sturdy organ. Arch Surg. 2003;138:475–81.
9. Nance FC, Cohn I. Surgical judgement in the management of stab wounds of the abdomen: a retrospective and prospective analysis based on a study of 600 stabbed patients. Ann Surg. 1969;170:569–80.
10. Pachter HL, Hofstetter SR. The current status of nonoperative management of adult blunt hepatic injuries. Am J Surg. 1995;169:442–54.
11. Carrillo EH, Platz A, Miller FB, et al. Non-operative management of blunt hepatic trauma. Br J Surg. 1998;85:461–8.
12. Kozar RA, Moore FA, Moore EE, West M, Cocanour CS, Davis J, Biffl WL, McIntyre RC Jr. Western Trauma Association critical decisions in trauma: nonoperative management of adult blunt hepatic trauma. J Trauma. 2009; 67:1144–8.
13. Shanmuganathan K, Mirvis SE. CT evaluation of the liver with acute blunt trauma. Crit Rev Diagn Imaging. 1995;36:73–113.
14. Meel BL. Incidence and patterns of violent and/or traumatic deaths between 1993 and 1999 in the Transkei region of South Africa. J Trauma. 2004;57:125–9.
15. Mirvis S, Whitley N, Vainwright J, et al. Blunt hepatic trauma in adults: CT-based classification and correlation with prognosis and treatment. Radiology. 1989;171:27–32.
16. Croce M, Fabian T, Menke P, et al. Nonoperative management of blunt hepatic trauma is the treatment of choice for hemodynamically stable patients. Results of a prospective trial. Ann Surg. 1995;221:744–55.
17. Fabian TC, Bee TK. Ch 31. Liver and biliary tract trauma. In: Moore EE, Felliciano DV, Mattox KL, editors. Trauma. 5th ed. Pennsylvania Plaza: The McGraw-Hill, Companies, Inc; 2004. p. 637–58.
18. Richardson JD, Franklin GA, Lukan JK, et al. Evolution in the management of hepatic trauma: a 25-year perspective. Ann Surg. 2000;232:324–30.
19. Malhotra A, Fabian T, Croce M, et al. Blunt hepatic injury: a paradigm shift from operative to nonoperative management in the 1990's. Ann Surg. 2000; 231:804–13.
20. Brinquin L, Borne M, Debien B, Clapson P, Jault P. Traumatismes balistiques: les lesions abdomino-pelviennes. Paris: Elsevier; 2008. p. 533–41.
21. Leonard D, Rebiel N, Perez M, Duchamp C, Grosdidier G. The place of laparoscopy in the management of the patients with penetrating abdominal trauma. J Chir. 2007;144:421–4.
22. Kopelman TR, O Neil PJ, Macias LH, Cox JC, Mathews MR, Drachman DA. The utility of diagnostic in the evaluation of anterior abdominal stab wounds. Am J Surg. 2008;196:871–7.
23. Nagy KK, Roberts RR, Joseph KT, et al. Experience with over 2500 diagnostic peritoneal lavages. Injury. 2000;31:479–82.
24. Trunkey DD. Hepatic trauma: contemporary management. Surg Clin North Am. 2004;84:437–50.
25. Christmas AB, Wilson AK, Manning B, et al. Selective management of blunt hepatic injuris including nonoperative management is a safe and effective strategy. Surgery. 2005;138:606–11.
26. Durham R, Buckley J, Keegan M, et al. Management of blunt hepatic injuries. Am J Surg. 1992;164:477–81.

27. Hammond J, Canal D, Broadie T. Nonoperative management of adult blunt hepatic trauma in a municipal trauma center. Am Surg. 1992;58:551–6.

28. Arikan S, Kocakusak A, Yucel AF, Adas G, et al. A prospective comparison of the selective observation and routine exploration method for penetrating abdominal stab wounds with organ or omentum evisceration. J Trauma. 2005;58:526–32.

29. Buckman RJ, Piano G, Dunham C, et al. Major bowel and diaphragmatic injuries associated with blunt spleen or liver rupture. J Trauma. 1988;28: 1317–21.

30. Suleman ND, Rasoul HA. War injuries of the chest. Injury. 1985;16:382–4.

31. Clemens M, Wittrin G. Bilhämie und hämobilie nach Reitunfall, Vortrag 166. 1975. Tagung Nordwestdeutscher Chirurgen.

32. Markert DJ, Shanmuganathan K, Mirvis SE, et al. Budd-Chiari syndrome resulting from intrahepatic IVC compression secondary to blunt hepatic trauma. Clin Radiol. 1997;52:384–7.

33. Letoublon C, Chen Y, Arvieux C, et al. Delayed celiotomy or laparoscopy as part of the nonoperative management of blunt hepatic trauma. World J Surg. 2008;32:1189–93.

34. Miller PR, Croce MA, Bee TK, Malhotra AK, Fabian TC. Associated injuries in blunt solid organ trauma: implications for missed injury in nonoperative management. J Trauma. 2002;53:238–42.

35. Monneuse OJ, Barth X, Gruner L, et al. Les plaies pénétrantes de l'abdomen, conduite diagnostique et thérapeutique. À propos de 79 patients. Ann Chir. 2004;129:156–63.

36. Walt AJ, Wilson RF. Management of trauma: pitfalls and practice. Philadelphia: Lea Febiger; 1975. p. 348.

37. Croce M, Fabian T, Spiers S, et al. Traumatic hepatic artery pseudoaneurysm with hemobilia. Am J Surg. 1994;168:235–8.

38. Pearl LB, Trunkey DD. Compartment syndrome of the liver. J Trauma. 1999; 47:796–8.

List of Contributors

Michael Sugrue and Shaheel M Sahebally
Department of Surgery, Letterkenny Hospital and Donegal Clinical Research Academy, National University Ireland Galway, Letterkenny, Donegal, Ireland

Luca Ansaloni
Department of Surgery, Papa Giovanni XXIII Hospital, Bergamo, Italy

Martin D Zielinski
Department of Surgery, Mayo Clinic, Rochester, Minnesota, USA

Eva-Corina Caragounis, David Pazooki and Hans Granhed
Department of Surgery, Institute of Clinical Sciences, Sahlgrenska Academy, University of Gothenburg, Gothenburg, Sweden

Monika Fagevik Olsén
Department of Surgery, Institute of Clinical Sciences, Sahlgrenska Academy, University of Gothenburg, Gothenburg, Sweden
Department of Physical Therapy, Institute of Neuroscience and Physiology, Sahlgrenska Academy, University of Gothenburg, Gothenburg, Sweden

Offir Ben-Ishay, Mai Daoud, Zvi Peled, Eran Brauner, Hany Bahouth and Yoram Kluger
Department of General of Surgery, Division of Surgery Rambam Health Care Campus, 8 Ha'Aliyah St, Haifa 35254, Israel

Ken Leslie
Department of Surgery, University of Western Ontario, London Health Sciences Centre, University Hospital, 339 Windermere Road, London, ON N6A 5A5, Canada

Neil Parry
Department of Surgery, University of Western Ontario, London Health Sciences Centre, University Hospital, 339 Windermere Road, London, ON N6A 5A5, Canada
Department of Critical Care, London, On, Canada

Richard Hilsden, Bradley Moffat and Sarah Knowles
Department of Surgery, University of Western Ontario, London Health Sciences Centre, University Hospital, 339 Windermere Road, London, ON N6A 5A5, Canada
Schulich School of Medicine and Dentistry, Western University, London, ON, Canada

Hugo Teixeira Farinha, Emmanuel Melloul, Dieter Hahnloser, Nicolas Demartines and Martin Hübner
Department of Visceral Surgery, University Hospital of Lausanne (CHUV), Lausanne 1011, Switzerland

Kyu-Hyouck Kyoung
Department of Surgery, Ulsan University Hospital, University of Ulsan College of Medicine, 877 Bangeojinsunhwando-ro, Dong-gu, Ulsan, Republic of Korea

Suk-Kyung Hong
Division of Trauma and Surgical Critical Care, Department of Surgery, Asan Medical Center, University of Ulsan College of Medicine, 388-1 Pungnap-dong, Songpa-gu, Seoul, Republic of Korea

Yohei Kawatani, Yoshitsugu Nakamura, Hirotsugu Kurobe, Yuji Suda and Takaki Hori
Department of Cardiovascular Surgery, Chiba-Nishi General Hospital, 107-1 Kanegasaku, Matsudo-Shi 2702251, Chiba-Ken, Japan

Alain Chichom-Mefire, Tabe Alain Fon and Marcelin Ngowe-Ngowe
Department of Surgery, Faculty of Health Sciences, University of Buea and Regional Hospital Limbe, Yaoundé, Cameroon

Suhail Hakim, Khalid Ahmed, Gaby Jabbour, Ruben Peralta, Husham Abdelrahman, Ammar Al-Hassani and Hassan Al-Thani
Trauma Surgery Section, Hamad General Hospital, Doha, Qatar

Ahammed Mekkodathil
Clinical Research, Trauma Surgery Section, Hamad General Hospital, Doha, Qatar

Ayman El-Menyar
Clinical Research, Trauma Surgery Section, Hamad General Hospital, Doha, Qatar
Clinical Medicine, Weill Cornell Medical College, Doha, Qatar

Syed Nabir
Department of Radiology, Hamad General Hospital, Doha, Qatar

Lewis E. Jacobson and Argenis J.Herrera
Department of Surgery, St. Vincent Indianapolis Hospital, 2001 West 86th Street, Indianapolis, IN 46260, USA

Mary Ziemba-Davis
St. Vincent Neuroscience Institute, 8333 Naab Road, Indianapolis, IN 46260, USA

Michal Grivna
Institute of Public Health, College of Medicine and Health Sciences, UAE University, Al Ain, United Arab Emirates

Hani O. Eid and Fikri M. Abu-Zidan
Trauma Group, Department of Surgery, College of Medicine and Health Sciences, UAE University, Al Ain, United Arab Emirates

Alan L. Beal
North Memorial Medical Center, 3300 Oakdale Ave N, Robbinsdale, MN 55431, USA

Steven V. Turner, Christopher A. Beal and Greg A. Beilman
University of Minnesota, Minnesota, USA

Mark N. Ahrendt, Eric D. Irwin, John W. Lyng and Matthew T. Byrnes
North Memorial Medical Center, Minnesota, USA

Keqin Luo, Huibao Long, Bincan Xu and Yanling Luo
Department of Emergency, SunYat-Sen memorial Hospital, Sun Yat-Sen University, 107 yan-jiangxi Road, Guangzhou 510120, China

Suvi Kaarina Rasilainen
Department of Abdominal Surgery, Jorvi Hospital, Turuntie, 150 Espoo, Finland

Mentula Panu Juhani and Leppäniemi Ari Kalevi
Department of Abdominal Surgery, Helsinki University Central Hospital, Helsinki, Finland

Eszter Mán, Tibor Németh, Tibor Géczi, Zsolt Simonka and György Lázár
Department of Surgery, University of Szeged, Szőkefalvi-Nagy Béla u. 6, H-6720 Szeged, Hungary

Takehito Yamamoto
Department of Surgery, Kitano Hospital, The Tazuke Kofukai Medical Research Institute, 2-4-20 Ogimachi, Kita-ku, Osaka 530-8480, Japan

Ryosuke Kita, Hideyuki Masui, Hiromitsu Kinoshita, Yusuke Sakamoto, Kazuyuki Okada, Junji Komori, Akira Miki, Kenji Uryuhara, Hiroyuki Kobayashi, Hiroki Hashida, Satoshi Kaihara and Ryo Hosotani
Kobe City Medical Center General Hospital, 2-1-1 Minatojima-Minamimachi, Chuoku, Kobe 650-0047, Japan

Toshiyuki Itamoto, Yuji Takakura, Takahisa Suzuki, Satoshi Ikeda and Takashi Urushihara
Department of Gastroenterological Surgery, Hiroshima Prefectural Hospital, 5-54, Ujinakanda, Minami-ku, Hiroshima 734-00041, Japan

Yuki Imaoka
Department of Gastroenterological Surgery, Hiroshima Prefectural Hospital, 5-54, Ujinakanda, Minami-ku, Hiroshima 734-00041, Japan
Department of Gastroenterological and Transplant Surgery, Applied Life Sciences, Institute of Biomedical and Health Sciences, Hiroshima University, 1-2-3, Kasumi, Minami-ku, Hiroshima 734-8551, Japan

Hao-wei Kou, Hong-Shiue Chou, Hsu-huan Chou and Song-Fong Huang
Department of Surgery, Chang Gung Memorial Hospital, Linkou, Taiwan, Republic of China

Ming-Chin Yu
Department of Surgery, Chang Gung Memorial Hospital, Linkou, Taiwan, Republic of China
College of Medicine, Chang Gung University, Guishan, Taoyuan, Taiwan, Republic of China

Chao-Wei Lee
Department of Surgery, Chang Gung Memorial Hospital, Linkou, Taiwan, Republic of China
College of Medicine, Chang Gung University, Guishan, Taoyuan, Taiwan, Republic of China
Graduate Institute of Clinical Medical Sciences, Chang Gung University, Guishan, Taoyuan, Taiwan, Republic of China

Chun-Hsing Wu
Graduate Institute of Clinical Medical Sciences, Chang Gung University, Guishan, Taoyuan, Taiwan, Republic of China

Hsin-I Tsai
Graduate Institute of Clinical Medical Sciences, Chang Gung University, Guishan, Taoyuan, Taiwan, Republic of China
Department of Anesthesiology, Chang Gung Memorial Hospital, Linkou, Taiwan, Republic of China

Chih-Hsiang Chang
Division of Nephrology, Kidney Research Center, Chang Gung Memorial Hospital, Linkou, Taiwan, Republic of China

Jun Ke
Department of Gastroenterology, Dongfang Hospital, Xiamen University, Fuzhou, Fujian 350025, China

Weihang Wu, Nan Lin, Weijin Yang, Zhicong Cai, Wei Wu and Yu Wang
Department of General Surgery, Dongfang Hospital, Xiamen University, Fuzhou, Fujian 350025, China

Dongsheng Chen
Department of Anesthesiology, Dongfang Hospital, Xiamen University, Fuzhou, Fujian 350025, China

C. Wetterauer, J. Ebbing, A. Halla and H. H. Seifert
Department of Urology, University Hospital Basel, Spitalstr. 21, 4031 Basel, Switzerland

R. Kuehl and S. Erb
Division of Infectious Diseases and Hospital Epidemiology, University Hospital Basel, University Basel, Basel, Switzerland

A. Egli
Division of Clinical Microbiology, University Hospital Basel, University Basel, Basel, Switzerland
Applied Microbiology Research, Department of Biomedicine, University Basel, Basel, Switzerland

D. J. Schaefer
Department of Plastic, Reconstructive, Aesthetic and Hand Surgery, University Hospital Basel, University Basel, Basel, Switzerland

Francesco M. Labricciosa
Department of Biomedical Science and Public Health, School of Hygiene and Preventive Medicine, Faculty of Medicine and Surgery, Università Politecnica delle Marche, Ancona, Italy

Massimo Sartelli
Department of Surgery, Macerata Hospital, Macerata, Italy

Sofia Correia and Milton Severo
Epidemiology Research Unit (EPIUnit), Instituto de Saúde Pública, Universidade do Porto (ISPUP), Porto, Portugal
Departamento de Ciências da Saúde Pública e Forenses e Educação Médica, Faculdade de Medicina, Universidade do Porto, Porto, Portugal

Ana Azevedo
Epidemiology Research Unit (EPIUnit), Instituto de Saúde Pública, Universidade do Porto (ISPUP), Porto, Portugal
Departamento de Ciências da Saúde Pública e Forenses e Educação Médica, Faculdade de Medicina, Universidade do Porto, Porto, Portugal
Centro de Epidemiologia Hospitalar, Centro Hospitalar São João, Porto, Portugal

Lilian M. Abbo
Infection Prevention and Antimicrobial Stewardship Jackson Health System, University of Miami Miller School of Medicine, Miami, FL, USA

Luca Ansaloni and Federico Coccolini
General Surgery Department, Papa Giovanni XXIII Hospital, Bergamo, Italy

Carlos Alves
Unit of Prevention and Control of Infections and Antimicrobial Resistance (UPCIRA), Centro de Epidemiologia Hospitalar, Centro Hospitalar São João, Porto, Portugal

Renato Bessa Melo
Department of General Surgery, Centro Hospitalar São João, Porto, Portugal

Gian Luca Baiocchi
Department of Clinical and Experimental Sciences, University of Brescia, Brescia, Italy

José-Artur Paiva
Department of Emergency and Intensive Care, Centro Hospitalar São João, Porto, Portugal
Department of Medicine, Faculdade de Medicina, Universidade do Porto, Porto, Portugal

Fausto Catena
Department of Emergency Surgery, Maggiore Hospital, Parma, Italy

G. Cocorullo, N. Falco, T. Fontana, R. Tutino, L. Licari, G. Salamone, G. Scerrino and G. Gulotta
General and Emergency Surgery–Policlinico P. Giaccone, University of Palermo, Via Liborio Giuffrè, 5, Palermo, Italy

A. Mirabella
General and Emergency Surgery–Villa Sofia Hospita, Palermo, Italy

Jeffrey Kerby and Patrick Bosarge
Division of Acute Care Surgery, Department of Surgery, University of Alabama at Birmingham, Birmingham, AL, USA

Parker Hu
Division of Acute Care Surgery, Department of Surgery, University of Alabama at Birmingham, Birmingham, AL, USA
Division of Acute Care Surgery, Department of Surgery, University of Alabama at Birmingham, 701 19th Street South, 112 Lyons-Harrison Research Building, Birmingham, AL 35294, USA

Rindi Uhlich and Frank Gleason
Department of Surgery, University of Alabama at Birmingham, Birmingham, AL, USA

Vincent P. Anto, Joshua B. Brown, Andrew B. Peitzman, Brian S. Zuckerbraun, Matthew D. Neal, Gregory Watson, Raquel Forsythe, Timothy R. Billiar and Jason L. Sperry
Division of General Surgery and Trauma, Department of Surgery, University of Pittsburgh Medical Center, 200 Lothrop Street, Pittsburgh, PA 15213, USA

Chia-Peng Chang and Chun-Nan Lin
Department of Emergency Medicine, Chang Gung Memorial Hospital, No.6, Sec. W., Jiapu Rd, Puzi City, Chiayi County 613, Taiwan

Cheng-Ting Hsiao and Wen-Chih Fann
Department of Emergency Medicine, Chang Gung Memorial Hospital, No.6, Sec. W., Jiapu Rd, Puzi City, Chiayi County 613, Taiwan
Department of Medicine, Chang Gung University, Taoyuan, Taiwan

Michal Grivna
Institute of Public Health, College of Medicine and Health Sciences, UAE University, Al-Ain, United Arab Emirates

Hanan M. Al-Marzouqi, Maryam R. Al-Ali and Nada N. Al-Saadi
Medical Student, College of Medicine and Health Sciences, UAE University, Al-Ain, United Arab Emirates

Fikri M. Abu-Zidan
Department of Surgery, College of Medicine and Health Sciences, UAE University, Al-Ain, United Arab Emirates

Wei Wang and He-Ping Xiang
Department of Emergency Surgery, The Second Affiliated Hospital of Anhui Medical University, 678 Furong Road, Hefei 230601, Anhui Province, People's Republic of China

Hui-Ping Wang
Hematology department, The Second Affiliated Hospital of Anhui Medical University, Hefei 230601, Anhui Province, People's Republic of China

Li-Xin Zhu
Central lab of the First Affiliated Hospital of Anhui Medical University, Hefei 230022, Anhui Province, People's Republic of China

Xiao-Ping Geng
Department of General Surgery, The Second Affiliated Hospital of Anhui Medical University, Hefei 230601, Anhui Province, People's Republic of China

Hiroyuki Otsuka, Toshiki Sato, Keiji Sakurai, Hiromichi Aoki, Takeshi Yamagiwa, Shinichi Iizuka and Sadaki Inokuchi
Department of Emergency and Critical Care Medicine, Tokai University School of Medicine, 143 Shimokasuya, Isehara city, Kanagawa Prefecture 259-1193, Japan

Panuwat Lertsithichai
Department of Surgery, Faculty of Medicine Ramathibodi Hospital, Mahidol University, Bangkok, Thailand

Chumpon Wilasrusmee and Napaphat Poprom
Department of Surgery, Faculty of Medicine Ramathibodi Hospital, Mahidol University, Bangkok, Thailand
Section for Clinical Epidemiology and Biostatistics, Faculty of Medicine Ramathibodi Hospital, Mahidol University, Bangkok, Thailand

Ammarin Thakkinstian
Section for Clinical Epidemiology and Biostatistics, Faculty of Medicine Ramathibodi Hospital, Mahidol University, Bangkok, Thailand

Patarawan Woratanarat
Section for Clinical Epidemiology and Biostatistics, Faculty of Medicine Ramathibodi Hospital, Mahidol University, Bangkok, Thailand
Department of Orthopedics, Faculty of Medicine Ramathibodi Hospital, Mahidol University, Bangkok, Thailand

Boonying Siribumrungwong
Department of Surgery, Faculty of Medicine Thammasat University Hospital, Thammasat University, Pathumthani, Thailand

Samart Phuwapraisirisan
Department of Surgery, Phukhieo Hospital, Chaiyaphum, Thailand

John Attia
School of Medicine and Public Health, The University of Newcastle, Newcastle, NSW, Australia

Ari Leppäniemi and Panu Mentula
Department of Gastrointestinal Surgery, Helsinki University Central Hospital, Helsinki, Finland

Henna E. Sammalkorpi
Department of Gastrointestinal Surgery, Helsinki University Central Hospital, Helsinki, Finland
University of Helsinki, Medical Faculty, Helsinki, Finland

Eila Lantto
Department of Radiology, Helsinki University Central Hospital, Helsinki, Finland

Giuseppe Salamone, Leo Licari, Giovanni Guercio, Sofia Campanella, Nicolò Falco, Gregorio Scerrino, Sebastiano Bonventre, Girolamo Geraci, Gianfranco Cocorullo and Gaspare Gulotta
Department of Surgical, Oncological and Oral Science, University of Palermo, Policlinico P.Giaccone. Via Liborio Giuffré 5, 90127 Palermo, Italy

S. Buci, M. Torba, Gj. Bushi and K. Kagjini
Service of General Surgery, Trauma University Hospital, Tirana, Albania

A. Gjata
Department of Surgery, UHC "Mother Teresa", Tirana, Albania

I. Kajo
Department of Internal Medicine, Trauma University Hospital, Tirana, Albania

Index

www.ingramcontent.com/pod-product-compliance
Lightning Source LLC
Chambersburg PA
CBHW080516200326
41458CB00012B/4234